AF614725

Methods in Molecular Biology

Series Editor
John M. Walker
School of Life Sciences
University of Hertfordshire
Hatfield, Hertfordshire, AL10 9AB, UK

For further volumes:
http://www.springer.com/series/7651

Systemic Lupus Erythematosus

Methods and Protocols

Edited by

Paul Eggleton

University of Exeter Medical School, Exeter, Devon, UK

Frank J. Ward

Section of Immunology and Infection, Division of Applied Medicine, Institute of Medical Sciences, University of Aberdeen, Aberdeen, UK

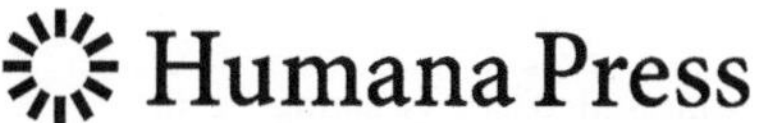

Editors
Paul Eggleton
University of Exeter Medical School
Exeter, Devon, UK

Frank J. Ward
Section of Immunology and Infection
Division of Applied Medicine
Institute of Medical Sciences
University of Aberdeen
Aberdeen, UK

ISSN 1064-3745 ISSN 1940-6029 (electronic)
ISBN 978-1-4939-0325-2 ISBN 978-1-4939-0326-9 (eBook)
DOI 10.1007/978-1-4939-0326-9
Springer New York Heidelberg Dordrecht London

Library of Congress Control Number: 2014931083

Printed on acid-free paper

Humana Press is a brand of Springer
Springer is part of Springer Science+Business Media (www.springer.com)

Dedication

This book is dedicated to our children, Buzzy and Hannah Eggleton and Aidan, Thomas, and Finlay Ward-Leggat.

Foreword

Systemic lupus erythematosus (SLE) is a complex autoimmune disease in which environmental factors such as prior infection, hormonal and chemical agents, UV light, and perhaps even diet have a strong epigenetic influence on any existing genetic disposition. This complexity is reflected in the broad range of symptoms and clinical manifestations that combine to render lupus very difficult to characterize and manage on an individual basis. Monitoring the disease is frustratingly difficult, furthering the need for appropriate, robust biomarkers to assess SLE disease activity before, during, and after treatment. The disease itself requires detailed scrutiny of the immune system, and in this volume, professors Isenberg and Ahearn (*Chapters 1* and *2*) emphasize some of the challenges ahead but also highlight the progress made on developing new biomarkers of the disease. Protocols from the emerging field of proteomics and high-throughput multiplex antibody arrays to delineate disease activity biomarkers in the serum proteome of SLE patients are also described (*Chapter 6*).

The measurement of several clinically relevant autoantibodies associated with lupus disease is important for monitoring disease activity. In this volume we provide methods from leading clinical laboratories to quantify antinuclear and antiphospholipid antibodies (*Chapters 3* and *8* and *17*). We have also provided a protocol to conduct an outline meta-analysis to systematically assess if a particular antibody measurement is a reasonable predictor of disease activity in SLE (*Chapter 19*).

Many of the "self-antigens" that become autoantigenic in SLE patients are present in high abundance as intracellular (nuclear, cytoplasmic, and membrane components) or extracellular components (e.g., complement proteins including C1q, C2, C4). The breakdown of immune tolerance to host components so that they are perceived as "foreign" is becoming an increasingly productive area of lupus and other autoimmune disease research. It appears highly likely that the increases in oxidative and nitrosative stress that evokes production of reactive oxygen and nitrogen species observed in SLE patients result in post-translational modifications of host molecules. This has the effect of provoking the immune system into attacking host rather than foreign tissue. We provide detailed methods describing how to modify host proteins by reactive oxygen and nitrogen species (*Chapter 12*) and also how to quantify markers of oxidative damage in patient serum (*Chapter 14*).

An important pathological association with SLE disease is the increased production of immune cell effector cytokines such as interferon (IFN)-alpha, which plays a pivotal role during the development of SLE, and a method for measuring IFN and other cytokines is described (*Chapter 10*).

The granular proteins released in weblike structures (NETs) from neutrophils are implicated as a source of autoantigens in SLE, and a protocol is described to allow isolation and characterization of the potential autoantigens contained within neutrophil nets (*Chapter 11*).

One consequence of anti-nucleoprotein autoantibodies in SLE is the formation of pro-inflammatory immune complexes, which may become insoluble and deposited in fine capillaries such as the glomeruli of lupus patients. The ability to measure pathogenic immune complex formation and their relative concentrations is important, as they are directly associated with particular disease pathologies, such as nephritis. We provide a method to measure immune complex formation in SLE patients (*Chapter 4*).

Both autoreactive B cells and T cells are implicated in SLE pathology, and a number of therapeutic biologics in the form of human or humanized monoclonal antibodies or antibody fragments have been developed to treat SLE. Some of these novel biologics rely on complement- and antibody-dependent cytotoxicity (CDC and ADCC, respectively) to eliminate autoreactive immune cells, but there is very little detailed information in the literature of how to perform ADCC. Therefore, a chapter is provided here, which describes three methods of killing cells by ADCC (*Chapter 5*). A further chapter also provides details of isolation, polarization, and expansion of autoantigen-specific $CD4^+$ T helper cells (*Chapter 18*). The development of new and novel antibody-based therapeutics to specifically eliminate subsets of autoreactive T or B cells is a strategy being pursued in the SLE therapeutic development field. We present a chapter (*Chapter 7*) that describes how to target immune cells using antibody variable fragments linked to death receptors to allow detection and elimination of lymphocytes, independent of CDC and ADCC mechanisms.

Another novel form of therapeutic relies on the use of synthetic peptides derived from protein autoantigens to selectively suppress the autoimmune response. A series of detailed protocols are provided here to develop such therapeutics (*Chapter 13*). The development of any new or novel therapeutics or indeed a means of understanding the complex immune processes in SLE requires murine models. A number of spontaneous models have been available for a number of decades, but in this volume detailed protocols are provided to generate inducible models of SLE to characterize and target particular elements of lupus disease in these models (*Chapter 9*).

The regulatory mechanisms of SLE disease are complex, but a recent, productive area of research is the application and measurement of microRNAs or miRNAs associated with disease activity. Many miRNAs have been shown to play a role in regulating SLE disease, particularly in SLE blood and renal tissue, described in two chapters here (*Chapters 15* and *16*).

Together, this range of protocols reflects the diversity and enthusiasm of current research in SLE and will provide an invaluable reference for anyone with an interest in this area.

This book would not have been possible without the wonderful effort and hard work of all the contributors from around the world who have a common passion to develop methods to aid our understanding of SLE pathology, which in turn helps alleviate the suffering and disease symptoms of SLE patients. Through the contributors' kindness, they have passed on their knowledge to help other researchers advance our understanding of immune mechanisms of SLE and develop the means to help prevent this debilitating disease. We would also like to thank all of the SLE patients, who have provided blood and other tissue samples to allow this research focus on their disease. We would like to acknowledge the support of one group of lupus patients in particular, who over the years have taken a keen interest in SLE research and actively supported the research of PE and the education of the medical students at the University of Exeter Medical School and Peninsula College of Medicine and Dentistry—namely, the Devon and Cornwall Lupus Group. We would also like to thank Susan Westoby of Exeter University Medical School who has helped coordinate the production of this book.

Exeter, Devon, UK *Paul Eggleton*
Aberdeen, UK *Frank J. Ward*

Preface

Systemic lupus erythematosus (SLE) is an autoimmune disease that affects five to six million people worldwide. Autoantibodies are generated and directed against multiple organs, including the heart, brain, lungs, kidney, and skin. The diagnosis of SLE can be a long and slow process due to the manifestation of a diverse set of symptoms, which include psychological, cardiovascular, musculoskeletal, and nephrology complications. Molecular biological techniques are being rapidly developed and adapted to provide insight into the molecular mechanisms of this multisystem autoimmune disease. SLE can take a number of years to diagnose, the disease can lead to the release of a multitude of inflammatory cytokines, and breakdown of immune tolerance can exasperate disease activity, leading to immune complex formation between host proteins and autoantibodies ultimately leading to organ pathology. This volume describes a number of genetic, biochemical, and immunological techniques that are advancing our understanding of the pathology, breakdown of the immune system, and therapeutic challenges of SLE in both humans and animal models. The volume should appeal to biomedical and clinical scientists in a number of pathology disciplines at the doctoral and postdoctoral level.

Exeter, Devon, UK *Paul Eggleton*
Aberdeen, UK *Frank J. Ward*

Contents

Contributors

JOSEPH M. AHEARN, M.D. • *Asthma Allergy and Autoimmunity Institute, Pittsburgh, PA, USA; Lupus Center of Excellence, Pittsburgh, PA, USA; Temple University School of Medicine, Pittsburgh, PA, USA*

CRISTIANO ALESSANDRI • *Dipartimento di Medicina Interna e Specialità Mediche, Sapienza Università di Roma, Policlinico Umberto I, Rome, Italy*

PEDRO CORREIA AZEVEDO • *Internal Medicine Department, Hospital Garcia de Orta, EPE, Almada, Portugal*

ROBERT N. BARKER • *Section of Immunology and Infection, Division of Applied Medicine, Institute of Medical Sciences, University of Aberdeen, Aberdeen, UK*

ALKA BHATIA, M.D. • *Department of Experimental Medicine and Biotechnology, Post Graduate Institute of Medical Education & Research PGIMER, Chandigarh, India*

CARL A.K. BORREBAECK • *Department of Immunotechnology and CREATE Health, Lund University, Lund, Sweden*

EDWIN BREMER • *Department of Surgery, Translational Surgical Oncology, University Medical Center Groningen, University of Groningen, Groningen, The Netherlands*

JEAN-PAUL BRIAND • *Immunopathology and Therapeutic Chemistry, CNRS, Institut de Biologie Moléculaire et Cellulaire, Strasbourg, France*

ANTONELLA CAPOZZI • *Dipartimento di Medicina Sperimentale, Sapienza Università di Roma, Policlinico Umberto I, Rome, Italy*

CARMELO CARMONA-RIVERA • *Systemic Autoimmunity Branch, Intramural Research Program, National Institute of Arthritis and Musculoskeletal and Skin Diseases, National Institutes of Health, Bethesda, MD, USA*

JIEJING CHEN • *Nephrology Department, Guilin 181st Hospital, Guangxi Key laboratory of Metabolic Diseases Research, Guilin, Guangxi, China*

FABRIZIO CONTI, M.D. • *Dipartimento di Medicina Interna e Specialità Mediche, Sapienza Università di Roma, Policlinico Umberto I, Rome, Italy*

ISABEL COTTRELL • *University of Exeter Medical School, Exeter, Devon, UK*

MARY K. CROW • *Division of Rheumatology, Hospital for Special Surgery, New York, NY, USA*

LEKH N. DAHAL • *Antibody and Vaccine Group, Cancer Sciences Unit, Faculty of Medicine, Tenovus Research Laboratory, Southampton General Hospital, University of Southampton, Hampshire, UK*

YONG DAI • *Clinical Medical Research Centre, Second Clinical Medical School of Jinan University (Shenzhen People's Hospital), Shenzhen, Guangdong, China*

PAUL EGGLETON • *University of Exeter Medical School, Exeter, Devon, UK*

HÉLÈNE GAZZANO-SANTORO • *Analytical Development and Quality Control, Genentech Inc., South San Francisco, CA, USA*

TAMER A. GHEITA • *Rheumatology and Clinical Immunology Department, Faculty of Medicine, Cairo University, Cairo, Egypt*

IAN GILES • *Centre for Rheumatology, University College London, London, UK*

WIJNAND HELFRICH • *Department of Surgery, Translational Surgical Oncology, University Medical Center Groningen, University of Groningen, Groningen, The Netherlands*
YIANNIS IOANNOU • *Arthritis Research UK Centre for Adolescent Rheumatology, London, UK; Adolescent and Adult Rheumatology, UCL/UCLH/GOSH, London, UK*
DAVID A. ISENBERG, M.D. • *University College Hospital, London, UK*
MARIANA J. KAPLAN, M.D. • *Systemic Autoimmunity Branch, Intramural Research Program, National Institute of Arthritis and Musculoskeletal and Skin Diseases, National Institutes of Health, Bethesda, MD, USA*
SANAA A. KENAWY • *Rheumatology and Clinical Immunology Department, Faculty of Medicine, Cairo University, Cairo, Egypt*
ASMA KHAN • *University of Exeter Medical School, Exeter, Devon, UK*
KYRIAKOS A. KIROU • *Division of Rheumatology, Hospital for Special Surgery, New York, NY, USA*
YASHWANT KUMAR, M.D., D.N.B. • *Department of Immunopathology, PGIMER, Chandigarh, India*
CHAU-CHING LIU • *Asthma Allergy and Autoimmunity Institute, Pittsburgh, PA, USA; Lupus Center of Excellence, Pittsburgh, PA, USA; Temple University School of Medicine, Pittsburgh, PA, USA*
FUHUA LIU • *Clinical Medical Research Centre, Second Clinical Medical School of Jinan University (Shenzhen People's Hospital), Shenzhen, Guangdong, China*
MARI LLIGUICOTA • *Division of Rheumatology, Hospital for Special Surgery, New York, NY, USA*
SUSAN MANZI • *Asthma Allergy and Autoimmunity Institute, Pittsburgh, PA, USA; Lupus Center of Excellence, Pittsburgh, PA, USA; Temple University School of Medicine, Pittsburgh, PA, USA*
SIDRA MAQSOOD • *University of Exeter Medical School, Exeter, Devon, UK*
FRANCESCO MARTINELLI • *Dipartimento di Medicina Interna e Specialità Mediche, Sapienza Università di Roma, Policlinico Umberto I, Rome, Italy*
AARON S. MILLER • *Analytical Development and Quality Control, Genentech Inc., South San Francisco, CA, USA*
ROBERTA MISASI • *Dipartimento di Medicina Sperimentale, Sapienza Università di Roma, Policlinico Umberto I, Rome, Italy*
LAURENCE MOREL • *Department of Pathology, Immunology & Laboratory Medicine, University of Florida, Gainesville, FL, USA*
SYLVIANE MULLER • *Immunopathology and Therapeutic Chemistry, CNRS, Institut de Biologie Moléculaire et Cellulaire, Strasbourg, France*
GRAINNE MURPHY • *Department of Rheumatology, University College London, London, UK*
MIKHAIL OLFERIEV • *Division of Rheumatology, Hospital for Special Surgery, New York, NY, USA*
MINGLIN OU • *Nephrology Department, Guilin 181st Hospital, Guangxi Key laboratory of Metabolic Diseases Research, Guilin, Guangxi, China*
CHARIS PERICLEOUS • *Centre for Rheumatology, University College London, London, UK*
SERENA RECALCHI • *Dipartimento di Medicina Sperimentale, Sapienza Università di Roma, Policlinico Umberto I, Rome, Italy*
WESTLEY H. REEVES • *Division of Rheumatology and Clinical Immunology, Department of Medicine, University of Florida, Gainesville, FL, USA*
VERA M. RIPOLL • *Centre for Rheumatology, University College London, London, UK*
BRENT J. RYAN • *Department of Physiology and Anatomy, University of Oxford, Oxford, UK*

NICOLAS SCHALL • *Immunopathology and Therapeutic Chemistry, CNRS, Institut de Biologie Moléculaire et Cellulaire, Strasbourg, France*

MAURIZIO SORICE • *Dipartimento di Medicina Sperimentale, Sapienza Università di Roma, Policlinico Umberto I, Rome, Italy*

FRANCESCA ROMANA SPINELLI • *Dipartimento di Medicina Interna e Specialità Mediche, Sapienza Università di Roma, Policlinico Umberto I, Rome, Italy*

GUNNAR STURFELT • *Section of Rheumatology, Department of Clinical Sciences, Skånes University Hospital, Lund University, Lund, Sweden*

WEIGUO SUI • *Clinical Medical Research Centre, Second Clinical Medical School of Jinan University (Shenzhen People's Hospital), Shenzhen, Guangdong, China*

MAX L. TEJADA • *Analytical Development and Quality Control, Genentech Inc., South San Francisco, CA, USA*

JEMMA THORNES • *University of Exeter Medical School, Exeter, Devon, UK*

GUIDO VALESINI • *Dipartimento di Medicina Interna e Specialità Mediche, Sapienza Università di Roma, Policlinico Umberto I, Rome, Italy*

FRANK J. WARD • *Section of Immunology and Infection, Division of Applied Medicine, Institute of Medical Sciences, University of Aberdeen, Aberdeen, UK*

MARK H. WENER, M.D. • *Department of Laboratory Medicine, University of Washington, Seattle, WA, USA; Rheumatology Division, Department of Medicine, University of Washington, Seattle, WA, USA*

CHRISTER WINGREN • *Department of Immunotechnology and CREATE Health, Lund University, Lund, Sweden*

YUAN XU • *Division of Rheumatology and Clinical Immunology, Department of Medicine, University of Florida, Gainesville, FL, USA*

LEILANI ZEUMER • *Department of Pathology, Immunology, and laboratory Medicine, University of Florida, Gainesville, FL, USA*

Chapter 1

Pathology of Systemic Lupus Erythematosus: The Challenges Ahead

Pedro Correia Azevedo, Grainne Murphy, and David A. Isenberg

Abstract

Many studies have explored the pathology of systemic lupus erythematosus (SLE), an autoimmune rheumatic disorder with a striking female predominance. Numerous autoimmune phenomena are present in this disease, which ultimately result in organ damage. However, the specific cellular and humoral mechanisms underlying the immune dysfunction are not yet fully understood.

It is postulated that autoimmunity is based on the interaction of genetic predisposition, hormonal and environmental triggers that result in reduced tolerance to self-tissues. These phenomena could occur because of altered antigen presentation, abnormalities in B cell responses, increases in the function of T-helper cells, abnormal cytokine production, exaggerated effector responses, or loss of regulatory T cells or B cells. Abnormalities in all of these components of the immune response have been implicated to varying degrees in the pathogenesis of SLE.

This chapter will attempt to provide a "state-of-the-art" review of the evidence about the mechanisms underlying the pathology of SLE.

Key words Autoimmunity, Systemic lupus erythematosus, Pathology, Cellular and humoral mechanisms, Organ damage, Autoantibodies, Immunology, Genetics

1 Introduction

Systemic lupus erythematosus (SLE) is a multisystem autoimmune rheumatic condition with a notable predilection to affect females during the childbearing years [1]. It has diverse clinical presentations ranging from photosensitivity, alopecia, and arthritis to internal organ involvement, including nephritis and CNS disease. It is an important condition to include in the differential diagnosis of patients with any of these clinical presentations, particularly in females aged between 15 and 50 years. Scientifically, SLE is an intriguing condition to study given the involvement of all components of the immune

The authors Pedro Correia Azevedo and Grainne Murphy contributed equally to this project and should be considered co-first authors.

Paul Eggleton and Frank J. Ward (eds.), *Systemic Lupus Erythematosus: Methods and Protocols*, Methods in Molecular Biology, vol. 1134, DOI 10.1007/978-1-4939-0326-9_1, © Springer Science+Business Media New York 2014

system and the intricate interactions between the arms of the innate and adaptive defenses.

Estimates of prevalence vary according to the reference population with rates of ~40 per 100,000 persons noted in Northern European cohorts which increases to >200 per 100,000 persons among black populations [2]. Although the prognosis has improved dramatically with advances in dialysis, in renal transplantation, and in the therapeutics of SLE, it still carries a significant increase in mortality [3]. This is largely attributable to greater rates of infection and active lupus (including lupus nephritis) in patients <35 years and a later increase associated with cardiovascular risk.

Our understanding of the molecular mechanisms which underlie SLE has led an increase in therapeutic options. In this chapter, we outline the current knowledge of the pathogenesis of SLE including the role of genetics, hormones, and cellular and humoral components of the immune system in the evolution of SLE.

2 Genetics of SLE

The role of genetics in lupus is corroborated by the 25 % concordance observed among monozygotic twins compared to 2 % concordance in dizygotic twins [4]. Over 40 different genes have been implicated in SLE by association studies. Studies in families with multiple members affected by lupus have identified eight susceptibility loci (Table 1). Among these are genes encoding components of the complement cascade, an essential arm of the innate immune response. In fact, genetic defects in molecules involved in the removal of anti-DNA-nucleosome complexes, such as complement, though rare, are among the strongest genetic factors predisposing to SLE. Deficiencies of C1q, C2, or C4 are well-described risk factors for a lupus-like disease as the null alleles causing deficiency occur more frequently in patients with lupus than in healthy individuals, even within the same family [5]. Complete C4 deficiency is rare, but associated with a dramatic 75 % incidence of a condition resembling SLE (the skin and joint manifestation are similar, but renal involvement and a positive ANA and anti-dsDNA antibodies are less frequently present) [6]. The mechanism underlying this increased risk is likely mediated by a defect in the complement-mediated clearance of apoptotic debris which has been proposed as a central mechanism in the induction of autoimmunity by increasing the "load" of autoantigens and thus aiding the development of pathogenic autoantibodies.

Because of their role in antigen presentation and subsequent T cell activation, the major histocompatibility complex (MHC) molecules have been targeted for study in SLE. Class I MHC molecules are known to protect the organism against intracellular pathogens, while class II protect against extracellular pathogens;

Table 1
Susceptibility loci with confirmed linkage to systemic lupus erythematosus

Cytogenetic location	Candidate genes with the loci	Immune response
1q23	CRP	Innate
	FCGR2A	Innate
	FCGR2B	Adaptive
	FCGR3A	Adaptive
	FCGR3B	Adaptive
1q25-31		
1q41-42	PRP	Adaptive
	TLR5	Innate
2q35-37	PDCD1	Adaptive
4p16-15.2		
6p11-21	MHC class II: DRB1	Adaptive
	MHC class III: TNF(alpha)	Adaptive
	C2, C4	Innate
12q24		
16q12-13	OAZ	Adaptive

thus, MHC class II diseases are usually associated with systemic autoimmunity characteristic antibodies such as rheumatoid arthritis. Mutations within the MHC complex may contribute to autoimmunity by facilitating the recognition of self-antigens by T cells. In SLE, HLA-DR3 has been associated with both lupus nephritis (LN) and anti-dsDNA antibodies, while a number of risk alleles of HLA DR2/DR3 have also been identified [7]. Other genetic loci associated with aberrations in innate immunity have been identified and are summarized in Table 2 [8].

Genome-wide association studies (GWAS) are used in many conditions to identify common genetic variants that may be associated with disease. This approach is noncandidate-driven and commonly focuses on associations between single nucleotide polymorphisms (SNPs) and a particular disease. Such genetic studies have also implicated other components of the immune response, including genes implicated in the IFN pathway, a cytokine strongly associated with SLE. Moreover, two independent studies confirming the genetic association of SLE, IRF5, MHC, PTPN22, FCγRIIA, and STAT4. IRF5 and STAT4 risk alleles showed a multiplicative interaction resulting in an odds ratio of 1.82 [9–11].

Table 2
GWAS have identified more than 30 SLE risk alleles

Main known function of gene	Genes associated with SLE
Dendritic cell function and IFN signaling	IRF5, STAT4, SPP1, IRAK1, TREX1, TNFAIP3, TNIP1, PRDM1, PHRF1, TYK2, SLC15A4, TLR8
T cell function and signaling	PTPN22, TNFSF4, PDCD1, IL10 BCL6, IL16, TYK2, PRL, STAT4, RASGRP3
B cell function and BCR signaling	BANK1, BLK, LYN, BCL6, RASGRP3
Immune-complex processing and innate immunity	ITGAM, C1QA, C2, C4A, C4B, FCGR2A, FCGR3B, KLK173, KLRG1, KIR2DS4
Cell cycle, apoptosis, and cellular metabolism	CASP10, NMNAT2, PTTG1, MSH5, PTPRT, UBE2L3, ATG5, RASGRP3
Transcriptional regulation	JAZF1, UHRF1BP1, BCL6, MECP2, ETS1, IKZF1
Other genes	PXK, ICA1, XKR6, SCUBE1

The majority of loci encode gene products in immune regulation pathways

Other proponents suggest a chromosomal hypothesis for SLE. The recognition that men with Klinefelter's syndrome have a greater likelihood of developing SLE lends support to this "sex chromosome" theory. Men with an XXY genotype have a tenfold higher risk of developing SLE than those with an XY genotype [12]. Interestingly, females with Turners syndrome (XO) are, conversely, protected from disease. In humans, the issue is more complex given the phenomenon of lyonization (the random inactivation of one X chromosome in somatic cells), a process now known to be incomplete. It has been suggested that skewing of this X inactivation, with preferential inactivation in certain tissues, may predispose to the development of autoimmune disease [13].

3 Environment

A number of environmental factors, notably ultraviolet radiation, have been implicated in SLE pathogenesis. Indeed, a photosensitive rash is one of ACR criteria for the classification of SLE [14]. Interestingly, sunlight is also essential for vitamin D production, which is receiving increasing attention in the field of immunology in relation to its ability to modulate the immune response. Evidence suggests that the circadian rhythm of vitamin D levels, especially during winter, is associated with increased disease activity in both SLE and rheumatoid arthritis [15].

Some drugs are known to induce a lupus-like disease, which primarily manifests as articular and cutaneous symptoms; the most common agents implicated in this phenomenon are procainamide, hydrazine, quinidine and more recently TNF alpha blockers [16].

Like many immune mediated disorders, an infectious trigger has been sought in SLE. Some patients describe a viral-like illness preceding either disease onset or a flare. Epstein-Barr virus (EBV) has been implicated as a potential culprit in this regard. Temporally, EBV infection has been shown to be associated with disease onset, and, in studies of juvenile SLE, EBV antibodies were present in 99 % and EBV-DNA was present in 100 % of children and young adults with lupus, significantly more prevalent than in the healthy controls [17]. Viruses are particularly of interest as their DNA and RNA are essential in the production of type I IFN, a cytokine closely related to SLE disease severity [18]. Exogenous IFN, when used therapeutically, particularly in the fields of cancer and treatment of viral infections, has been implicated as an additional cause of drug-induced lupus with the formation of autoantibodies in 4–19 % and the development of lupus-like symptoms in 0.15–0.7 % of patients. This is postulated to be due to a break in peripheral tolerance mediated by the activation of myeloid dendritic cells (mDCs) in response to excess IFN-αβ [19].

4 Hormonal

The notable increase in SLE incidence and prevalence in women of childbearing years (female/male, 9:1) has lead to intense interest in the role of hormones in the pathogenesis of SLE. Moreover, disease flares have been reported at times of rapid hormonal changes, such as in pregnancy, the puerperium, and, occasionally, following the use of exogenous estrogen-containing contraceptives and hormone-replacement therapy. Some have reported altered estrogen metabolism in men and women with SLE, with, particularly, an increase in 16α-hydroxylation of estrone [20]. While others also describe biochemical hypoandrogenism in men with SLE, it is not clear whether this is a greater reflection of concomitant corticosteroid therapy. Nonetheless, androgen therapy may alleviate the course of certain SLE manifestations [21, 22].

These clinical data are supported by laboratory evidence of an immunomodulatory role for estrogen and other sex hormones.

Both the innate and adaptive immune systems are susceptible to the influence of endogenous sex hormones. Estradiol is capable of altering cytokine production from lymphocytes, as well as their surface cytokine repertoire [23]. Supporting Th2 polarization, estrogen increases production of IFN-γ, IL-4, IL-10, as well as TNF-α, IL-1, and IL-5. Both estrogen and prolactin can also promote the failure of immune tolerance and autoantibody secretion through stimulation of autoreactive B cells [24, 25]. At an innate immune level, estrogen increases the secretion of a number of cytokines by dendritic cells and enhances the stimulatory effect of dendritic cells on T lymphocytes [26]. However, the results of clinical trials of hormonal therapies for SLE have not demonstrated a significant benefit.

5 Cytokines

Cytokines are key effector molecules and play important roles in systemic inflammation, immunomodulation, and tissue damage. A number of cytokines are upregulated in SLE. Moreover, certain cytokines have been proposed as potential biomarkers of disease activity suggesting that their therapeutic targeting may be of benefit in SLE. Here we focus on a number of cytokines which have received increasing attention in lupus pathophysiology.

5.1 Interleukin 6 (IL-6)

IL-6 is a pleiotropic molecule, primarily secreted by monocytes, endothelial cells, and fibroblasts [27]. Its many functions include the synthesis of acute phase reactants, osteoclastic differentiation, and, notably in SLE, the maturation of B lymphocytes into plasma cells and augmentation of immunoglobulin secretion [28]. Evidence implicating IL-6 in SLE comes from both human and murine studies of disease.

Patients with SLE have increased serum levels of IL-6 which correlate with both disease activity and anti-dsDNA antibodies [29]. Both renal and CNS lupus have been specifically associated with increased IL-6 in urine and CSF, respectively [30, 31]. Histologically, IL-6 expression is enhanced in glomeruli and tubules further supporting its role in tissue injury [32].

Thus, IL-6 may be an integral promoter of LN and a potential therapeutic target. Indeed, inhibition of IL-6 at a preclinical level (NZB/W) leads to reduction in proteinuria and anti-DNA antibodies and improved survival [33]. This has prompted the application of the currently available anti-IL-6 monoclonal antibody, tocilizumab, in the treatment of SLE with modest success in a preliminary trial [34].

5.2 Interleukin-10 (IL-10)

IL-10 is a monocyte- and lymphocyte-derived cytokine with both pro- and anti-inflammatory roles. Through its inhibitory effects on the activation of antigen presenting cells and expression of co-stimulatory molecules, it inhibits T cell activation and TNF-α secretion [35]. On a proinflammatory note and of relevance to SLE, IL-10 augments B cell proliferation and immunoglobulin class switching, thus increasing autoantibody production. It has been detected in intrarenal cells in patients with LN [36], and the binding of anti-dsDNA antibodies and immune complexes to FcγRII can trigger its secretion [37, 38]. Early clinical studies on its inhibition have shown some improvement in patients with SLE, primarily in cutaneous and joint symptoms [39].

5.3 Type 1 Interferon (IFN)

The type 1 IFN was one of the first cytokines implicated in SLE. In patients with this disease, serum levels are increased and correlate with both disease activity and anti-dsDNA titers [40]. Additionally, PBMCs from patients with SLE express IFN-inducible genes which also correlate with the disease state [41]. The therapeutic inhibition of IFN in other disease states, such as cancer and viral infections, can lead to the development of both autoantibodies and, in some, an SLE-like syndrome [42].

There are several different mechanisms proposed for the role of IFN in SLE. Although potentially produced by any leukocyte, plasmacytoid DCs are the most active secretors of IFN [43]. Enhanced IFN secretion from DCs can result from the enhanced antigen presentation on DC activation by immune complexes in patients with SLE. IFN may then feedback and increase the expression of autoantigen and promote the maturation of DCs [44] in addition to upregulating surface MHC classes I and II [45]. This interaction results in the generation of the Th1 response classically associated with SLE. Furthermore, modulation of B cell function which includes increased antibody production and class switching occurs in the context of enhanced type 1 IFN [46]. Finally, genetic evidence supports a role for IFN in the pathogenic mechanism of SLE with mutations in the IRF5 and STAT4 transcription factors associated with higher serum IFN levels and SLE [47, 48].

5.4 Interleukin 17 (IL-17)

IL-17 is a proinflammatory cytokine produced by a subset of CD4+ T cells, the Th17 population, which has recently been the subject of intense interest in many inflammatory conditions. In conjunction with IL-21 and IL-22 also produced by the Th17 cell, IL-17 can stimulate B lymphocytes and has been implicated in SLE pathogenesis [49]. Serum levels of Il-17 are increased in patients with SLE and correlate with disease activity [50]. This cytokine and its parent cell seem of particular relevance to LN where an aberrantly active Il-23/IL-17 axis in mice has been associated with nephritis induction [51] and in human studies where Th17 cell infiltration has been detected in biopsy specimens from LN [52].

5.5 B Lymphocyte Stimulator (BLyS)

BlyS is a member of the TNF superfamily and is essential in the survival of most B cells beyond the transitional 1 stage [53]. A closely related cytokine, APRIL, shares many of the biological functions and can bind to all 3 receptors, with which BLyS interacts (BCMA, TACI, and BAFF-R). In addition to supporting B cell survival, BLyS can also upregulate cytokine production and co-stimulatory molecules on DCs which express its receptors. BLyS exists in a transmembrane and soluble form, cleaved from the surface of myeloid cells by a furin protease [54]. A member of the TNF ligand family, its release is upregulated by IFN and IL-10. Of pathogenic relevance to SLE, BLyS is a powerful stimulator of B cell proliferation and immunoglobulin secretion [55].

In humans, circulating levels of BLyS are elevated in serum and correlate with anti-dsDNA antibodies [56]. Belimumab, a fully humanized monoclonal antibody that binds soluble BLyS, is now an approved and licensed treatment for SLE (by the Food and Drug Administration and European Medicines Agency). It mainly met its primary endpoints in two clinical trials (which focused on SLE patients with articular and cutaneous manifestations) [57].

5.6 Tumor Necrosis Factor α (TNF-α)

The role of TNF-α in SLE pathogenesis is more contentious. TNF-α is mainly produced by activated macrophages, CD4+ lymphocytes, and NK cells. There is some evidence suggesting that it may be protective, as the administration of TNF-α to the lupus-prone NZB/W F1 mouse delays disease development [58]. Moreover, the inhibition of TNF-α therapeutically, as in rheumatoid arthritis, has been associated with the induction of anti-dsDNA antibodies in some patients, with lupus developing in a very small minority [59]. Contradictory evidence has implicated TNF-α in supporting the disease state; TNF-α mRNA is high in renal biopsy specimens from patients with LN [32], and in a small series a reduction of both articular symptoms and proteinuria in patients with SLE who were administered the TNF inhibitor, infliximab, was noted [60]. The reason for these differences is unclear but may reflect an alteration in the pro- and anti-inflammatory roles that TNF-α can play dependent on its receptor binding. More research is required to clarify whether TNF-α plays a critical part in the cytokine dysfunction implicated in SLE.

6 The Role of T Cells

Abnormalities in various subsets of T cells have been reported in autoimmunity, although the mechanism and functional consequences of such changes remain unclear. SLE is traditionally described as a T-helper cell type 2 (Th2)-mediated disease, but it is now known that other T-helper (Th) subsets, such as Th17 cells and T-regulatory (Treg) cells, are of importance and likely contribute to the immune disturbance in this disease.

It is now well known that not all autoantibodies are pathogenic. In relation to dsDNA antibodies, tissue damage is more strongly associated with high-affinity IgG antibodies than either those of low affinity or IgM anti-dsDNA antibodies [61, 62]. The production of such pathogenic high-affinity molecules occurs in an antigen-driven fashion, a process facilitated by T cell help. Thus, B lymphocytes, which are co-stimulated by both T cells and antigen, undergo continuous selective pressure generating a population of B cells which display and secrete high-affinity immunoglobulin for the stimulating antigen [8]. Indirectly T cells also influence B cell responses through the soluble mediators they produce. T cell-derived cytokines, such as TNF-α, IFN-γ, and IL-10, stimulate B cell division, facilitate immunoglobulin class switching, and promote production of more high-affinity autoantibodies which have been implicated in the tissue damage observed in lupus. This process of generating high-affinity antibodies may also occur through a qualitative difference in T cells in patients with SLE [63]. Isolated stimulated T cells from patients with SLE can produce cytokines following interaction with a number of histone-derived peptides as outlined by Lu et al. [64], a process which does not occur in healthy controls. The histones constitute the protein core of the nucleosome, and this aberrant response in SLE patients may allow T-helper cells to stimulate autoreactive B cells specific for nucleosome-derived antigenic epitopes, yielding high-affinity anti-nucleosome antibodies which may be of pathogenic importance in lupus [65].

The Th17 subset of T-helper cells has received increasing attention in many inflammatory disorders, including SLE. Characterized by their secretion of IL-17, Th17 cells have been reported at increased frequency and detected at the site of end-organ damage in SLE. Serum levels of IL-17 are increased in SLE and correlate with disease activity in some studies [66]. Supporting evidence also comes from genetic studies where some of the described genetic risks for SLE have been shown to be of importance in the formation or maintenance of the Th17 population. IRF5 acts as a transcription factor for both IL-6 and the p40 subunit of IL-23, cytokines which are critical in the generation of the Th17 response [67]. Other genetic loci within the IRF8 gene, a repressor of Th17 cell differentiation, and in the IL-21 gene and its receptor have also been implicated in SLE, suggesting that further characterization of the role of the Th17 axis may yield interesting targets for future therapeutic intervention [68, 69].

Finally, Treg cells have been shown to be altered in patients with SLE. Both human and murine studies have reported a deficiency in number and/or function of these cells, which act to suppress the activation of both T-helper cells and B cells [70]. Treg cells isolated from patients with active SLE have been shown to be less effective in suppressing T cell proliferation and IFN-γ production in comparison with cells from healthy controls or patients with inactive lupus. In SLE, intrinsic defects in Treg cells may also exist which include a greater susceptibility to cell-mediated death via CD95 and reduced expression of FOXP3, a transcription factor that promotes Treg cells. Complicating matters is the additional evidence that effector T cells may be more resistant to the suppressive effect of Treg cells in SLE. This phenomenon was independent of disease activity and highlights the complexity underlying the immune dysfunction in lupus [71].

7 The Role of B Cells and Autoantibodies in SLE

7.1 B Cells

Multiple B cell abnormalities have been reported in SLE, which facilitate the aberrant immune response and, as a consequence, result in the formation of antibodies targeting self-antigens. It remains unclear as to whether these alterations in B cell function are as a result of defects at a central "checkpoint" level or arise in the periphery from abnormal selection. There is some evidence to suggest that defects in early negative selection exist, resulting in the persistence of naïve B cells expressing self-reactive B cell receptors [72]. However, it has been shown that autologous stem cell transplantation in SLE is successful, but relapse coincides with the reestablishment of immune memory [73], suggesting that autoreactivity is dependent on acquired abnormalities after antigen exposure, and selection.

The repertoire of circulating B cells is also altered in SLE with a skewing toward increased frequencies of pre-immune B cells, memory cells, and plasma cells. On further phenotyping, the circulating memory cells have been shown to include a population of antigen-experienced post-switched memory B cells [74]. These are less susceptible to immunosuppression and can be activated rapidly by TLR agonists or cytokine combinations, independent of antigen or T cells (same). There is also a quantitative difference in the $CD27^{+}$ population of plasma cells/plasmablasts in SLE [75, 76]. This expansion in active disease may reflect as activated immune system which responds to rituximab therapy [77]. Of further interest, GWAS have demonstrated an association between SLE and polymorphisms in the PDRM-1 gene [78]; this encodes Blimp-1, a transcription factor required for plasma cell differentiation further highlighting the importance of B cells in SLE pathogenesis.

The regulatory B cell population has also emerged as an interesting population in SLE. In SLE distinct populations of regulatory B cells have been identified. These can secrete IL-10 and can suppress Th1 and Th2 functions [79]. These cells, although present at similar levels to healthy controls, have been shown to lack full functionality in SLE. Further research is required to define the exact phenotype and role of regulatory B cells in SLE. Furthermore, it has been shown that B cell-mediated expansion and activation of invariant natural killer T (iNKT) cells is defective in SLE, a phenomenon corrected by the treatment with rituximab, demonstrating an additional role for B cells in SLE pathogenesis [80].

7.2 Autoantibodies

A significant majority of SLE patients have circulating autoantibodies with >95 % having antinuclear antibodies. Although many other autoantibodies exist, their precise role in pathogenesis has not fully been elucidated. Histologically the kidneys and skin have been most intensively studied in SLE, and both demonstrate inflammation and deposition of both complement and autoantibodies. The first description of anti-dsDNA antibodies in relevant tissue lesions published in 1967 focused on renal biopsy specimens of patients with lupus nephritis [81]. These antibodies are now known to be highly specific for lupus, present in 60–70 % of SLE patients and in <0.5 % of the healthy population [82]. In a select group of patients, the titer of anti-dsDNA antibodies correlates with disease activity. Furthermore, in patients with clinically quiescent disease and elevated titers of anti-dsDNA antibodies, 80 % of patients will have clinically active disease in the ensuing 5 years [83].

Renal biopsy specimens have also demonstrated the deposition of a number of other antibodies. These include anti-Ro (ribonucleoprotein complex), anti-La (RNA-binding protein), C1q (subunit of C1 complement component), and Sm (nuclear particle with several different polypeptides) [84]. Whether these antibodies are directly pathogenic or are deposited following the release of nuclear antigens post-apoptosis is not known.

Specific associations of particular autoantibodies with clinical manifestations of SLE are well reported. To this end, anti-Ro antibodies and anti-nucleosome antibodies are implicated in cutaneous lupus [85]. Anti-NMDA antibodies may be of pathogenic relevance to CNS lupus as the administration of serum from patients with anti-dsDNA and anti-NMDA antibodies to mice resulted in cognitive impairment and hippocampus damage [86]. Finally, the hematological manifestations of lupus, which include autoimmune hemolytic anemia and thrombocytopenia, are mediated by antibodies targeting red cell and platelet antigens, respectively [87, 88]. Other autoantibodies that may be of pathological relevance to SLE are summarized in Table 3.

The mechanism by which autoantibodies mediate tissue destruction is still debated. Most studies pertain to anti-dsDNA antibodies and their role in LN. Two theories exist. The first is that circulating anti-dsDNA antibodies bind to circulating nucleosomes released by apoptotic cells [89]. These complexes then settle in the basement membrane of renal glomeruli, fix complement, and initiate glomerulonephritis. In support of this, IgG antibodies co-localize with chromatin in LN, and anti-nucleosome antibodies are found both in the circulation and at the site of tissue damage in SLE [90, 91]. The second theory implicates autoantibodies more directly in the pathogenesis of LN. It is suggested that anti-dsDNA or anti-nucleosome antibodies cross-react with proteins in the kidney with an ensuing inflammatory response.

8 Conclusion

The complexity of the immunopathogenesis of SLE is confirmed by the numerous abnormalities described within the cells and mediators of both the innate and adaptive immune systems. The relative

Table 3
Autoantibodies prevalence and related main clinical effects in systemic lupus erythematosus

Antigen	Prevalence (%)	Main clinical effects
Anti-double-stranded DNA	70–80	Kidney and skin disease
Nucleosomes	60–90	Kidney and skin disease
Ro (SSA)	30–40	Kidney and skin disease, fetal heart problems
La (SSB)	15–20	Fetal heart problems
Sm	10–30	Kidney disease
snRNPs[a]	15–25	Raynaud's, puffy fingers, myositis, hypergammaglobulinemia
NMDA[b] receptor	33–50	Brain disease
Phospholipids[c]	20–30	Thrombosis, pregnancy loss
α-Actinin	20	Kidney disease
Ribosomes P0, P1, P2	4–12	Hepatic and central nervous system manifestations (psychosis)
C1q	40–50	Kidney disease
Rheumatoid factor	30–40	(unspecific)

[a]snRNPS—small nuclear ribonucleoproteins [spliceosomes, U1-RNP (70 kD, A, C)]
[b]NMDA—*N*-methyl-D-aspartate
[c]Phospholipids—cardiolipin, β2-glycoprotein-1, prothrombin

importance of distinct cell subtypes and how they interact remains debated and incompletely understood. It is, however, through the identification of biological pathways to disease that new therapeutic targets can be defined. The relatively recent introduction of rituximab, belimumab, and limited trials with other anti-cytokine therapies, such as tocilizumab, highlights the expansion of therapeutic options in SLE. While therapeutics have evolved significantly and have certainly contributed to the improved mortality observed in SLE patients, from a mean 4-year survival of 50 % in the 1950s to a 15-year survival rate of 85 % today, it is clear that a greater understanding of the immunologic disturbance driving the immune response in SLE will improve this figure even further.

References

1. Lu LJ, Wallace DJ, Ishimori ML, Scofield RH, Weisman MH (2010) Male systemic lupus erythematosus: a review of sex disparities in this disease. Lupus 19:119–129
2. Johnson AE, Gordon C, Palmer RG, Bacon PA (1995) The prevalence and incidence of systemic lupus erythematosus in Birmingham, England: relationship to ethnicity and county of birth. Arthritis Rheum 38:551–558
3. Gladman DD, Urowitz MB (2007) Prognosis, mortality and morbidity in systemic lupus erythematosus. In: Wallace DJ, Hahn BH (eds) Dubois' Lupus erythematosus, 7th edn. Lippincott Williams & Wilkins, Philadelphia, pp 1333–1353

4. Sullivan KE (2000) Genetic of systemic lupus erythematosus: clinical implications. Rheum Dis Clin North AM 26:229–256
5. Walport MJ (2002) Complement and systemic lupus erythematosus. Arthritis Res 4(Suppl 3): S279–S293
6. Yang Y, Chung EK, Wu YL, Savelli SL, Nagaraja HN, Zhou B et al (2007) Gene copy-number variation and associated polymorphisms of complement component C4 in human systemic lupus erythematosus (SLE): low copy number is a risk factor for and high copy number is a protective factor against SLE susceptibility in European Americans. Am J Hum Geneti 80:1037–1054
7. Graham RR, Ortmann W, Rodine P, Espe K, Langefeld C, Lange E et al (2007) Specific combinations of HLA-DR2 and DR3 class II haplotypes contribute graded risk for disease susceptibility and autoantibodies in human SLE. Eur J Hum Genet 15:823–830
8. Rahman A, Isenberg D (2008) Systemic lupus erythematosus. N Eng J Med 358:929–939
9. Harley JB, Alarcón-Riquelme ME, Criswell LA, Jacob CO, Kimberly RP, Moser KL et al (2008) Genome-wide association scan in women with systemic lupus erythematosus identifies susceptibility variants in ITGAM, PXK, KIAA1542 and other loci. Nat Genet 40:204–210
10. Graham RR, Kozyrev SV, Baechler EC, Reddy MV, Plenge RM, Bauer JW et al (2006) A common haplotype of interferon regulatory factor 5 (IRF5) regulates splicing and expression and is associated with increased risk of systemic lupus erythematosus. Nat Genet 38:550–555
11. Sigurdsson S, Nordmark G, Goring HHH, Lindroos K, Wiman AC, Sturfelt G et al (2005) Polymorphisms in the tyrosine kinase 2 and interferon regulatory factor 5genes are associated with systemic lupus erythematosus. Am J Hum Gen 76:528–537
12. Stern R, Fishman J, Brusman H, Kunkel HG (1977) Systemic lupus erythematosus associated with Klinefelter's syndrome. Arthritis Rheum 20:18–22
13. Chanchoub G, Uz E, Maalej A (2009) Analysis of skewed X chromosome inactivation in females with rheumatoid arthritis and autoimmune thyroid diseases. Arthritis Res Ther 11:R106
14. Hochberg MC (1997) Updating the American college of rheumatology revised criteria for the classification of systemic lupus erythematosus. Arthritis Rheum 40:1725
15. Cutolo M, Pizzorni C, Sulli A (2011) Vitamin D endocrine system involvement in autoimmune rheumatic diseases. Autoimmun Rev 11:84–87
16. Patel D, Richardson B (2013) Drug-induced lupus: etiology, pathogenesis, and clinical aspects. In: Wallace DJ, Hahn BH (eds) Dubois' Lupus erythematosus, 8th edn. Elsevier, Philadelphia, pp 484–494
17. James JA, Kaufman KM, Farris AD, Taylor-Albert E, Lehman TJ, Harley JB (1997) An increased prevalence of Epstein-Barr virus infection in young patients suggests a possible etiology for systemic lupus erythematosus. J Clin Invest 100:3019–3026
18. Netea MG, van der Meer JWH (2001) Mechanisms of disease—immunodeficiency and genetic defects of pattern-recognition receptors. N Eng J Med 364:60–70
19. Ronnblom LE, Alm GV, Oberg KE (1991) Autoimmunity after alpha-interferon therapy for malignant carcinoid-tumors. Ann Intern Med 115:178–183
20. Lahita RG, Bradlow HL, Kunkel HG, Fishman J (1979) Alterations of estrogen metabolism in systemic lupus erythematosus. Arthritis Rheum 22:1195–1198
21. Fromer JL (1950) The use of testosterone in chronic lupus erythematosus. Preliminary report. Lahey Clin Bul 8:13–17
22. Agnello V, Pariser K, Gell J, Gelfand J, Turksoy RN (1983) Preliminary observations on danazol therapy of systemic lupus erythematosus. Effects on DNA antibodies, thrombocytopaenia and complement. J Rheum 10:682–687
23. Zen M, Ghiradello A, Iaccarino L, Tonon M, Campana C, Arienti S et al (2010) Hormones, immune response and pregnancy in healthy women and pregnancy. Swiss Med Weekly 140:187–201
24. Cohen-Solal JF, Jeganathan V, Grimaldi CM, Peeva E, Diamond B (2006) Sex hormones and SLE: influencing the fate of autoreactive B cells. Curr Top Microbiol Immunol 305: 67–88
25. Grimaldi CM, Cleary J, Dagtas AS, Moussai D, Diamond B (2002) Estrogen alters thresholds for B cell apoptosis and activation. J Clin Invest 109:1625–1633
26. Siracusa MC, Overstreet MG, Housseau F, Scott AL, Klein SL (2008) 17 beta-oestradiol alters the activity of conventional and IFN-producing killer dendritic cells. J Immunol 180:1423–1431
27. Hiran T (1998) IL-6 and its receptor. Int Rev Immunol 6:249–284
28. Tackey E, Lipsky P, Illei G (2004) Rationale for interleukin-6 blockade in systemic lupus erythematosus. Lupus 13:339–343
29. Linker-Israeli M, Deans R, Wallace DJ, Prehn J, Ozeri-Chen T, Klinenberg JR (1991)

Elevated levels of endogenous IL-6 in systemic lupus erythematosus: a putative role in pathogenesis. J Immunol 147:117–123

30. Tsai CY, Wu TH, Yu CL, Lu JY, Tsai YY (2000) Increased excretions of β2-microglobulin, IL-6 and IL-8 and decreased excretion of Tamm-Horsfall glycoprotein in urine of patients with active lupus nephritis. Nephron 85:207–214
31. Hirohata S, Kanai Y, Mitsuo A, Tokano Y, Hashimoto H (2009) Accuracy of cerebrospinal fluid IL-6 testing for diagnosis of lupus psychosis. A multicentre retrospective study. Clin Rheumatol 28:1319–1323
32. Herrera-Esparza R, Barbosa-Cisneros R, Villalobos-Hurtado R, Avalos-Diaz E (1998) Renal expression of IL-6 and TNF-α genes in lupus nephritis. Lupus 7:154–158
33. Mihara M, Takagi N, Takeda Y, Ohsugi Y (1998) IL-6 receptor blockade inhibits the onset of autoimmune kidney disease in NZB/Wfl mice. Clin Exp Immunol 112:397–402
34. Illei G, Yarboro C, Shirota Y, Daruwalla J, Tackey E, Takada K et al (2006) Tocilizumab (humanized anti-IL6 receptor antibody) in patients with systemic lupus erythematosus(SLE): safety, tolerability and preliminary efficacy. Arthritis Rheum 54:4043
35. Llorente L, Zou W, Levy Y, Richaud-Patin Y, Wijdenes J, Alcocer-Varela J et al (1995) Role of Interleukin-10 in the B lymphocyte hyperactivity and autoantibody production of human systemic lupus erythematosus. J Exp Med 181:839–844
36. Uhm WS, Na K, Song GW, Jung SS, Lee T, Park MH et al (2003) Cytokine balance in kidney tissue from lupus nephritis patients. Rheumatology (Oxford) 42:935–938
37. Ronnelid J, Tejde A, Mathsson L, Nilsson-Ekdahl K, Nilsson B (2003) Immune complexes from SLE sera induce IL-10 production from normal peripheral blood mononuclear cells by an FcγRII dependent mechanism: implications for a possible vicious cycle maintaining B cell hyperactivity in SLE. Ann Rheum Dis 62:37–42
38. Sun KH, Yu CL, Tang SJ, Sun GH (2000) Monoclonal anti-double stranded DNA autoantibody stimulates the expression of IL-1β, IL-6, IL-8, IL-10 and TNF-α from normal human mononuclear cells involving in the lupus pathogenesis. Immunology 99:352–360
39. Llorente L, Richaud-Patin Y, Garcia-Padilla C, Claret E, Jakez-Ocampo J, Cardiel MH et al (2000) Clinical and biologic effects of anti-interleukin-10 monoclonal antibody administration in systemic lupus erythematosus. Arthritis Rheum 43:1790–1800
40. Bengtsson G, Sturfelt G, Truedsson L, Blomberg J, Alm G, Vallin H et al (2000) Activation of type 1 Interferon system in systemic lupus erythematosus correlates with disease activity but not with antiretroviral antibodies. Lupus 9:664–671
41. Baechler EC, Batliwalla FM, Karypis G, Gaffney PM, Ortmann WA, Espe KJ et al (2003) Interferon-inducible gene expression signature in peripheral blood cells of patients with severe lupus. Proc Natl Acad Sci U S A 100:2610–2615
42. Ioannou Y, Isenberg DA (2000) Current evidence for the induction of autoimmune rheumatic manifestations by cytokine therapy. Arthritis Rheum 43:1431–1442
43. Fitzgerald-Bocarsly P, Dai J, Singh S (2008) Plasmacytoid dendritic cells and type 1 IFN: 50 years of convergent history. Cytokine Growth Factor Rev 19:3–19
44. Lovgren T, Eloranta ML, Bave U, Alm GV, Rönnblom L (2004) Induction of interferon-α production in plasmacytoid dendritic cells by immune complexes containing nucleic acid released by necrotic or late apoptotic cells and lupus IgG. Arthritis Rheum 50:1861–1872
45. Baccala R, Hoebe K, Kono DH, Beutler B, Theofilopoulos N (2007) TLR-dependent and TLR-independent pathways of Type 1 interferon induction in systemic autoimmunity. Nat Med 13:543–551
46. Le Bon A, Thompson C, Kamphuis E, Durand V, Rossmann C, Kalinke U et al (2006) Cutting edge: enhancement of antibody responses through direct stimulation of B and T cells by type 1 IFN. J Immunol 176:2074–2078
47. Niewold TB, Kelly JA, Flesch MH, Espinoza LR, Harley B, Crow MK (2008) Association of the IRF5 risk haplotype with high serum interferon-α activity in systemic lupus erythematosus patients. Arthritis Rheum 58:2481–2487
48. Remmers EF, Plenge RM, Lee AT, Graham RR, Hom G, Behrens TW et al (2007) STAT4 and the risk of rheumatoid arthritis and systemic lupus erythematosus. N Engl J Med 357:977–986
49. Hin Yap D, Neng Lai K (2010) Cytokines and their roles in the pathogenesis of systemic lupus erythematosus: from basics to recent advances. J Biomed 2010:365083. doi:10.1155/2010/365083. Epub 2010 May 6
50. Wong CK, Lit LC, Tam LS, Li EK, Wong PT, Lam CW (2008) Hyperproduction of IL-23 and IL-17 in patients with systemic lupus erythematosus: implications for Th-17 mediated inflammation in auto-immunity. Clin Immunol 127:385–393

51. Zhang Z, Kyttaris VC, Tsokos GC (2009) The role of IL-23/IL-17 axis in lupus nephritis. Journal Immunol 183:3160–3169
52. Crispin JC, Oukka M, Bayliss G, Cohen RA, Van Beek CA, Stillman IE et al (2008) Expanded double-negative T cells in patients with systemic lupus erythematosus produce IL-17 and infiltrate the kidneys. Journal Immunol 181:8761–8766
53. Mackay F, Schneider P (2009) Cracking the BAFF code. Nat Rev Immunol 9:491–502
54. Nardelli B, Belvedere O, Roschke V, Moore PA, Olsen HS, Migone TS et al (2001) Synthesis and release of B-lymphocyte stimulator from myeloid cells. Blood 97:198–204
55. Moore PA, Belvedere O, Orr A, Pieri K, LaFleur DW, Feng P et al (2001) BLyS: member of the tumor necrosis factor family and B lymphocyte stimulator. Science 293:2111–2114
56. Cheema GS, Roschke V, Hilbert DM, Stohl W (2001) Elevated serum B lymphocyte stimulator levels in patients with systemic immune-based rheumatic diseases. Arthritis Rheum 44:1313–1319
57. Navarra SV, Guzmán RM, Gallacher AE, Hall S, Levy RA, Jimenez RE et al (2011) Efficacy and safety of belimumab in patients with active systemic lupus erythematosus: a randomised, placebo-controlled, phase 3 trial. Lancet 377(9767):721–731
58. Jacob CO, Mcdevitt HO (1988) Tumour necrosis factor-alpha in murine autoimmune lupus nephritis. Nature 331:356–358
59. Mohan AK, Edwards ET, Cote TR, Siegal JN, Braun MM (2002) Drug-induced systemic lupus erythematosus and TNF-alpha blockers. Lancet 360:646
60. Aringer M, Graninger WB, Steiner G, Smolen JS (2004) Safety and efficacy of tumor necrosis factor alpha blockade in systemic lupus erythematosus: an open label study. Arthritis Rheum 50:3161–3169
61. Ravirajan CT, Rahman MA, Papadaki L, Griffiths MH, Kalsi J, Martin AC et al (1998) Genetic, structural and functional properties of an IgG DNA-binding monoclonal antibody from a lupus patient with nephritis. Eur J Immunol 28:339–350, Erratum: Eur J Immunol 1999; 29: 3052
62. Okamura M, Kanayama Y, Amastu K, Negoro N, Kohda S, Takeda T et al (1993) Significance of enzyme linked immunosorbent assay (ELISA) for antibodies to double stranded and single stranded DNA in patients with lupus nephritis: correlation with severity of renal histology. Ann Rheum Dis 52:14–20
63. Rahman A (2004) Autoantibodies, lupus and the science of sabotage. Rheumatology (Oxford) 43:1326–1336
64. Lu L, Kaliyaperumal A, Boumpas DT, Datta SK (1999) Major peptide autoepitopes for nucleosome-specific T cells of human lupus. J Clin Invest 104:345–355
65. Kang HK, Chiang MY, Liu M, Ecklund D, Datta SK (2011) The histone peptide H471-94 is more effective than a cocktail of peptides epitopes in controlling lupus: immunoregulatory mechanisms. J Clin Immunol 31: 379–394
66. Apostolidis SA, Lieberman LA, Kis-Toth K, Crispin JC, Tsokos GC (2011) The dysregulation of cytokine networks in systemic lupus erythematosus. J Interferon Cytokine Res 31:769–779
67. Gigante A, Gasperini ML, Afeltra A, Barbano B, Margiotta D, Cianci R et al (2011) Cytokines expression in SLE nephritis. Eur Rev Med Pharmacol Sci 15:15–24
68. Cunninghame Graham DS, Morris DL, Bhangale TR, Criswell LA, Syvänen AC, Rönnblom L et al (2011) Association of NCF2, IKZF1, IRF8, IFIH1, and TYK2 with systemic lupus erythematosus. PLoS Genet 7:e1002341
69. Sawalha AH, Kaufman KM, Kelly JA, Adler AJ, Aberle T, Kilpatrick J et al (2008) Genetic association of interleukin-21 polymorphisms with systemic lupus erythematosus. Ann Rheum Dis 67:458–461
70. Sakaguchi S, Yamaguchi T, Nomura T, Ono M (2008) Regulatory T cells and immune tolerance. Cell 133:775–787
71. Buckner JH (2010) Mechanisms of impaired regulation by CD4(+)CD25(+)FOXP3(+) regulatory T cells in human autoimmune diseases. Nat Rev Immunol 10:849–859
72. Yurasov SV, Wardermann H, Hammersen J, Pascual V, Meffre E, Nussenzweig MC (2004) Autoreactive B cells and immune tolerance alterations in peripheral blood of patients with systemic autoimmunity. Pediatr Res 292A
73. Alexander T, Thiel A, Rosen O, Massenkeil G, Sattler A, Kohler S et al (2009) Depletion of autoreactive immunologic memory followed by autologous hematopoietic stem cell transplantation in patients with refractory SLE induced long term remission through de novo generation of a juvenile and tolerant immune system. Blood 113:214–223
74. Nimmerjahn F, Ravetch JV (2007) Fc-receptors as regulators of immunity. Adv Immunol 96:179–204

75. Medina F, Segundo C, Campos-Caro A, González-García I, Brieva JA (2002) The heterogeneity shown by human plasma cells from tonsil, blood and bone marrow reveals graded stages of increasing maturity, but local profiles of adhesion molecule expression. Blood 99:2154–2161
76. Odendahl M, Jacobi A, Hansen A, Feist E, Hiepe F, Burmester GR et al (2000) Disturbed peripheral B lymphocyte homeostasis in systemic lupus erythematosus. J Immunol 165: 5970–5979
77. Anolik JH, Aringer M (2005) New treatments for SLE: cell-depleting and anti-cytokine therapies. Best Pract Res Clin Rheumatol 19:859–878
78. Gateva V, Sandling JK, Hom G, Taylor KE, Chung SA, Sun X et al (2009) A large-scale replication study identifies TNIP1, PRDM1, JAZF1, UHRF1BP1 and IL10 as risk loci for systemic lupus erythematosus. Nat Genet 41:1228–1233
79. Blair PA, Norena LY, Flores-Borja F, Rawlings DJ, Isenberg DA, Ehrenstein MR et al (2010) CD19(+)CD24(hi)CD38(hi) B cells exhibit regulatory capacity in healthy individuals but are functionally impaired in systemic lupus erythematosus patients. Immunity 32:129–140
80. Bosma A, Abel-Gadir A, Isenberg DA, Jury EC, Mauri C (2012) Lipid-antigen presentation by CD1d(+) B cells is essential for the maintenance of invariant natural killer T cells. Immunity 36:477–490
81. Koffler D, Schur PH, Kunkel HG (1967) Immunological studies concerning the nephritis of systemic lupus erythematosus. J Exp Med 126:607–624
82. Isenberg DA, Shoenfeld Y, Walport M, Mackworth-Young C, Dudeney C, Todd-Pokropek A et al (1985) Detection of cross-reactive anti-DNA antibody idiotypes in the serum of systemic lupus erythematosus patients and of their relatives. Arthritis Rheum 28:999–1007
83. Ng KP, Manson JJ, Rahman A, Isenberg DA (2006) Association of anti-nucleosome antibodies with disease flare in serologically active clinically quiescent patients with systemic lupus erythematosus. Arthritis Rheum 55:900–904
84. Mannik M, Merrill CE, Stamps LD, Wener MH (2003) Multiple autoantibodies form the glomerular immune deposits in patients with systemic lupus erythematosus. J Rheumatol 30:1495–1504
85. Sontheimer RD, Maddison PJ, Reichlin M, Jordan RE, Stastny P, Gilliam JN (1982) Serologic and HLA associations in subacute cutaneous lupus erythematosus, a clinical subset of lupus erythematosus. Ann Intern Med 97:664–671
86. Kowal C, Degiorgio LA, Lee JY, Edgar MA, Huerta PT, Volpe BT et al (2006) Human lupus autoantibodies against NMDA receptors mediate cognitive impairment. Proc Natl Acad Sci U S A 103:19854–19859
87. Quisimoro FP (2007) Other serologic abnormalities in systemic lupus erythematosus. In: Wallace DJ, Hahn BH (eds) Dubois' Lupus erythematosus, 7th edn. Lippincott Williams and Wilkins, Philadelphia, pp 527–550
88. Pujol M, Ribera A, Vildarell M, Ordi J, Feliu E (1995) High prevalence of platelet autoantibodies in patients with systemic lupus erythematosus. Br J Haematol 89:137–141
89. Berden JH, Licht R, van Bruggen MC, Tax WJ (1999) Role of nucleosomes for induction and glomerular binding of autoantibodies in lupus nephritis. Curr Opin Nephrol Hypertens 8:299–306
90. Kalaaji M, Fenton KA, Mortensen ES, Olsen R, Sturfelt G, Alm P et al (2007) Glomerular apoptotic nucleosomes are central target structures for nephritogenic antibodies in human SLE nephritis. Kidney Int 71:664–672
91. Kalaaji M, Mortensen E, Jorgensen L, Olsen R, Rekvig OP (2006) Nephritogenic lupus antibodies recognize glomerular basement membrane-associated chromatin fragments released from apoptotic intraglomerular cells. Am J Pathol 168:1779–1792

Chapter 2

The Lupus Biomarker Odyssey: One Experience

Joseph M. Ahearn, Susan Manzi, and Chau-Ching Liu

Abstract

The last decade has witnessed an explosion in efforts to discover and validate lupus biomarkers. The currently steep trajectory of this progress is unprecedented. However, advances in the lupus biomarker field remain fewer and slower than physicians, patients, and pharmaceutical companies have hoped for. This chapter will review the challenges confronted by physicians and scientists in pursuit of lupus biomarkers and will present our experience on this path and specific efforts to surmount some of the obstacles in this endeavor. A comprehensive review of the current landscape in lupus biomarker research has recently been published elsewhere (Ahearn et al. Transl Res 159:326–342, 2012; Liu et al. Ther Adv Musculoskelet Dis 5:210–233, 2013; Liu and Ahearn Best Pract Res Clin Rheumatol 23:507–523, 2009; Liu et al. Curr Opin Rheumatol 17:543–549, 2005).

Key words Systemic lupus erythematosus, Biomarkers, Complement, Flow cytometry, CB-CAPs

1 Introduction

There is an urgent need for lupus biomarkers for several reasons. First, SLE is commonly misdiagnosed, even by experienced rheumatologists. The diagnosis requires interpretation of complex criteria developed by the American College of Rheumatology, as no single test is sufficiently sensitive and specific to be diagnostic. It has been generally held that many individuals with a positive test for ANA alone are misdiagnosed as lupus, despite many patients with other diseases and even healthy individuals also testing positive for ANA. Although anti-dsDNA is highly specific for lupus and a positive test essentially guarantees an accurate lupus diagnosis, the majority of patients with lupus test negative for anti-dsDNA at a given point in time. Published studies document that even experienced rheumatologists misdiagnose lupus. In one report, of 263 patients referred with a presumptive diagnosis of lupus, 125 were found to be misdiagnosed and of these 76 were ANA-positive but did not have an autoimmune disease [5]. Second, the course of SLE in a given patient is characterized by unpredictable flares and

Paul Eggleton and Frank J. Ward (eds.), *Systemic Lupus Erythematosus: Methods and Protocols*, Methods in Molecular Biology, vol. 1134, DOI 10.1007/978-1-4939-0326-9_2, © Springer Science+Business Media New York 2014

remissions. Again, there is no laboratory test with reliable capacity to identify or predict a disease flare. Third, the lack of biomarkers has impeded efforts to evaluate new SLE therapeutics in clinical trials. Pharmaceutical companies, with potential therapies in the pipeline and in hand, may be reluctant to invest in clinical trials because response to therapy cannot be determined with confidence or trials that are completed may fail for the same reason. Fourth, biomarker discovery and development are a critical link between pathogenic mechanisms and therapeutics. In some cases, discovery of molecular and cellular mechanisms (e.g., those involving interferon) may lead to identification of candidate biomarkers that may in turn suggest potential therapeutic targets and provide direction for drug development. The capacity of the innovative therapeutics to interfere with the targeted pathogenic mechanisms can then be evaluated with those same biomarkers that led to the drug discovery.

2 Challenges to Lupus Biomarker Discovery and Validation

The disappointing pace of lupus biomarker development, even compared with similar efforts in other diseases, is at least partly due to challenges unique to SLE. First, the extraordinary clinical heterogeneity of lupus, most likely due to distinct and overlapping pathogenic mechanisms, requires precision medicine to pair the patient not only with the right therapeutic but also with the biomarker(s) that will accurately reflect the disease process in that same patient. If all patients with lupus are evaluated as a single group for efficacy of a single biomarker, no difference might be observed compared with the control group(s) although the biomarker might be highly valuable among a subset of patients for diagnosis, monitoring or predicting response to a specific therapeutic intervention. Second, because lupus is frequently misdiagnosed, it is possible that the "lupus" subjects in a particular biomarker investigation may not actually have the disease. Third, studies of lupus biomarkers for disease activity are extremely challenging because there is no clear "gold standard" by which the potential biomarkers can be evaluated. If a study is designed to demonstrate an impact on clinical care of lupus patients, it must be superior to what is currently in use. The numerous complex disease activity indices used by lupus aficionados are not employed in routine clinical practice yet these may be the standards to which novel biomarkers for monitoring patients are held for validation and acceptance. Fourth, laboratory assays for lupus diagnosis and monitoring that have been used for decades, such as anti-dsDNA, serum C3/C4, and ANA, have never been standardized or validated themselves, yet these are the standards to which emerging biomarkers are typically compared. This dilemma regarding the utility of ANA testing has recently been thoughtfully considered [6]. Frequent false-positive results with the traditional indirect immunofluorescence ANA assay and recent false-negative results with higher-throughput ANA technologies further emphasize the need for advances and standardization in lupus diagnostics and beyond. In addition to these obstacles that may be particularly relevant to the development of lupus biomarkers, another challenge common to many biomarker discovery strategies includes the reality that humans are not rodents and many advances made with animal models of human disease cannot be directly translated to humans because of different genetics, biology, pathophysiology, or other interspecies differences. Additional challenges to biomarker validation in general include considerations of time and temperature, shipping, freeze-thawing, and other quality control issues that are essential but not always rigorously evaluated in development.

3 Biomarker Discovery Strategies

The two general strategies employed in biomarker development are the technology-driven versus the candidate biomarker approaches. Technology-driven approaches capitalize on the power of recent and rapidly developing genomic, proteomic, metabolomic, peptidomic, and microarray technologies to compare various sets of biologic samples to identify meaningful differences. Many such efforts are not necessarily driven by specific hypotheses beyond predicting that differences will be identified when comparing serum, plasma, urine, DNA, RNA, etc. from two or more groups of study subjects. The alternate strategy is to focus on specific molecular and/or cellular pathways, usually because prior discoveries have suggested them as fertile sources to mine for biomarkers. Of course, these two approaches are not mutually exclusive. For example, a microarray study might identify a promising signature that is then specifically mined for candidate molecular biomarkers. Alternatively, the knowledge that a specific molecular and cellular pathway is involved in a disease might lead to targeted proteomic characterization of these pathways in serum or plasma from patients versus control subjects. Regardless of which general approach is taken, the biomarker discovery journey typically progresses through sequential stages of conceptualization, identification, development, and validation. The remainder of this chapter will describe our efforts for the past decade during which we took a candidate-driven approach from conceptualization to validation focused on cell-bound complement activation products (CB-CAPs) as lupus biomarkers for diagnosis, monitoring, stratification, and precision (personalized) medicine. Hopefully, lessons learned from our experience may help guide future efforts in the field as the lupus biomarker odyssey has just begun.

4 CB-CAP Conceptualization

The compelling rationale for mining the complement system for lupus biomarkers has been thoroughly described previously [7–11] and will be recapitulated here. The complement system is a highly complex group of plasma and membrane-bound proteins that form three distinct pathways (classical, alternative, and lectin-dependent) evolved primarily to protect against invasion of foreign pathogens. The classical pathway is the major effector mechanism for antibody-mediated immune responses. Because antibody/immune complex-triggered activation of the complement system is believed to play an important role in the pathogenesis of SLE, measurement of serum C3 and C4 has traditionally been the "gold standard" for monitoring disease activity in SLE patients. Decreased C3 and C4 levels are considered to be markers of inflammation and increased SLE disease activity. However, there are several drawbacks in this approach. First, there is a wide range of variation in serum C3 and C4 levels among healthy individuals, and this range overlaps with the range observed in SLE patients. Second, standard laboratory tests measure the concentration of parental C3 and C4 molecules rather than products of activation. Third, acute phase response during inflammation may lead to an increase in C4 and C3 synthesis, which can balance the activation and increased consumption of these proteins. Fourth, partial deficiencies of C4, which are commonly present in the general population and in SLE patients, may result in lower than normal serum C4 levels because of decreased synthesis rather than increased complement activation and/or active SLE. As a result of these complexities, there have been conflicting conclusions regarding the value of serial measurement of serum C3 and C4 in monitoring disease activity in SLE patients. Some studies have found these assays valuable in this regard, while others have found C3 and C4 levels to remain normal during SLE flares. These conflicting results suggest that current standard tests, based on serum levels of the native form of complement proteins, are inadequate to accurately and promptly detect SLE disease flares. During the past several years, other investigators have explored the potential for measurement of soluble complement activation products such as C3a and C4d to serve as biomarkers in SLE. Despite some intriguing observations, serum levels of complement activation products have not replaced measurement of native C3 and C4 as gold standards.

Together, these prior observations led to the hypothesis that complement activation products (CAPs) during the course of lupus pathogenesis may covalently bind to surfaces of circulating cells, potentially rendering the cells dysfunctional. As such, CB-CAPs might serve as lupus biomarkers to guide clinical care of patients while also participating directly in lupus pathogenesis through a novel molecular-cellular pathway.

5 CB-CAP Identification

Efforts during the past decade have led to the CB-CAP technology platform, which currently consists of a panel of assays designed to identify C4d and C3d complement activation products that have been deposited on essentially any circulating cell type. Cell types and cell subsets are identified by routine flow cytometric gating practices and the use of cell-specific phenotypic surface markers, while CB-CAPs are simultaneously identified with anti-C4d and anti-C3d monoclonal antibodies (Fig. 1).

5.1 E-C4d: The First CB-CAP

Initial efforts to prove the CB-CAP hypothesis were focused on the erythrocyte [12] because normal erythrocytes are known to bear constitutively low levels of C4d and are unique in this regard among circulating human cells. An initial study showed that abnormally high levels of C4d are deposited on the surface of erythrocytes (E-C4d) in patients with SLE as compared with healthy

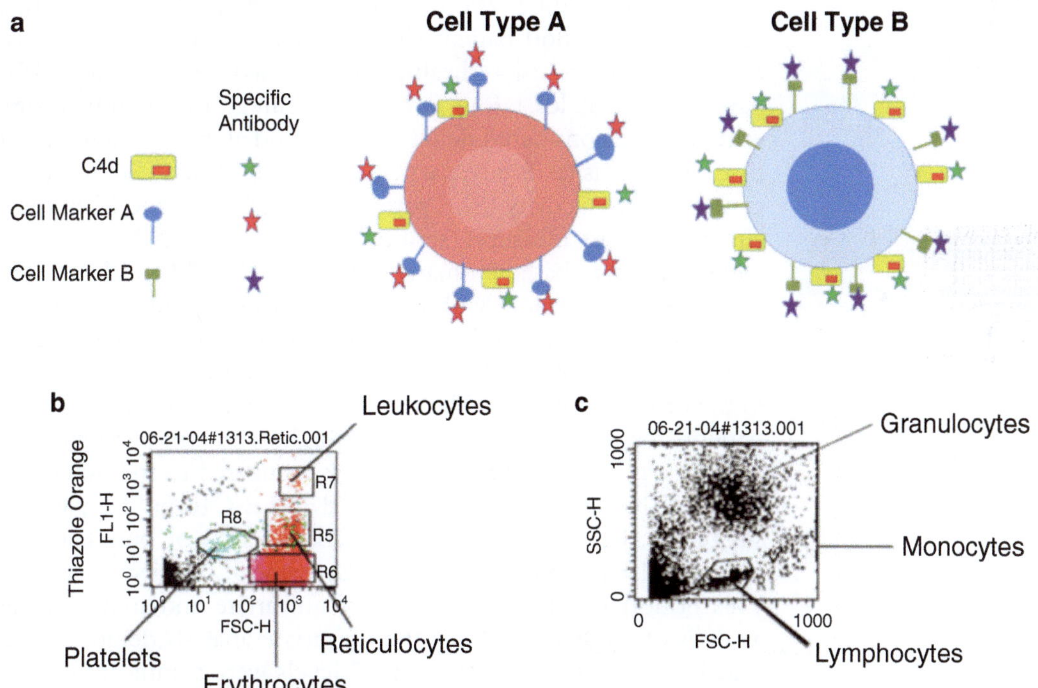

Fig. 1 Flow cytometric assay of CB-CAPs. (**a**) Schematic illustration of the multicolor staining of circulating cells for cell type-specific surface markers and surface-bound CAPs (e.g., C4d). (**b**) A representative dot plot shows the identification of reticulocytes (gate R5) and erythrocytes (gate R6) by thiazole orange staining (*Y*-axis). Contaminating leukocytes and platelets present in the samples can be differentiated from reticulocytes and erythrocytes based on the thiazole orange staining intensity and forward scattering property. (**c**) A representative dot plot demonstrates the identification of lymphocytes, monocytes, and granulocytes. These cell types are also differentiated by using mAbs specific for different cell lineages added to the cell suspension (e.g., anti-CD3, anti-CD19, etc.). The latter staining pattern is not shown here

subjects and patients with other diseases. As a diagnostic marker for SLE, E-C4d was 72 % sensitive and 79 % specific in differentiating SLE from other inflammatory diseases.

It was also noted during these studies of erythrocytes that E-C4d levels in the same SLE patient examined on different days varied considerably, suggesting that changes in E-C4d levels in SLE patients might reflect fluctuation in disease activity. We pursued this hypothesis through both cross-sectional and longitudinal studies [13]. In the initial longitudinal study, we analyzed the erythrocyte-based markers as disease activity biomarkers in patients with SLE using a regression formulation in which each patient's evolving clinical status was regressed on each of the biomarkers. The Systemic Lupus Activity Measure (SLAM), and the SLE Disease Activity Index (SLEDAI), were used as the clinical measures to assess disease activity in these patients. In addition to the CB-CAP biomarkers, we also tested the more traditional markers of disease activity for SLE, serum C3 and C4, and anti-dsDNA. Briefly, 156 patients with SLE, 290 patients with other diseases, and 256 healthy individuals were followed prospectively over a 5-year period (2001–2005), encompassing 1,005 patient-visits (SLE patients), 660 patient-visits (patients with other diseases), and 395 subject-visits (healthy individuals). All of these 156 patients met at least four American College of Rheumatology criteria to be considered definitive SLE, and all had a minimum of three study visits. Study participants were closely followed for clinical disease activity (SLE patients, using SLAM and SLEDAI), clinic laboratory measures (serum C3, C4, anti-dsDNA, and ESR), and erythrocyte-based biomarker measures (E-C3d and E-C4d).

As we had previously observed, SLE patients had higher levels of E-C4d than did the healthy controls and patients with other diseases. Levels of E-C3d were also higher in the SLE group than in the other two groups. The variances within patient and between patients for E-C3d and E-C4d were high, while the variability for E-CR1 was low in the SLE patients as compared to the other two groups. The high variability of E-C3d and E-C4d in SLE patients suggested that levels of these biomarkers vary not only between different SLE patients but also within the same SLE patient over time. This notion was further verified by univariate and multivariable analysis of covariance. While the univariate analysis demonstrated that E-C4d, E-C3d, and serum C3 levels were significantly associated with SLAM and SLEDAI (all $p<0.001$), the multivariate analysis showed that only E-C4d remained significant predictors of SLE disease activity even after adjusting for serum C3, C4, and anti-dsDNA antibody.

5.2 E-C4d as a Time Capsule of Lupus Disease Activity

These E-C4d data strongly supported the possibility that E-C4d levels may reflect disease activity in SLE patients, leading to the E-C4d "time capsule" hypothesis as follows. Human erythrocytes survive in the circulation for approximately 120 days. While erythrocytes circulating during a disease flare (i.e., increased complement activation) may have an increased amount of C4d deposited on their surface, erythrocytes emerging from the bone marrow after the flare has subsided (i.e., diminished complement activation) may have a low ("remission") level of surface C4d. Considering that erythrocytes of different ages ranging from 1 day old to 120 days old are present in the circulation at any given time, we postulated that detection of erythrocyte subpopulations expressing distinct levels of C4d at a specific time point should theoretically reveal, much like time capsules, SLE disease activity during the preceding 120 days.

To verify this hypothesis, we performed experiments examining the C4d levels on age-fractionated erythrocytes. The most well-established methodology for separating human erythrocytes of different ages is density gradient fractionation. This technique is based on the concept that the buoyant density of erythrocytes increases with cell age. Briefly, erythrocytes derived from 0.25 ml of freshly drawn blood were washed in PBS containing EDTA (to avoid cell clumping), resuspended in 0.5 ml isotonic buffer, and centrifuged through a continuous Percoll gradient (0–50 % Percoll; 1–1.15 g/ml density; GE Healthcare Biosciences). Erythrocyte fractions were sequentially collected from the bottom of the gradient and washed two times with PBS to remove residual Percoll. Levels of C4-derived products on age-fractionated erythrocytes and unfractionated erythrocytes from the same individual (SLE patient or healthy control) were assayed by flow cytometry and quantitated as SMFI. SMFI data of the whole set of fractions derived from each patient and control were analyzed collectively to obtain the overall pattern of the differential E-C4d levels on old versus young erythrocytes. Three general patterns of E-C4d levels among age-fractionated erythrocytes were identified. Figure 2 shows the data obtained from three representative SLE patients respectively. The first pattern demonstrates high E-C4d levels on the older erythrocytes (Fig. 2, left upper panel patient #1043); the second pattern demonstrates constant E-C4d levels on all fractions regardless of the age of erythrocytes (Fig. 2, left middle panel patient #1014); the third pattern showed demonstrates high E-C4d levels on the youngest erythrocytes (Fig. 2, left lower panel patient #1066). We speculated that these different E-C4d patterns may represent, respectively, a previously active, a stable (or chronically active), and a recently activated disease state. Collectively, these data provide support for the "time capsule" hypothesis indicating that the levels of C4d on erythrocytes of SLE patients may contribute informative clues to remote, current, and imminent disease activity.

5.2.1 Method: Erythrocyte CB-CAP Assays

Blood was collected in Vacutainer™ tubes containing EDTA as an anticoagulant (Becton Dickinson) and used for experiments within 24 h after collection. After partitioning by centrifugation at 800 × *g*,

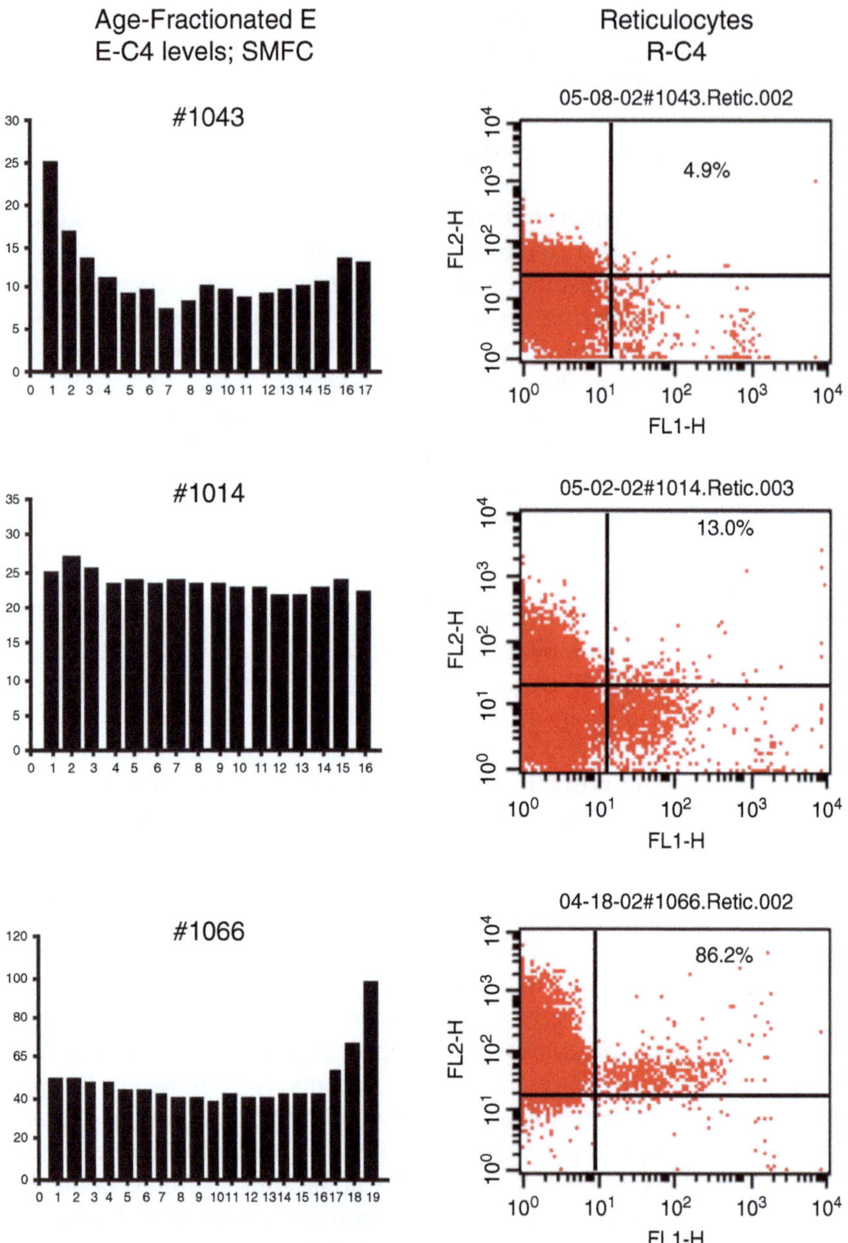

Fig. 2 Three general patterns of E-C4d deposition on age-fractionated erythrocytes. The EC4d levels (SMFI) of all fractions of erythrocytes of each of three patients are presented as a bar graph on the *left*. The *X*-axes are the numbered fractions with 1 being the oldest fraction. The *Y*-axes are the MFI of C4d determined by flow cytometry. C4d deposition on reticulocytes of the same patient analyzed on the same day is shown as a dot blot on the *right*. *Numbers* in the dot blots represent the percentage of C4d+ reticulocytes

the plasma was removed for storage and the blood cell portion diluted in phosphate buffered saline (PBS). Erythrocytes in the diluted blood were washed with PBS, resuspended in PBS, and aliquotted for antibody staining using mouse anti-human C4d monoclonal antibodies (mAb) (reactive with native C4, C4b, iC4b, and C4d; from Quidel), mouse anti-human C3d mAb (reactive with native C3, C3b and C3d), or the isotype-matched mouse IgG control. Additional studies have demonstrated that the erythrocyte surface antigens reactive with these two mAbs are indeed C4d and C3d, not the native molecules or other activation products. Fluorescein isothiocyanate (FITC)-conjugated goat anti-mouse IgG $F(ab')_2$ (Jackson ImmunoResearch Laboratories, Inc.) at a concentration of 10 μg/ml was used as the secondary antibody. Stained cells were analyzed using a FACSCalibur™ flow cytometer (Becton Dickinson Immunocytometry Systems) in conjunction with CellQuest Software. Erythrocytes were electronically gated based on forward and side scatter properties to include only single cells. Levels of surface-bound C4d and C3d on gated cells were expressed as specific mean fluorescence intensity: C4d- or C3d-specific mean fluorescence minus the isotype control mean fluorescence.

5.3 Reticulocyte-Bound C4d as a Biomarker for Ongoing SLE Disease Activity

These "time capsule" studies led to a focus on the reticulocyte as a potential "instant messenger" of lupus disease activity [14]. As mentioned above, erythrocytes ranging from 1 day old to 120 days old are present in the circulation at any given time point. The E-C4d levels on such a heterogeneous population may theoretically represent a cumulative result of complement activation/binding during the preceding 120 days, confounding the differential diagnosis of ongoing disease activation versus an earlier SLE flare. To overcome this problem, we established another assay examining the level of complement C4-derived activation products bound to reticulocytes (R-C4d). These cells are the youngest erythrocytes that emerge from the bone marrow, and they circulate in the blood for approximately 1 day before fully maturing into erythrocytes. We speculated that a high level of C4d identified on reticulocytes may indicate ongoing complement activation and reflect the degree of SLE disease activity on that day. Indeed, upon examining the presence of C4-derived products on reticulocytes of SLE patients, a wide spectrum of R-C4d ranging from undetectable to high levels was detected (Figs. 2 and 3). As noted above, during our studies of age-fractionated erythrocytes of SLE patients, high E-C4d levels were detected on younger erythrocytes, but not older erythrocytes, in some patients (Fig. 2, left lower panel patient #1066). Interestingly, reticulocytes of these same patients also exhibited high R-C4d levels (Fig. 2, right lower panel patient #1066). Moreover, preliminary inspection suggested a correlation between the R-C4d levels and clinical disease activity. These initial studies supported our hypothesis that reticulocytes may serve as "instant messengers" by carrying products of complement activation to reflect ongoing disease activity in SLE patients.

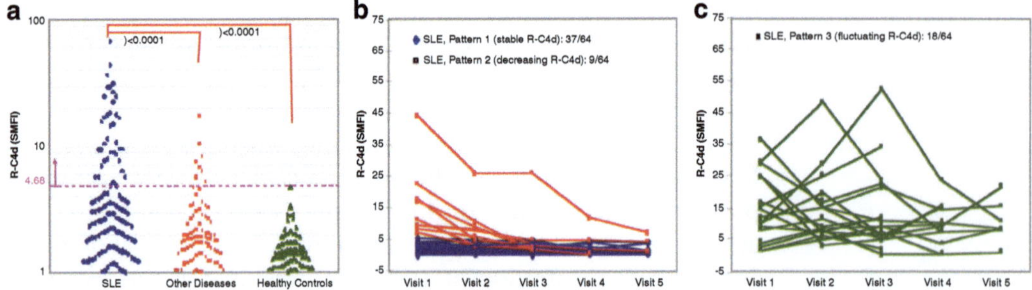

Fig. 3 Reticulocyte-C4d levels are significantly elevated in patients with SLE and fluctuate over time. (**a**) Reticulocytes from patients with SLE have significantly higher levels of C4d than those from patients with other diseases or healthy controls. Shown on the *Y*-axis is the C4d-specific median fluorescence intensity for reticulocytes from 156 patients with SLE, 140 patients with other diseases, and 159 healthy controls. The *pink line* represents an empirically determined cutoff point. Numbers of SLE patients, patients with other diseases, and healthy controls with R-C4d higher than this point are shown in *pink* in the *X*-axis legend (see text for details). (**b** and **c**) R-C4d levels fluctuate in a significant fraction of patients with SLE. Shown are R-C4d levels of 64 patients with SLE examined at three to five different study visits. In 37 patients, R-C4d remained stably low. In nine patients, R-C4d was elevated at the first visit but decreased in subsequent visits. Significant fluctuation of R-C4d was observed in 18 patients

To date, we have analyzed, in both cross-sectional and prospective fashions, R-C4d levels in 156 patients with SLE, 140 patients with other autoimmune diseases, and 159 healthy individuals. The R-C4d levels were found to be significantly higher in SLE patients than in patients with other autoimmune diseases or healthy controls. Moreover, during longitudinal observation, the R-C4d levels in a significant fraction of SLE patients varied considerably over time (Fig. 3), suggesting that fluctuations in R-C4d levels coincide with changes in disease activity. In addition, within the SLE patient population, the level of R-C4d appears to be proportionate to the clinical disease activity in a given SLE patient, i.e., patients with higher R-C4d levels have higher disease activity scores. These results strongly suggest that R-C4d levels, in contrast to E-C4 levels, reflect more precisely and promptly ongoing disease activity in an SLE patient, supporting the role for reticulocytes as "instant messengers" of SLE disease activity.

5.3.1 Method: Reticulocyte CB-CAP Assays

A two-color immunofluorescence staining method was employed to examine the levels of C4- and C3-derived CAPs on reticulocytes. Briefly, 10 μl of the erythrocyte suspension (containing reticulocytes), was incubated sequentially with (1) anti-human C4d or anti-C3d mAb or isotype-matched mouse IgG control followed by a phycoerythrin (PE)-conjugated anti-mouse IgG antibody and (2) thiazole orange (a supravital dye emitting green fluorescence; Retic-Count™ reagent; Becton Dickinson). All mAbs were used at a concentration of 10 μg/ml. After staining, cells were analyzed using a FACSCalibur™ cytometer and CellQuest Software. Reticulocytes were identified by thiazole orange staining as well as forward and side scatter properties.

5.4 Platelet-Bound C4d as a Biomarker for Stratification in SLE

The erythrocyte studies, as mentioned above, were initially conducted because normal red blood cells are known to be unique in their C4d-positive phenotype, despite not bearing any receptors for C4d. Demonstration of the utility of E-C4d and RC4d as lupus biomarkers suggested that cells other than those in the erythroid lineage might also carry the CB-CAP phenotype. Therefore, our attention turned to the platelet [15].

In view of the biological role of platelets in hemostasis, coagulation, and thrombosis, we postulated that abnormal CB-CAPs on platelets may serve as a useful biomarker for SLE patients who are at increased risk of cardiovascular and cerebrovascular events. Using flow cytometric analysis, P-C4d measure was shown to be a specific (98 %) diagnostic assay for SLE. Moreover, this study showed that P-C4d correlated with a history of neurological event ($p = 0.006$) and positive antiphospholipid antibody tests ($p = 0.013$), a clinical manifestation, and a known risk factor for thrombotic complications of SLE, respectively. This observation suggested that P-C4d may represent a stratification biomarker capable of identifying a unique set of SLE patients with increased risk for developing cerebrovascular and neurologic complications.

Most recently, PC4d was also shown to be associated with stroke and with all-cause mortality in SLE patients [16]. In this study, a cohort of 356 consecutive patients with SLE was followed from 2001 to 2009. Seventy SLE patients (19.7 %) were positive for P-C4d. P-C4d was associated with all-cause mortality (hazard ratio 7.52, 95 % confidence interval/CI 2.14–26.45, $p = 0.002$) after adjusting for age, ethnicity, sex, cancer, and anticoagulant use. Patients with positive P-C4d were also more likely to have had vascular events compared to those who were P-C4d negative (35.7 % versus 18.2 %, $p = 0.001$). Specifically, P-C4d was associated with ischemic stroke (odds ratio 4.54, 95 % CI 1.63–12.69, $p = 0.004$) after adjusting for age, ethnicity, and antiphospholipid antibodies. These observations suggest that PC4d may be a clue to a unique relationship shared by complement activation, the thrombocyte, cerebrovascular disease, and perhaps worse outcome for patients with SLE.

5.4.1 Method: Platelet CB-CAP Assays

Immediately after collection, an aliquot of the blood was diluted using Ca^{2+}/Mg^{2+}-free PBS and divided into equal-volume portions and stained for different molecules. Platelets were distinguished from other blood cells based on the expression of CD42b (GPIb) using a PE-conjugated anti-CD42b antibody (BD Biosciences). The presence of platelet-associated CAPs was examined by a dual-color staining procedure using, in conjunction with PE anti-CD42b, a mouse anti-human C4d mAb (or anti-C3d mAb, or isotype-matched mouse IgG control) labeled with Alexa Fluor 488 (Invitrogen/Molecular Probes).

5.5 Lymphocyte CB-CAPs

Extending the panel of CB-CAPs from the erythroid to the megakaryocyte lineage suggested that all circulating cells might potentially have the capacity to carry CB-CAPs, and the myeloid cells were characterized as such [17]. Flow cytometric analysis of C4d on (T-C4d) and (B-C4d) cells demonstrated that both T-C4d and B-C4d levels are significantly and specifically elevated in SLE patients, as compared with healthy controls and patients with other diseases. Initial studies demonstrated that T-C4d and B-C4d are, respectively, 56 % sensitive and 80 % specific and 60 % sensitive and 82 % specific in differentiating SLE patients from patients with other diseases reflecting potential value as lupus diagnostic biomarkers.

In addition, levels of C4d bound to T and B cells of the same patients were strongly correlated ($r = 0.708$; data not shown). Based on T-C4d and B-C4d levels, with those greater than the "mean plus 2 SD of the levels in healthy controls" defined as the "high" phenotype, the SLE patients could be classified into four subgroups: T-C4d^{Low}/B-C4d^{Low} (37.0 %), T-C4d^{High}/B-C4d^{Low} (5.8 %), T-C4d^{Low}/B-C4d^{High} (14.3 %), and T-C4d^{High}/B-C4d^{High} (42.9 %). Interestingly, we noticed that SLE patients with the T-C4d^{High}/B-C4d^{High} phenotypes were younger but had longer disease duration than did patients with the other phenotypes such that the T-C4d^{High}/B-C4d^{High} phenotype of a given SLE patient may be suggestive of earlier onset disease.

We also observed that, in contrast to the constant T-C4d levels in healthy individuals, T-C4d levels in a given SLE patient examined on different days vary significantly (Fig. 4), suggesting a potential for T-C4d as a biomarker for tracking SLE disease activity over time.

5.5.1 Method: Lymphocyte, Monocyte, and Granulocyte CB-CAP Assays

To simultaneously enrich mononuclear cells (lymphocytes and monocytes) and polynucleated granulocytes, we developed a simple method as an alternative to the conventional isolation of peripheral blood mononuclear cells by Ficoll-Paque gradient centrifugation. Briefly, 5 ml of blood was collected into an EDTA-containing Vacutainer™ tube (Becton Dickinson). After low-speed centrifugation, the buffy coat consisting of leukocytes was carefully transferred into a fresh tube and contaminating erythrocytes were hypotonically lysed. The leukocyte suspension was washed extensively with PBS to remove lysed erythrocytes, resuspended, divided into equal-volume portions, and stained for different cell surface markers and C4- or C3-derived CAPs. Lymphocytes, monocytes, and granulocytes were distinguished based on their unique features of forward (size)/side (granularity) scattering and expression of

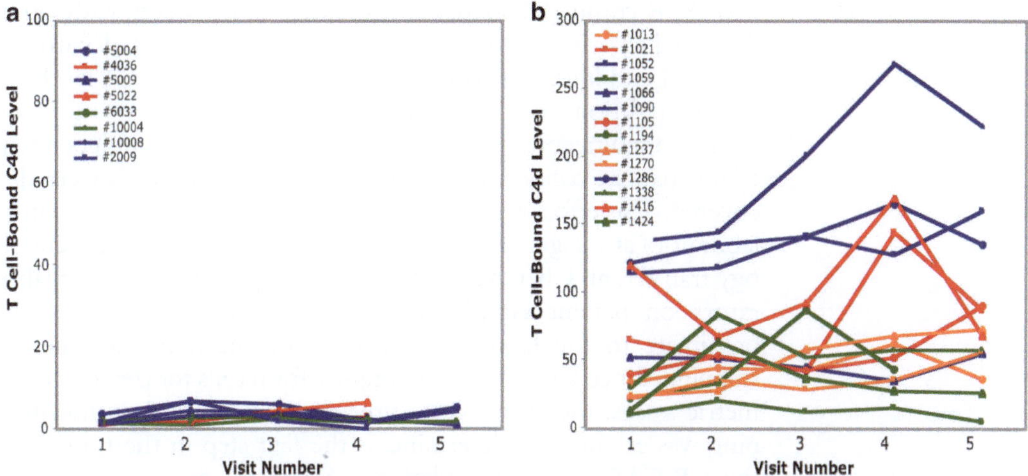

Fig. 4 T cell-bound C4d levels in SLE patients fluctuate over time but remain stable in patients with other diseases and healthy controls. Shown in (**a**) are T-C4d levels of patients with Sjogren's syndrome, rheumatoid arthritis, or inflammatory myopathy or of healthy controls examined at four or five different visits. Shown in (**b**) are T-C4d levels of 14 SLE patients examined at five visits. *Y*-axis: specific median fluorescence intensity

characteristic surface molecules. Granulocytes were differentiated from mononuclear cells by forward/side scatter properties through electronic gating. The presence of CAPs on cells was examined by three-color or four-color flow cytometric analysis, in which mAbs reactive with lineage-specific cell surface markers (e.g., CD3, CD4, CD8 for T cells, CD19 for B cells, and CD14 for monocytes; from BD Biosciences) were used in conjunction with either an anti-human C4d mAb (Quidel) or an anti-human C3d mAb (Quidel). All mAbs were used at a concentration of 10 μg/ml. After staining, cells were analyzed using a FACSCalibur™ cytometer and CellQuest Software. To ensure the specificity of the primary antibody, leukocyte aliquots from each patient stained with mouse IgG of appropriate isotypes were routinely included in all experiments.

5.6 Validation of the CB-CAP Technology Platform

A biomarker platform can be defined as a group of selected biomarkers, the assays to detect them, and algorithms to interpret and translate the results. Prior to being implemented for clinical decision-making and patient care, a biomarker platform requires carefully conducted validation studies in well-characterized patient cohorts. The validated biomarker platform should be accurate, stable, reliable, and sensitive to measure its intended application such as disease presence (diagnosis), activity (monitoring) subsets (stratification), and/or theranostics (precision or personalized medicine).

Single-center validation of CB-CAPs as lupus biomarkers for both diagnosis and monitoring has been reported by Yang et al. who demonstrated significant elevation of EC4d levels in patients with SLE compared to healthy subjects and patients with other diseases [18]. In addition, EC4d levels were correlated with the SLEDAI and inversely correlated with serum C3 and C4 levels.

In addition to these independent single-center validation studies, a multicenter validation effort was conducted independent of our patient cohort and laboratories where the assays were discovered. This effort required transfer of the technology to a central laboratory at Exagen Diagnostics, San Diego. Prior to the technology transfer, all CB-CAP studies had been performed in our laboratory on patient samples that had been obtained in a clinic proximate to the laboratory, without the need for commercial shipping. Since CB-CAP assays require fresh cells for the flow cytometric assays, the influence of time and temperature during shipping was essential to determine as the first step in the transfer of the CB-CAP technology platform. Samples were obtained from study subjects on day 0, split into two aliquots, and assayed immediately for levels of E-C4d, P-C4d, B-C4d, R-C4d, and T-C4d. The second aliquot of each sample was shipped overnight at ambient temperature to our own laboratory and assayed on day 1. The results of the paired assays performed on each sample were compared and shown to generate nearly identical results, indicating that overnight shipping of whole blood samples at ambient temperature would not compromise the integrity of the CB-CAP assays (Fig. 5). Following this quality control study, Kalunian et al. completed the CAPITAL study, a multicenter validation of CB-CAPs as diagnostic lupus biomarkers [19]. This study was conducted at 14 sites in the United States by investigators with lupus expertise. An assay panel consisting of E-C4d, B-C4d, anti-mutated citrullinated vimentin antibody (anti-MCV), ANA, and anti-dsDNA was evaluated in a cross-sectional study of 593 well-characterized subjects (210 SLE patients, 178 patients with other rheumatic diseases, and 205 healthy subjects). An algorithm was generated to calculate an index score, which was 80 % sensitive for SLE and 87 % specific versus other rheumatic diseases. An ongoing companion study focused on validation of CB-CAPs as biomarkers for monitoring disease activity in patients with SLE was launched in 2012. The success of the multicenter CAPITAL validation study coincided with the commercial launch of the Avise SLE test (Exagen Diagnostics, San Diego) that contains the same assay panel, including EC4d and BC4d, as that validated in the CAPITAL study.

6 The CB-CAP Signature

Collectively, these data clearly demonstrated that CAPs generated during systemic or local activation of the complement system in patients with SLE are capable of binding to essentially all circulating blood cells. However, it remained to be determined whether CAP

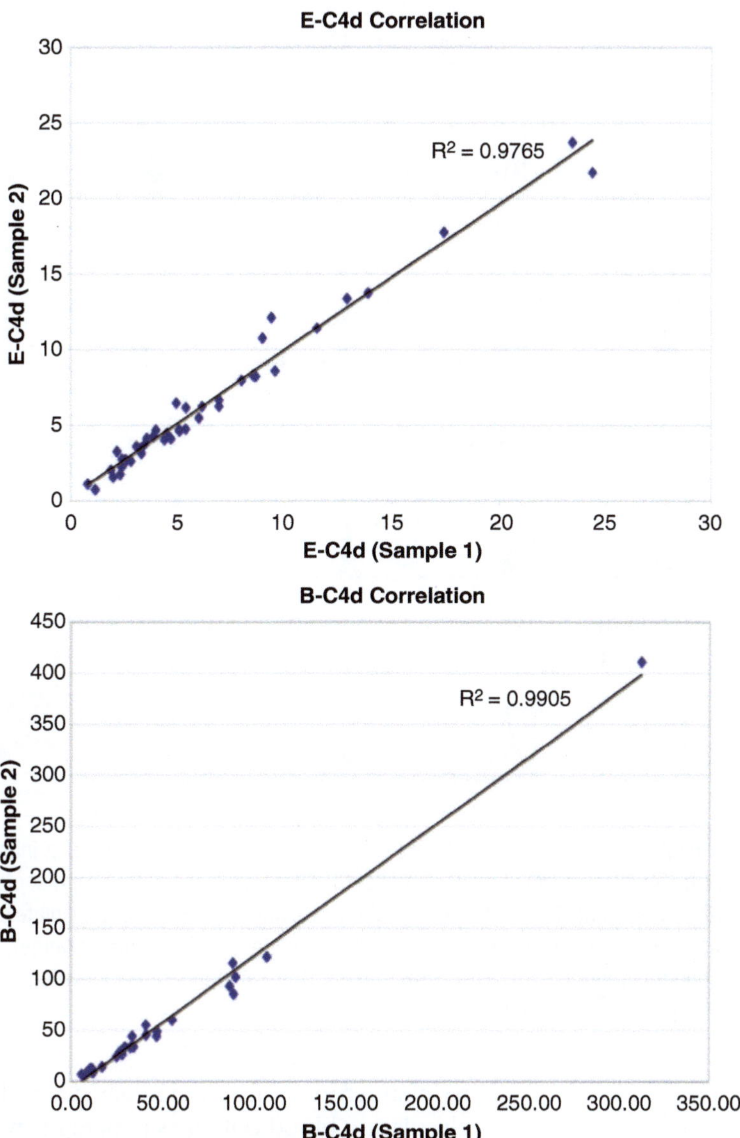

Fig. 5 Shipping stability of CB-CAPs. CB-CAP levels remain stable after overnight shipment of blood samples. Aliquots of the blood sample derived from the same patient were analyzed for CB-CAPs on the day of blood drawn (sample 1) or the next day after overnight shipment (sample 2). Shown are the comparisons of E-C4d and B-C4d levels on the blood sample pairs prepared from 53 patients. The correlation between the datasets of sample 1 and sample 2 was evaluated using the Pearson correlation coefficient calculation. Note the excellent correlation coefficients for both the E-C4d and B-C4d comparison

deposition occurs nonspecifically and indiscriminately on all cells in a given patient as a result of systemic complement activation or whether specific cell types are targeted and these targets differ among individual patients. Therefore, we conducted a pilot study

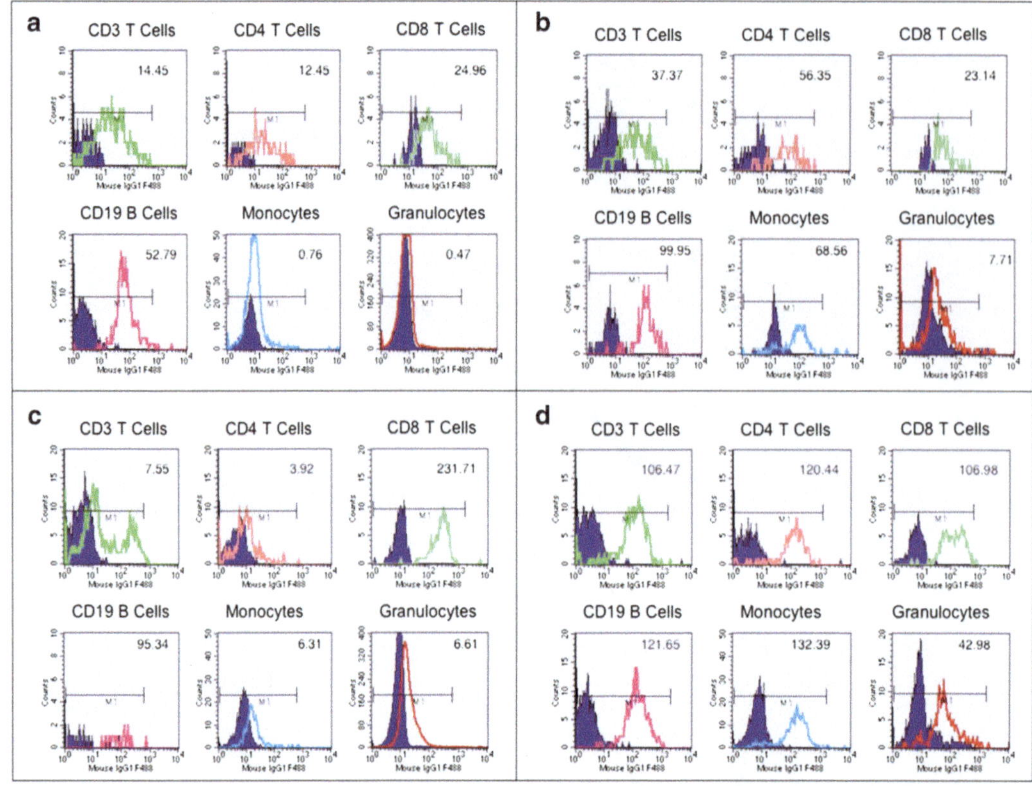

Fig. 6 CAPs bind to circulating blood cells in cell type-specific patterns in individual SLE patients. Shown are the CB-C4d histograms of the differential CB-CAP signatures of four representative SLE patients. The levels of erythrocyte-bound C4d (E-C4d), reticulocyte-bound C4d (R-C4d), and platelet-bound C4d (P-C4d) of these patients are, respectively, 4.46, 1.10, 0.00 (patient A; all within normal range), 12.16, 5.08, 9.23 (patient B; all in abnormal range), 7.59, 2.36, 3.96 (patient C; R-C4d moderately elevated, P-C4d elevated), and 6.57, 1.30, 30.10 (patient D; P-C4d highly abnormal)

to characterize simultaneously C4d deposition on a panel of circulating blood cell types in patients with SLE. The results demonstrated that high levels of C4d were not necessarily present concurrently on erythrocytes, platelets, lymphocytes, monocytes, and granulocytes of a given SLE patient on a particular day (Fig. 6). Moreover, the cell type-specific pattern/signature (not absolute level) of C4d deposition appeared to remain stable in a given patient over time. Together, these observations indicate that a patient-dependent, cell lineage-specific mechanism is responsible for an individual's CB-CAP signature. It is not simply due to indiscriminate complement activation that affects all cells in the circulation simultaneously and equally. These observations led us to conclude that CB-CAP signatures are highly characteristic of lupus patients and to propose the model shown in Fig. 7. This model is based upon the hypothesis that CB-CAP signatures may provide value as lupus biomarkers beyond the value contributed by each

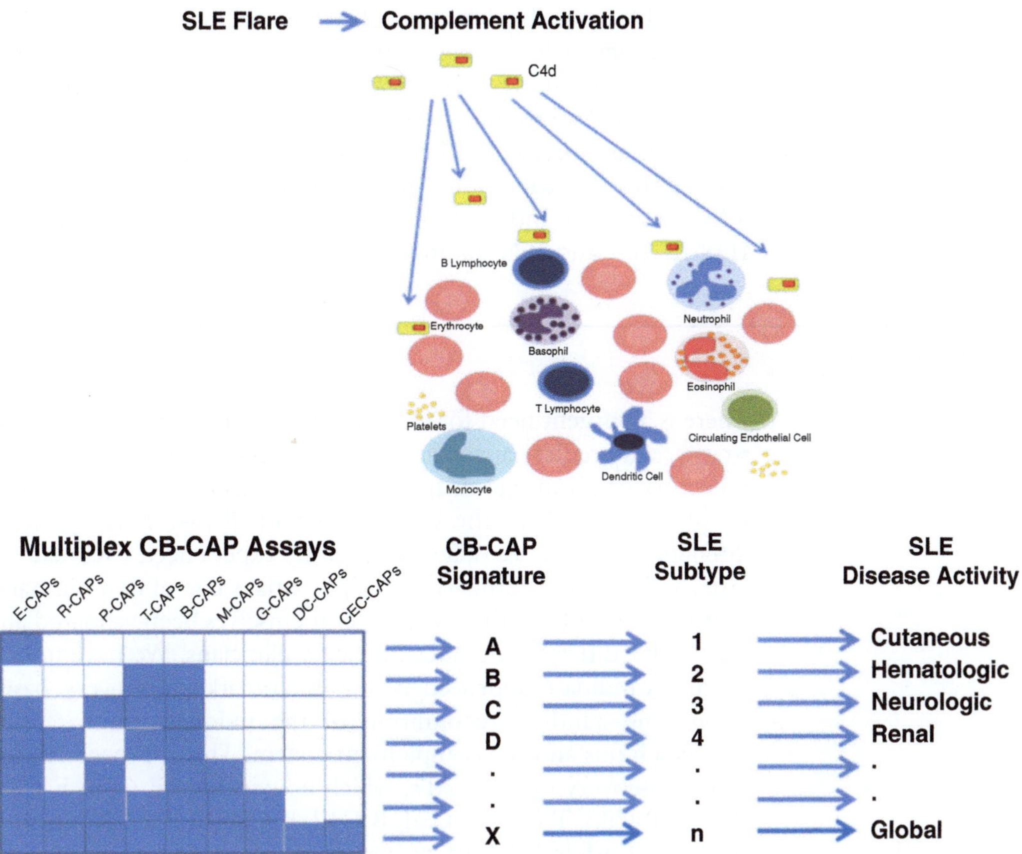

Fig. 7 The CB-CAP signature. Patient-specific patterns of CB-CAP deposition on distinct lineages and subsets of circulating cells may ultimately be proven to correlate with and/or predict clinical stratification, autoantibody profiles, or response to specific therapies

individual CB-CAP. Studies are in progress to determine if CB-CAP signatures might serve as biomarkers for lupus diagnosis, monitoring, prediction of flare, stratification, and/or response to specific therapies.

7 CB-CAPs in Lupus Pathogenesis

The collective findings described above also led to the hypothesis that CB-CAPs, upon binding to circulating cells, may lead to dysfunction of these cells and in turn contribute to a wide range of pathophysiologic mechanisms in patients with SLE. CB-CAP deposition may not only serve as lupus biomarkers but they may also contribute to tissue damage and the disease process. This hypothesis has been confirmed by two studies to date. First, Kyttaris and colleagues have shown that deposition of E-C4d leads to calcium-dependent cytoskeletal changes in RBC that render them less deformable, possibly impairing their capacity to flow through capillaries and deliver oxygen to tissues [20]. The second demonstration that CB-CAP deposition leads to cellular dysfunction was reported by Tsokos and colleagues who demonstrated that C3d fragments are localized to lipid rafts in T cells of patients with SLE and contribute to cellular dysfunction by modulating calcium influx responses and significantly increasing production of IL-2, IL-4, IL-17, and IFN-gamma [21].

8 Conclusion

There is an urgent need for lupus biomarkers to diagnose, monitor, stratify, and predict patient flares and response to therapy. The steep trajectory of advance in this field is unprecedented yet still impeded by obstacles such as the complexities of disease heterogeneity, difficulties in accurate diagnosis even by experienced rheumatologists, and required comparisons of potential value of new biomarkers to gold standards that have never themselves been validated and standardized despite decades of use by clinicians. We have undertaken a candidate approach to lupus biomarker discovery based upon long-standing recognition of the uniquely intimate link between lupus and the complement system. This approach has led to the discovery of CB-CAPs, which now include E-C4d, E-C3d, P-C4d, P-C3d, T-C4d, T-C3d, B-C4d, B-C3d, and E-CR1, among others. E-C4d and B-C4d, as part of the Avise SLE panel, are the first lupus biomarkers to be successfully validated in a multicenter study, and other CB-CAPs have shown promise as biomarkers for diagnosis, stratification, monitoring, and precision medicine. In addition to their value as lupus biomarkers, deposition of CB-CAPs may also contribute to lupus pathogenesis by rendering cells dysfunctional and may thereby represent a potential target for therapeutic intervention.

References

1. Ahearn JM, Liu CC, Kao AH, Manzi S (2012) Biomarkers for systemic lupus erythematosus. Transl Res 159:326–342
2. Liu CC, Kao AH, Manzi S, Ahearn J (2013) Biomarkers in systemic lupus erythematosus: challenges and prospects for the future. Ther Adv Musculoskelet Dis 5:210–233
3. Liu CC, Ahearn JM (2009) The search for lupus biomarkers. Best Pract Res Clin Rheumatol 23:507–523
4. Liu CC, Manzi S, Ahearn JM (2005) Biomarkers for systemic lupus erythematosus: a review and perspective. Curr Opin Rheumatol 17:543–549
5. Narain S, Richards HB, Satoh M, Sarmiento M, Davidson R, Shuster J (2004) Diagnostic accuracy for lupus and other autoimmune diseases in the community setting. Arch Intern Med 164:2435–2441
6. Fritzler M (2011) The antinuclear antibody test: last or lasting gasp? Arthritis Rheum 63:19–22
7. Liu CC, Manzi S, Kao AH, Navratil JS, Ahearn JM (2010) Cell-bound complement biomarkers for systemic lupus erythematosus: from benchtop to bedside. Rheum Dis Clin North Am 36:161–172

8. Calano SJ, Shih PB, Liu CC, Kao AH, Navratil JS, Manzi S et al (2006) Cell-bound complement activation products (CB-CAPs) as a source of lupus biomarkers. Adv Exp Med Biol 586:381–390
9. Liu CC, Danchenko N, Navratil JS, Nilson SE, Manzi S, Ahearn JM (2005) Mining the complement system for lupus biomarkers. Clin Appl Immunol Rev 5:185–206
10. Liu CC, Manzi S, Danchenko N, Ahearn JM (2004) New advances in measurement of complement activation: lessons of systemic lupus erythematosus. Curr Rheumatol Rep 6:375–381
11. Liu CC, Ahearn JM, Manzi S (2004) Complement as a source of biomarkers in systemic lupus erythematosus: past, present and future. Curr Rheumatol Rep 6:85–88
12. Manzi S, Navratil JS, Ruffing MJ, Liu CC, Danchenko N, Nilson SE et al (2004) Measurement of erythrocyte C4d and complement receptor 1 in systemic lupus erythematosus. Arthritis Rheum 50:3596–3604
13. Kao AH, Navratil JS, Ruffing MJ, Liu CC, Hawkins D, McKinnon KM et al (2010) Erythrocyte C3d and C4d for monitoring disease activity in systemic lupus erythematosus. Arthritis Rheum 62:837–844
14. Liu CC, Manzi S, Kao AH, Navratil JS, Ruffing MJ, Ahearn JM (2005) Reticulocytes bearing C4d as biomarkers of disease activity for systemic lupus erythematosus. Arthritis Rheum 52:3087–3099
15. Navratil JS, Manzi S, Kao AH, Krishnaswami S, Liu CC, Ruffing MJ et al (2006) Platelet C4d is highly specific for systemic lupus erythematosis. Arthritis Rheum 54:670–674
16. Kao AH, McBurney CA, Sattar A, Lertratanakul A, Wilson NL, Rutman S et al (2013) Relation of platelet C4d with all-cause mortality and ischemic stroke in patients with systemic lupus erythematosus. Transl Stroke Res (in press)
17. Liu CC, Kao AH, Hawkins DM, Manzi S, Sattar A, Wilson N (2009) Lymphocyte-bound complement activation products as biomarkers for diagnosis of systemic lupus erythematosus. Clin Transl Sci 2:300–308
18. Yang DH, Chang DM, Lai JH, Lin FH, Chen CH (2009) Usefulness of erythrocyte-bound C4d as a biomarker to predict disease activity in patients with systemic lupus erythematosus. Rheumatology 48:1083–1087
19. Kalunian KC, Chatham WW, Massarotti EM, Reyes-Thomas J, Harris C, Furie RA et al (2012) Measurement of cell-bound complement activation products enhances diagnostic performance in systemic lupus erythematosus. Arthritis Rheum 64:4040–4047
20. Ghiran IC, Zeidel ML, Shevkoplyas SS, Burns JM, Tsokos GC, Kyttaris VC (2011) SLE serum deposits C4d on red blood cells, decreases red blood cell membrane deformability, and promotes nitric oxide production. Arthritis Rheum 63:503–512
21. Borschukova O, Paz Z, Ghiran IC, Liu CC, Kao AH, Manzi S et al (2012) Complement fragment C3d is colocalized within lipid rafts of T cells and promotes cytokine production. Lupus 21:1294–1304

Chapter 3

Detection of Antinuclear Antibodies in SLE

Yashwant Kumar and Alka Bhatia

Abstract

The antinuclear antibodies (ANA) also known as antinuclear factors (ANF) are unwanted molecules which bind and destroy certain structures within the nucleus. In systemic lupus erythematosus (SLE), they are produced in excess; hence their detection in the blood of patients is important for diagnosis and monitoring of the disease. Several methods are available which can be used to detect ANA; nevertheless, indirect immunofluorescence antinuclear antibody test (IF-ANA) is considered a "reference method" for their detection. Though IF-ANA is relatively easier to perform, its interpretation requires considerable skill and experience. The chapter therefore is aimed to provide comprehensive details to readers, not only about its methodology but also the result interpretation and reporting aspects of IF-ANA.

Key words SLE, Antinuclear antibody, Indirect immunofluorescence, Hep-2 cells, Immunofluorescence pattern

1 Introduction

Systemic lupus erythematosus (SLE) is a multiorgan autoimmune disease, which affects females more often than males. It can involve virtually any organ system and is associated with periods of relapse and remission. The SLE and other autoimmune rheumatic disorders, (ARD) i.e., rheumatoid arthritis, Sjogren's syndrome, scleroderma, Raynaud's disease, polymyositis, and mixed connective tissue disease, are characterized by production of autoantibodies against many intracellular components. Presence of antinuclear antibodies (ANA) in the blood/serum is a hallmark of SLE. They are valuable not only for its diagnosis but also in monitoring of disease progression [1, 2]. Hence, its detection has been formulated as one of the diagnostic criteria for SLE by American College of Rheumatology subcommittee [3].

ANA can be categorized as autoantibodies to DNA and histones (i.e., anti-dsDNA and anti-histone) and those against extractable nuclear antigens (ENA). The ENA comprise of Smith antigen (Sm), ribonucleoproteins (RNP), SS-A (Ro), SS-B (La), Scl-70,

Paul Eggleton and Frank J. Ward (eds.), *Systemic Lupus Erythematosus: Methods and Protocols*, Methods in Molecular Biology, vol. 1134, DOI 10.1007/978-1-4939-0326-9_3, © Springer Science+Business Media New York 2014

Jo-1, PM-Scl, centromere, nucleosomes, and many others [4]. Though, each ANA is closely associated with a particular ARD (e.g., anti-dsDNA and anti-Sm for SLE, anti-histones for drug induced SLE), there is considerable overlapping among them (e.g., anti-SS-A and anti-SS-B may be seen in Sjogren's syndrome, SLE, and also in mixed connective tissue disorder). Moreover, besides SLE and other ARD, ANA may also be seen in patients with severe burns, infections, malignancies, and even in healthy individuals [5]. Hence, a test utilized to detect ANA should be sensitive as well as specific enough to correctly identify, categorize, and segregate the diseased subjects from healthy individuals. Though a number of techniques have been invented over the years (indirect immunofluorescence, enzyme immunoassay, immunoblot, passive hemagglutination, immunodiffusion, counterimmunoelectrophoresis, and more recent antigen microarray, flow cytometry, and multiplexed immunoassays), none of them can be labeled as "perfect." All these methods have variable sensitivity and specificity and their own advantages as well as disadvantages [6].

So far, detection of ANA using indirect immunofluorescence (IF-ANA) is considered the "gold standard" screening test. But because of low specificity, it is recommended that all IF-ANA-positive samples should be analyzed further for more specific autoantibodies, i.e., dsDNA and ENA. For this reason an enzyme-linked immunosorbent assay for dsDNA (dsDNA ELISA) with or without immunoblot is used in addition to IF-ANA in many labs [7]. This is important as specific autoantibodies help in differentiation of SLE from other ARD. Also a positive IF-ANA test comprises only one factor in determination of SLE, and results of positive IF-ANA need to be correlated with clinical features of the patient, e.g., butterfly rashes, arthritis, pleurisy, blood abnormalities, kidney disease, etc. [8].

IF-ANA is cheaper, relatively easy to perform, and has good sensitivity. It recognizes the ANA in the blood of the patient, which adhere to reagent test cells (substrate), by producing distinct fluorescence patterns. In the past, various substrates like tissue sections, desquamated cells, chicken erythrocytes, and HeLa cells have been tried, but later tissue sections, e.g., rat liver or cell lines, became the standard substrate. After introduction of HEp-2 cells in 1975, the sensitivity of IF-ANA has increased further, and nowadays most of the labs use cultured human epithelial cells of laryngeal squamous cell carcinoma (Hep-2) as the standard substrate. These are available commercially as prefixed on glass slides and used more commonly than in-house preparation (a laborious process and requires maintenance of cultured cells). Besides the type of substrate, there are three other factors which affect the performance of IF-ANA: (1) fixative used for slide preparation, (2) fluorescein to protein ratio, and (3) immunoglobulin (Ig) subclass specificity of the conjugate. Some fixatives are known to destroy certain nuclear antigens, e.g., alcohol; fluorescein to protein ratio determines the sensitivity and nonspecific background staining of a conjugate, e.g., FITC; and Ig subclass reactivity influences the specificity to a disease, e.g., SLE. Nearly all clinically relevant ANA react to IgG irrespective of the presence of IgM and IgA, while in healthy individuals IF-ANA positivity is usually due to IgM and IgA only. Hence, conjugates specific for IgG are more disease specific [9, 10].

Though the IF-ANA is a simple technique, its interpretation requires considerable skill and experience. Hence besides procedural details the chapter also deals in the interpretation of results and reporting aspects of IF-ANA.

2 Materials

IF-ANA should be performed with a serum specimen only (*see* **Note 1**).

1. Pre-coated Hep-2 substrate slides (6 or 12 wells; *see* Fig. 1) [NOVA Lite Hep-2 substrate slides, INOVA Diagnostics, Inc. USA].
2. FITC-labeled antihuman IgG conjugate (Goat) in buffer containing Evans blue and 0.09 % sodium azide (*see* **Note 2**).
3. ANA-positive control (buffer containing 0.09 % sodium azide and human serum antibodies to Hep-2) (*see* **Note 3**).
4. ANA-negative control (buffer containing 0.09 % sodium azide and no human serum antibodies to Hep-2).
5. Phosphate-buffered saline (PBS) concentrate (40×), to be diluted in a ratio of 1:40 (i.e., 25 ml of PBS in 975 ml of distilled or deionized water and mixed thoroughly) used as wash buffer (*see* **Note 4**).
6. Mounting medium or buffered glycerol.
7. Coverslips (60 × 20 mm size).
8. Micropipettes to deliver 15–1,000 µl volume.

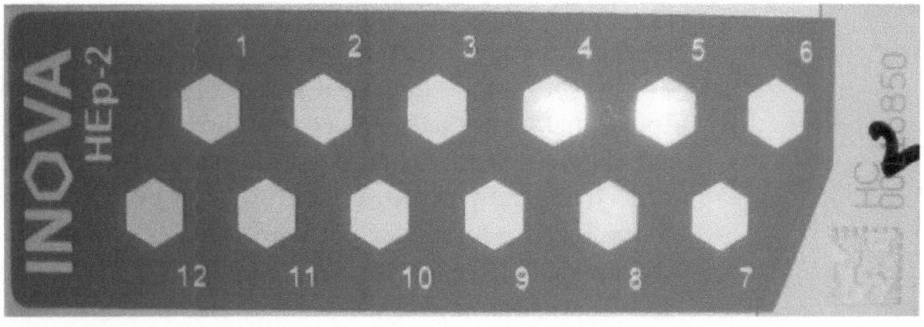

Fig. 1 A 12 wells, prefixed Hep-2 slide

9. Pipette tips, glass tubes, rack, plastic squeeze bottle, paper towel, and large Petri dish or glass container with lid (for moist chamber).
10. Distilled or deionized water.
11. Squeeze bottles or Pasteur pipettes.
12. Moist chamber.
13. 1 l container for diluting PBS.
14. Coplin jar.
15. Fluorescence microscope with 495 nm exciter and 515 nm barrier filter.

3 Methods

The procedures should be performed at room temperature (RT); hence bring all the reagents and samples to room temperature (18–25 °C) at least half an hour before use and mix well (*see* **Note 5**).

1. Label the clean glass tubes and arrange them in a rack along with positive and negative controls and samples to be tested.
2. Dilute patient samples in a ratio of 1:40 with diluted PBS buffer (i.e., 50 μl of serum in 1.95 ml of PBS buffer) by adding and mixing both in the each glass tube.
3. Allow the substrate slides to achieve RT prior to removal from its pouch. To prepare a moist chamber, soak a folded paper towel with tap water and keep it on flat bottom of a Petri dish and cover with lid. Now label the slide and place it in the moist chamber (*see* **Note 6**). Add one drop (20–25 μl) of the undiluted positive and negative controls to wells 1 and 2, respectively (*see* **Note** 7). Add one drop each of the diluted patient samples to remaining wells (*see* **Note 8**).
4. Incubate the slide for 30–35 min at 37 °C in the moist chamber. This is important to maintain the suitable humidity environment. Do not allow the substrate to dry out during the assay procedure.
5. After incubation, gently wash off the serum with diluted buffer. For washing the slide should be kept straight and vertical. Individual wells of the lower row should be washed first, then the slide should be turned upside down, and the wells of the other row (now on lower side) should be washed. This is to minimize the carryover between wells (*see* **Note 9**). Do not stream the buffer directly on to the wells as it may damage the substrate. Alternatively, slides may also be kept in a Coplin jar of diluted PBS buffer for up to 5 min (*see* **Note 10**).

6. Shake off the excess of PBS buffer. The margins and sides of the wells should be wiped out by paper towel to ensure that no carryover takes place during and after washing.
7. Keep the slides back in the moist chamber and immediately cover each well with a drop of fluorescent conjugate (*see* **Note 11**). Incubate further for 30–35 min.
8. Repeat **step 5**.
9. Place a coverslip on a paper towel. Apply a drop of mounting medium in its central part. Softly touch the reaction surface of the slide to the edge of coverslip and lift it. Immediately the media spreads over the slides without air bubble formation or entrapment.
10. For titration make serial twofold dilutions from the initial screening dilution for all positive samples diluted with PBS buffer (i.e., 1:80, 1:160, 1:320, or more if needed). Sometimes if there is strong clinical suspicion or in case of weak fluorescence intensity, undiluted sample or less dilution (e.g., 1:10 or 1:20) may be used.

4 Result Interpretation

After mounting the slide it should be examined immediately by an immunopathologist (*see* **Note 12**). The following parameters are evaluated while reporting and to be mentioned in the final report:

(a) Intensity of fluorescence
(b) Pattern of fluorescence
(c) Titer of a positive test
(d) Substrate used

4.1 Intensity of the Fluorescence

The positive samples are graded depending on the intensity of fluorescence as follows:

(a) ++++ (4+): Brilliant apple green fluorescence
(b) +++ (3+): Bright apple green fluorescence
(c) ++ (2+): Clearly distinguishable positive fluorescence
(d) + (1+): Lowest fluorescence intensity that enables nuclear and/or cytoplasmic staining to be clearly differentiated from the background fluorescence
(e) Negative: No immunofluorescence or feeble intensity making difficult to distinguish nuclear and cytoplasmic details

The intensity of the fluorescence is first assessed in negative and positive control wells. A positive control must show staining intensity ≥3+. A test sample is considered negative if staining intensity is less than or equal to negative control. A negative IF-ANA result essentially excludes possibility of active SLE. Fluorescence intensity of 3+ or more strongly favors an ARD, while in case of low intensity further confirmation should be done by ELISA or other suitable method.

4.2 Immunofluorescence Pattern

A variety of patterns are observed in a patient of ARD which give a clue to significance of ANA and type of ARD. While reporting following patterns may be seen (Fig. 2):

(a) Homogenous—a solid and uniform staining of nucleus with or without apparent masking of the nucleoli. Usually seen for nuclear antigens, i.e., dsDNA and ssDNA, and histones, and strong positivity is suggestive of SLE.

(b) Peripheral—A ringlike staining along the border of the nucleus (forming a rim) with weaker staining towards the center of the nucleus. Easily appreciated in a tissue section but may be difficult to appreciate in Hep-2 cells. Generally seen for dsDNA, ssDNA, histones, and DNP. Peripheral pattern is also commonly seen in SLE patients.

(c) Speckled—a fine or coarse granular appearance of the nucleus generally without fluorescent staining of the nuclei. Seen with Sm, RNP, Scl-70, SS-A, SS-B, etc. Suggestive but not specific for any particular ARD.

(d) Nucleolar—large, coarse granular staining within the nucleus. About one to six nucleoli may be visible. Usually favors ARD other than SLE.

(e) Centromeric—discrete granules usually in multiple of 46. Suggest ARD other than SLE.

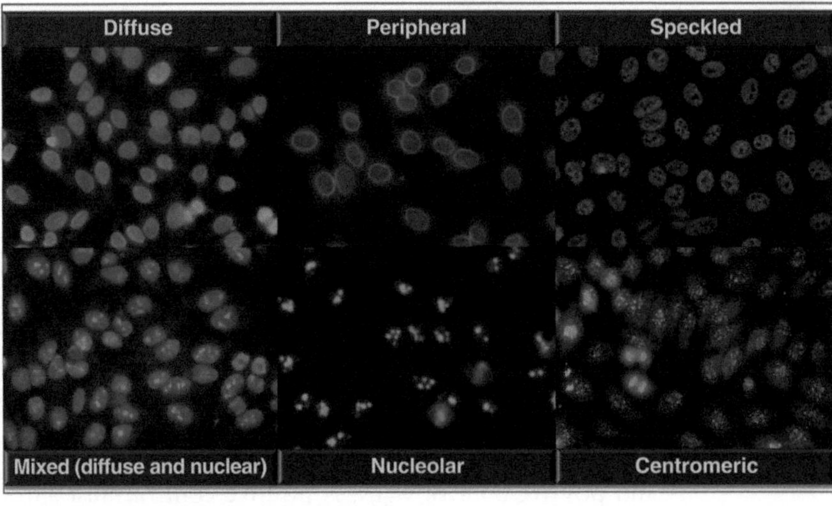

Fig. 2 Common and clinically significant IF-ANA patterns

(f) Mixed—a combination of any of the above patterns. May be seen in SLE, mixed connective tissue disorder, or an overlap syndrome (*see* **Note 13**).

4.3 Titer of the Positive Test

In our lab we use a titer of 1:40 and sometimes 1:20 for pediatric patients, though each lab planning to perform IF-ANA should standardize their own reporting titers (*see* **Note 14**).

4.4 Substrate Used

Despite Hep-2 cells used most widely, many labs still use other substrates, e.g., mouse kidney and rat liver, which have lesser sensitivity; hence it is imperative to report the type of substrate used by the lab.

A final report therefore should guide the clinician about the levels of ANA in the serum (titers and intensity of fluorescence), type of autoantibody (staining pattern), and sensitivity of the test (substrate use) (*see* **Note 15**).

5 Notes

1. Addition of anticoagulants or preservatives may adversely affect the results. After collection of blood sample, serum should be separated from the blood clot. Lipemic, hemolyzed, heat-treated specimen containing visible particles or microbially contaminated may give erroneous results; hence should be rejected. At RT, sample should be stored no longer than 8 h. If the test cannot be done within 8 h, refrigerate the sample at −20 °C or lower. Frozen samples must be mixed well after thawing and prior to testing.
2. Sodium azide, used as a preservative, is poisonous and may be toxic if ingested or absorbed through skin or eyes. Flush sinks with large volume of water to prevent azide build up.
3. Additional suitable control sera may be prepared by aliquoting pooled human serum specimens and storing at ≤−70 °C.
4. pH of PBS should be between 7.2 and 7.4; otherwise intensity of staining may be tainted.
5. All reagents and slides should be stored at 2–8 °C. Do not freeze.
6. Slides should be labeled with pencil only or with a permanent marker. Use of any other writing material may cause artifactual staining due to spillover.
7. Positive and negative controls should be run every time a test is performed to ensure that all reagents and procedures perform properly.
8. Samples and reagents should be added in each well in an orderly manner to avoid mix-up.

9. Incomplete or inefficient washing of wells may cause high background.
10. Coplin jars if used for slide washing should be free from all dye residues; otherwise it may lead to artifactual staining.
11. If kept for long the antihuman IgG conjugate may change in color due to exposure to light. However, the color change does not affect the assay performance.
12. A variety of external factors influence the sensitivity of the test, i.e., accuracy and reproducibility of pipetting technique, thoroughness of washing, length of incubation time during assay, type of fluorescence microscope used, the strength and age of bulb, filter system, magnification, gap between staining and reporting time, and the observer. If a band pass filter is used rather than 515 barrier filter, increased artifactual staining may be seen. If immediate reporting is not possible the slide should be refrigerated (at 4 °C). However, reporting should be done as soon as possible (preferably within few hours) as fading process starts soon after staining process is over.
13. Except for nucleolar and centromere patterns which are characteristic for autoantibodies against 4–6S RNA and centromere, other patterns are not specific for any particular autoantibody. Hence, a confirmatory testing (immunoblot, ELISA) for autoantibodies against other antigens, e.g., dsDNA and ENA, is recommended for speckled, homogenous, and mixed patterns.
14. IF-ANA pattern may change as the sample is tittered out to endpoint. This phenomenon is because of lower titer antibodies dropping below the sensitivity of the test as more dilute samples are tested.
15. IF-ANA is used as a screening test; hence a strongly positive IF-ANA with high titers though is suggestive but not diagnostic for SLE or any other ARD. IF-ANA-positive samples should always be correlated with clinical features of the patient and followed by a confirmatory test, i.e., dsDNA ELISA and an immunoblot if necessary.

References

1. Mutasim DF, Adams BB (2000) A practical guide for serologic evaluation of autoimmune connective tissue diseases. J Am Acad Dermatol 42:159–174, quiz 174–156
2. Rekvig OP, Kalaaji M, Nossent H (2004) Anti-DNA antibody subpopulations and lupus nephritis. Autoimmun Rev 3:1–6
3. Tan EM, Cohen AS, Fries JF, Masi AT, Mcshane DJ, Rothfield NF et al (1982) The 1982 revised criteria for the classification of systemic lupus erythematosus. Arthritis Rheum 25:1271–1277
4. Tan EM (1982) Autoantibodies to nuclear antigens (ANA): their immunobiology and medicine. Adv Immunol 33:167–240
5. Tan EM (1989) Antinuclear antibodies: diagnostic markers for autoimmune diseases and probes for cell biology. Adv Immunol 44:93–151
6. Kumar Y, Bhatia A, Minz RW (2009) Antinuclear antibodies and their detection

methods in diagnosis of connective tissue diseases: a journey revisited. Diagn Pathol 4:1

7. Egner W (2000) The use of laboratory tests in the diagnosis of SLE. J Clin Pathol 53: 424–432
8. Kavanaugh A, Tomar R, Reveille J, Solomon DH, Homburger HA (2000) Guidelines for clinical use of the antinuclear antibody test and tests for specific autoantibodies to nuclear antigens. American College of Pathologists. Arch Pathol Lab Med 124:71–81
9. Gonzalez EN, Rothfield NF (1966) Immunoglobulin class and pattern of nuclear fluorescence in systemic lupus erythematosus. N Engl J Med 274:1333–1338
10. Tonutti E, Visentini D, Bizzaro N (2007) Interpretative comments on autoantibody tests. Autoimmun Rev 6:341–346

Chapter 4

Tests for Circulating Immune Complexes

Mark H. Wener

Abstract

Antigen–antibody complexes in tissues play a central role in the pathogenesis of lupus. Some of the immune complexes are formed in situ, i.e., in the tissues. Others are present in the blood stream, and these circulating immune complexes may deposit in tissues and incite inflammatory mechanisms in those tissues. A variety of techniques are available to measure circulating immune complexes. The assays that have been most studied in SLE include approaches that rely on the interaction of immune complexes with complement proteins, and therefore bind to C1q or contain bound C3.

In the process of investigating circulating immune complexes, it was recognized that lupus patients generate serum autoantibodies directed against C1q and other complement proteins. Antibodies reacting with the collagen-like region of C1q are known to be closely linked both clinically and pathophysiologically to lupus nephritis. This chapter describes methods for detection of C1q-binding immune complexes via the C1q solid-phase assay and the related test for autoantibodies to C1q.

Key words C1q, Complement proteins, Collagen-like region, Globular head, Immune complexes, Lupus nephritis

Abbreviations

C1qSP	C1q solid-phase assay for immune complexes
C1qBA	C1q fluid-phase binding assay for immune complexes
AHG	Aggregated human IgG

1 Introduction

Historical Background and Rationale: Serum sickness resulting from repeated administration of horse antitoxins was hypothesized to be an immune complex disease by von Pirquet and Schick at the beginning of the twentieth century. Experimental serum sickness models of glomerulonephritis and vasculitis clarified the potential for circulating immune complexes (antigen–antibody complexes) to cause disease [1]. Immune complexes are responsible for the

Paul Eggleton and Frank J. Ward (eds.), *Systemic Lupus Erythematosus: Methods and Protocols*, Methods in Molecular Biology, vol. 1134, DOI 10.1007/978-1-4939-0326-9_4, © Springer Science+Business Media New York 2014

glomerulonephritis of SLE and also contribute to the pathogenesis of a variety of other manifestations of SLE.

Principles of Circulating Immune Complex Assays: Many assays for immune complexes have been developed, although relatively few techniques have been put into routine clinical use or have been adapted widely. The techniques employed for immune complex detection depend on a few general principles.

Recognition of Immune Complexes—Assays Based on Physical Properties: Because of their larger lattice, Fc-interactions, etc., immune complexes aggregate and precipitate more easily than normal immunoglobulins or most other proteins. This precipitation or aggregate formation can be enhanced by cold temperatures (e.g., forming cryoglobulins) or by the use of polyethylene glycol (PEG). PEG is thought to enhance the activity of antigen and antibody reactants by the principle of solvent exclusion, in which the PEG polymer allows water within its polymer space but excludes higher molecular weight antigens and antibodies. Thus, the interaction of immune reactants is enhanced, promoting precipitate formation. This precipitate can be detected visibly or the protein or immunoglobulin content of the precipitate can be measured to quantify the immune complex. Precipitation of immunoglobulins by PEG is relatively nonspecific, however, and depends on the concentration of immunoglobulins present in the specimen and the concentration of PEG employed [2].

Assays Based on Binding and Activation of Complement: Activation of the classical pathway of the complement system is dependent on the presence of IgG- or IgM-containing immune complexes; thus it is not surprising that interaction of immunoglobulins with complement has been used to detect circulating immune complexes. C1q initiates the classical pathway of complement activation and is the protein responsible for recognition of immune complexes. This property of recognizing immune complexes has been used in several assays, which depend on binding of immune complexes to C1q, which can then be detected in different ways. The C1q solid-phase (C1qSP) assay uses C1q present on a solid phase (typically a polystyrene microtiter plate or test tube), which is then incubated with serum containing immune complexes. The IgG that binds to the solid-phase C1q is detected by enzyme-linked antibodies to IgG. The C1q fluid-phase binding assay (C1qFPBA) takes advantage of both the immune complex recognition property of C1q and the enhancement of precipitate formation promoted by PEG. For the C1q fluid-phase assay, radiolabeled fluid-phase C1q incubates with immune complex-containing serum, and then PEG is added. C1q, which is not bound to other reactants, remains soluble, whereas bound C1q is precipitated under those conditions.

Several assays take advantage of the fact that C3 or C3 fragments become bound to immune complexes after complement activation [3]. Detection of immunoglobulins bound to C3 is presumptive evidence that the immunoglobulin is in the form of an immune complex. Recognition and binding of C3 can be accomplished by several different approaches. One approach employed cellular complement receptors, such as C3 receptors on B cells. The Raji cell line is a lymphoblastoid cell line expressing cell-surface C3b receptors (as well as receptors for C3d, C1q, and Fc). In the Raji cell assay, serum containing immune complexes is allowed to react with the Raji cell, and then cell bound immunoglobulins are detected using labeled antibodies to IgG [3]. Since the Raji cell assay requires maintenance of cell lines, it was largely replaced by assays in which the recognition of C3 is performed by purified and standardized antibodies to C3 fragments, rather than by the Raji cell.

Principles of Immune Complex Assays—Platform: A difference between assay techniques that has implications for both performance and interpretation of results depends on whether the assays involve solid-phase or fluid-phase binding of immune complexes for recognition and detection of the immune complex. The solid-phase techniques are generally "sandwich assays" with a recognition step in which immune complexes bind to the immune complex recognition moiety (e.g., C1q for the C1qSP), followed by a detection step in which antibodies directed against human immunoglobulins are used to detect the immune complexes bound on the solid phase. This detection step adds specificity to the assay and typically limits detection to the immunoglobulin class or classes recognized by the antisera used in the assays (e.g., IgG for the C1qSP). In contrast, fluid-phase assays typically employ a single molecule for both recognition and detection (e.g., ^{125}I-C1q for the C1qBA) and thus can detect immunoglobulins of multiple classes simultaneously. Unfortunately, other substances that bind to the detecting molecule can also influence assay results. For example, lipopolysaccharide and DNA, which bind to C1q, can alter results of the C1qBA [4]. In studies analyzing the material precipitated by polyethylene glycol in the PEG assay, many non-immunoglobulin serum proteins were precipitated. Furthermore, the addition of PEG to plasma or serum theoretically could cause precipitation of immunoglobulins present in abnormally high concentration, even if the immunoglobulins were not in the form of an immune complex. Although the PEG assays are relatively easy to perform, and use inexpensive reagents, they have potential problems with lack of specificity.

Specific Autoantibodies Detected as "Immune Complexes" in Immune Complex Assays: Another potential confounder in interpreting immune complex assays is that they can give positive results when antibodies directed against the recognition proteins bind to those

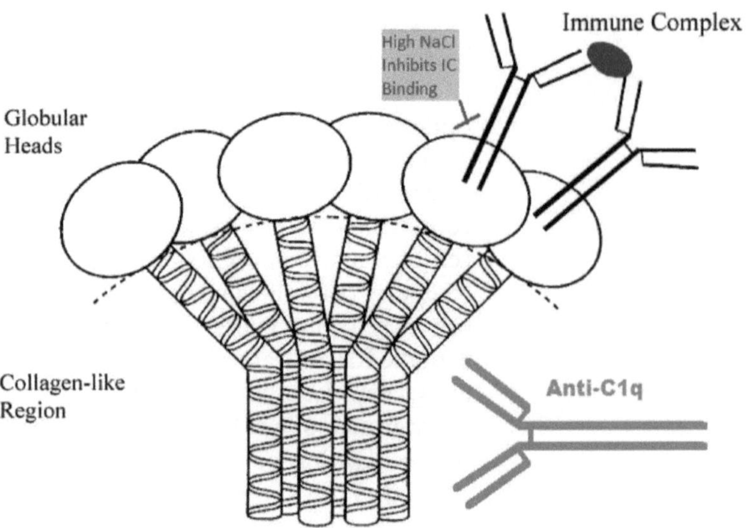

Fig. 1 C1q with bound immune complex and anti-C1q. C1q is shown with "bouquet of tulips" hexameric structure. Each C1q subunit has a globular protein head and a collagen-like region tail. Immune complexes bind via their Fc regions to the globular head region of C1q, an interaction that is inhibited by high ionic strength (high salt concentration). Autoantibodies to C1q bind via the F(ab) region to the collagen-like region of C1q

proteins as antibodies, rather than as immune complex interactions. For example, with the Raji cell assay, antilymphocyte antibodies from some patients with SLE could give a positive result, recognizing antigens on the Raji cell as targets [5]. Use of the C1qSP assay allows autoantibodies directed against C1q to bind and give positive results, even in the absence of immune complexes [6]. Similarly, autoantibodies to C3 components are frequently present in the sera of patients with SLE and related disorders [7] and could lead to positive results in immune complex assays based on recognition of C3. In these examples, the positive results are "false-positive" in that the results are not caused by immune complexes, yet clinically useful results may be obtained (see below). However, since the assays may become positive because of the presence of pathologic substances in addition to immune complexes, investigators employing these assays and using them to make conclusions about circulating immune complexes should confirm that immune complexes are responsible for the positive results observed.

Autoantibodies to C1q—Principles: The C1q protein consists of six subunits, each of which has a globular region and a collagen-like region (*see* Fig. 1). Autoantibodies to the collagen-like region (CLR) of C1q can be detected using the C1q solid-phase assay for immune complexes, and those antibodies are characteristic of patients with proliferative lupus nephritis [8]. The CLR can be prepared from C1q by limited pepsin digestion, followed by gel chromatography [9], but preparation of CLR is laborious. A simpler approach to measurement of anti-C1q has been used by many investigators [10]. In this approach, undigested C1q is used as the antigen, but the binding is performed in high salt (1.0 M NaCl) buffer, rather than usual normal saline. The binding of immune complexes to C1q, which involves interactions between Fc portions of IgG and the globular portion of C1q, is relatively inhibited in high ionic strength (high salt) concentrations. Thus, antibodies to C1q can bind, but immune complexes do not bind as well. This high salt approach may not be as specific as techniques involving isolated CLR as antigen, but is more easily adapted to existing C1qSP immune complex assays [6].

Clinical Applications: Problems in interpreting results of immune complex assays arise because of the multiplicity of different techniques available for detecting immune complexes, differences in results when using different techniques, lack of reproducibility between the same techniques performed in different laboratories, and lack of studies demonstrating clear clinical predictive value of immune complex measurements. The World Health Organization (WHO)/IUIS sponsored a working group which reviewed clinical immunology tests and concluded that immune complex detection was neither essential nor specific for any disease and that lack of detectable circulating immune complexes did not exclude the presence of immune complex-mediated diseases [11]. The working group also concluded that detection of immune complexes could be helpful in monitoring conditions such as rheumatoid arthritis and SLE, and in some malignancies such as acute leukemia, and that the most reliable methods were the C1q solid-phase test, the C1q fluid-phase binding test, the conglutinin assay, monoclonal rheumatoid factor inhibition test, and the Raji cell assay.

Numerous studies have suggested that immune complex assays based on C1q and C3 are positive in patients with SLE [4] and can be helpful in assessing disease activity in patients with SLE [12]. In studies of SLE, C3-dependent techniques serve as disease activity markers. The Raji cell assay has been shown to correlate with disease activity in several but not all studies of patients with SLE. Antilymphocyte antibodies in sera of patients with SLE may cause elevations in the Raji cell assay, potentially even in the absence of immune complexes [5]. C1qSP immune complex assays have been used to study patients with SLE and have shown that results reflect disease activity [13]. Changes in the C1qSP assay correlated with a clinician's decision to change therapy, and the clinical activity of SLE correlated better with the C1qSP than with the C1qBA [13].

Sera of patients with SLE contained autoantibodies to the collagen-like region of C1q, and these antibodies were detected using C1q solid-phase but not fluid-phase assay [8]. Among patients with SLE, anti-C1q antibodies are associated with lupus nephritis and are less commonly demonstrable in serum of patients with non-renal lupus [10, 14]. Rising concentrations of IgG anti-C1q are associated with flares of lupus nephritis [10, 15]. High levels of anti-C1q are associated with proliferative forms of lupus glomerulonephritis and subendothelial deposits of immune complexes [10, 14]. A positive test for anti-C1q is among the best predictors of lupus nephritis, and a negative test for anti-C1q in a given patient indicates a low probability of diffuse proliferative lupus nephritis [15]. In murine models of immune complex nephritis, anti-C1q was shown to serve as an amplifier of immune complex-mediated inflammation caused by a variety of different immune complexes [16]. These data indicate that one of the reasons for the clinical utility of the C1qSP assay in SLE is because of its ability to detect anti-CLR, in addition to its value as an assay for circulating immune complexes.

Quality Control, Standards, and Calibrators: Aggregated gamma globulin, chemically cross-linked immunoglobulin, and immune complexes of defined antigen–antibody composition have all been used as calibrators for immune complex assays by various investigators. Nonspecifically aggregated IgG has been most widely used.

Summary: A variety of immune complex assays have been developed over the last several decades. None should be considered diagnostic for any disorder. The presence of antibodies to the collagen-like region of C1q, often detected in the C1qSP assay, is a characteristic of active lupus with renal disease and also detects autoantibodies to C1q. The C1q SP assay for circulating immune complexes can be made somewhat more specific for anti-C1q detection by a slight modification, namely, using a higher concentration of salt in the buffer. This chapter provides information about the C1q solid-phase assay for immune complexes and the modification for detecting anti-C1q.

2 Materials

1. *Serum Samples*: The usual sample specimen is serum, which should be stored at −70 °C prior to assay (*see* **Note 1**).
2. *Aggregated Human γ-Globulin (AHG) Calibrator*: Prepare a solution of human γ-globulins. The preparation can be a relatively crude preparation of only partially purified material, e.g., Cohn fraction II, at a concentration of 5–6 mg/ml in 0.9 % w/v NaCl (*see* **Note 2**). Several hours may be required for this solubilization step. Heat with occasional stirring at 63 °C for 20 min. Immediately place in an ice bath until cool. Centrifuge at 1,500 × *g* for 15 min to remove precipitated solids and save the supernatant. Test for protein concentration. Dilute to a

concentration of ~5.0 mg/ml in sample buffer and store at –70 °C in 0.5 ml aliquots.

3. *C1q Isolation and Purification*: C1q can be isolated by a variety of techniques. These include differential solubility based on ionic strength, ion exchange chromatography and size exclusion gel chromatography, or IgG affinity chromatography [9]. Purified C1q can be purchased commercially, as well (e.g., Quidel; *see* **Note 3**). Before use in immune complex assays, the purity of C1q should be verified by one or more methods (*see* **Note 4**).

   For use in immune complex assays, C1q must retain functional activity. IgG-coated latex particles (rheumatoid factor reagents) can be used to document binding of C1q to IgG, and measurement of C1 hemolytic complement activity can be used as a sensitive and quantitative functional assay. C1q protein concentration is measured by radial immunodiffusion or similar immunochemical means or estimated by measuring absorbance using the extinction coefficient $\varepsilon_{\text{cm}}^{1\%} = 6.8$ at 280 nm [9]. For consistency, the activity of each new batch of C1q should be validated by comparing assay results using the new batch of C1q with results obtained by similar assays using previous batches of C1q. C1q can be stored at –70 °C and will retain its functional properties for many months.

4. *C1q Coating Buffer*: Phosphate buffered saline (*see* **Note 5**).

5. *Sample Buffers*

   (a) Sample buffer for C1q solid-phase immune complex assay: The serum sample buffer employed can be modified PBS. It should be at neutral pH (7.4), 0.15N NaCl, and should contain Tween20 (0.1 %) and protein (either 0.5 % bovine serum albumin or 2 % nonfat milk) to prevent nonspecific binding of serum IgG to the microtiter plate.

   (b) High salt sample buffer for anti-C1q assay: The buffer is the same as the sample buffer above except that additional NaCl is added to give a final concentration of 1.0 M NaCl.

6. *Microtiter Plate*: Microtiter plates from different vendors are available with a range of products that vary in the selectivity of protein coating and nonspecific binding, optimum pH of use, and mechanisms of coating. We employ MaxiSorp (Nunc, Inc.) plates for many of our studies.

7. *Enzyme-Linked Antihuman IgG*: The antihuman IgG should be specific for the gamma chain of IgG, so that only IgG is detected. Either peroxidase- or alkaline phosphatase-linked polyclonal antihuman IgG can be employed, with colorimetric substrate appropriate for the enzyme. We use alkaline phosphatase-conjugated goat antihuman IgG (Fc or gamma chain specific) (Sigma), with nitophenylphospate (NPP) as substrate.

3 Methods

3.1 C1q Solid Phase Assay for Immune Complexes

3.1.1 Preparation of C1q-Coated Microtiter Plates

To prepare C1q-coated microtiter plates, dilute an aliquot of C1q preparation in PBS (without Tween or other proteins) to the working concentration (typically 4–8 mg/ml). Add 220 μl of the dilution to each well of a microtiter plate leaving wells 1A and 1B blank. (These wells will serve to blank the microtiter plate reader at the end of the assay.) Cover the plate with plastic film. Incubate at 4 °C overnight (~18–20 h).

3.1.2 C1q Solid-Phase Immune Complex Procedure

1. Prepare six AHG standards, over a range of 1–1,500 ng/ml IgG, in sample buffer.
2. Prepare 1:100 dilutions of samples in sample buffer. Include negative control serum and at least two levels of positive control sera.
3. Empty the microtiter plate containing C1q. Wash by filling the wells with sample buffer and letting the plate stand for 5 min. Empty and repeat two more times for a total of three washes. Forcefully tap the plate as completely dry as possible (*see* **Note 6**).
4. Add 200 μl of each pre-diluted standard, control and sample to duplicate wells. Include blanks containing buffer only as a blank.
5. Cover the plate. Incubate for 60 min at 37 °C.
6. Empty the plate, tap dry, and wash three times with sample buffer.
7. Add 200 μl appropriate dilution (usually about 1:1,000) of the enzyme-linked antibody in wash buffer. Dilution can vary with each lot of reagent. Cover the plate. Incubate for 2 h at room temperature in moisture chamber.
8. Wash three times with sample buffer.
9. Add 200 μl of appropriate substrate to each well (including wells 1A and 1B), and incubate. Monitor the absorbance of the top standard and stop the reaction when its absorbance is ~1,000 OD units. Stop the reaction as appropriate for the enzyme used.
10. Read the OD of each well. Calculations to determine the concentration in samples are performed using the standard curve, using a four-parameter logistic equation, or using other appropriate curve-fitting algorithm. Results are reported in units of microgram AHG equivalents/ml.

3.1.3 Quality Control Procedures

When running assays repeatedly over time, run-to-run precision studies should be performed to achieve consistency. Each microtiter plate run must include a standard curve plus the following:

1. A reagent blank consisting of substrate only in uncoated wells 1A and 1B.
2. A buffer blank, where buffer alone is substituted for sample.

3. A normal serum control: Drawn from a single donor and aliquoted and stored at −70 °C.
4. Abnormal controls: Serum samples from patient pools giving elevated results of approximately 10–20 and 60–80 μg AHG equivalents/ml. These sera may be diluted in sample buffer to bring into an acceptable range prior to aliquoting. Store at −70 °C. The expected ranges for the normal and abnormal controls should be determined before use of the assay, ideally by running the assay controls 20 times and determining the mean and standard deviation of the value of the control. The coefficient of variation (calculated as "standard deviation/mean value") of each abnormal control is expected to be 20 % or less.
5. If a control specimen is more than three standard deviations from its mean or expected value, or two of the controls are two standard deviations or more from their mean/expected value, then the assay run should be reviewed, and the specimens in that assay run may need to be reassayed.

3.2 Autoantibodies to the Collagen-Like Region of C1q (Anti-CLR)

The assay is performed in the exact fashion as the C1q solid-phase immune complex assay, except that the samples are diluted in the high salt (1.0 M) sample buffer prior to incubating in the C1q-coated microtiter plate. A known positive serum can be used as a calibrator, or values can be reported as a *z*-score, i.e., as the number of standard deviations from the mean of 20 or more normal/reference sera.

4 Notes

1. *Sample treatment*: Repeat freeze-thaw cycles should be avoided. Heating of the sample to 56 °C ("decomplementing") is contraindicated due to the risk of aggregating IgG, leading to false-positive results.
2. *Calibrator treatment*: Avoid vigorous mixing, which may cause bubbles to form around the protein particles, thus inhibiting solubilization.
3. *Commercial sources*: A few commercial sources of immune complex assay kits have become available. While some have not had consistently satisfactory levels of performance [17], others have been used successfully in many laboratories. Commercial anti-C1q reagents have also become available, and they perform reasonably well [18].
4. *Affinity chromatography methods for checking C1q purity*: Immunoblotting using antibodies to human IgG is useful to verify that traces of IgG are not present in the C1q preparation. Removal of trace amounts of IgG can be achieved by passage over an anti-IgG or a *staphylococcal* protein A or protein G

affinity column (associated with some loss of C1q due to binding of C1q to IgG). Since native C1q is a glycoprotein that binds to concanavalin A by virtue of its glycosylation, the purity of C1q can also be improved by affinity chromatography on concanavalin A-agarose (Sigma), with elution of C1q using alpha-methylglucopyranoside (Sigma).

5. *Plate buffer selection*: A number of different buffers can be used to coat microtiter plates. Although some authorities prefer using alkaline buffers to promote binding, we find that typical inexpensive and stable phosphate buffered saline (PBS, 0.01 M phosphate, pH 7.4, NaCl 0.15 M) works effectively. PBS can be prepared in the lab from sodium phosphate salts, purchased as a concentrated tablet for preparation of standard volumes of buffer or purchased as a liquid solution.
6. *Plate drying*: Do not leave the coated wells standing dry for a prolonged period of time.

References

1. Dixon FJ (1963) The role of antigen-antibody complexes in disease. Harvey Lect 58:21–52
2. Cooper KM, Moore M (1983) Critical aspects of immune complex assays employing polyethylene glycol. J Immunol Methods 60: 289–303
3. Theofilopoulos AN, Dixon FJ (1979) The biology and detection of immune complexes. Adv Immunol 28:89–220
4. Lambert PH, Dixon FJ, Zubler RH, Agnello V, Cambiaso C, Casali P et al (1978) WHO collaborative study for evaluation of 18 methods for detecting immune-complexes in serum. J Clin Lab Immunol 1:1–15
5. Cooper KM, Moore M (1983) Reactivity of low molecular weight material in cellular immune complex assays. Clin Exp Immunol 52:407–416
6. Kohro-Kawata J, Wener MH, Mannik M (2002) The effect of high salt concentration on detection of serum immune complexes and autoantibodies to C1q in patients with systemic lupus erythematosus. J Rheumatol 29:84–89
7. Durand CG, Burge JJ (1984) A new enzyme-linked immunosorbent assay (ELISA) for measuring immunoconglutinins directed against the third component of human complement. Findings in systemic lupus erythematosus. J Immunol Methods 73:57–66
8. Uwatoko S, Mannik M (1988) Low-molecular weight C1q-binding immunoglobulin G in patients with systemic lupus erythematosus consists of autoantibodies to the collagen-like region of C1q. J Clin Invest 82:816–824
9. Reid KB (1982) C1q. Methods Enzymol 82(Pt A):319–324
10. Siegert CE, Daha MR, Swaak AJ, Van Der Voort EA, Breedveld FC (1993) The relationship between serum titers of autoantibodies to C1q and age in the general population and in patients with systemic lupus erythematosus. Clin Immunol Immunopathol 67:204–209
11. Bentwich Z, Bianco N, Jager L, Houba V, Lambert P, Knaap W (1982) Use and abuse of laboratory tests in clinical immunology: critical considerations of eight widely used diagnostic procedures. Report of a joint IUIS/WHO meeting on assessment of tests used in clinical immunology. Clin Immunol Immunopathol 24:122–138
12. Lloyd W, Schur PH (1981) Immune complexes, complement, and anti-DNA in exacerbations of systemic lupus erythematosus (SLE). Medicine (Baltimore) 60:208–217
13. Abrass CK, Nies KM, Louie JS, Border WA, Glassock RJ (1980) Correlation and predictive accuracy of circulating immune complexes with disease activity in patients with systemic lupus erythematosus. Arthritis Rheum 23:273–282
14. Wener MH, Uwatoko S, Mannik M (1989) Antibodies to the collagen-like region of C1q in sera of patients with autoimmune rheumatic diseases. Arthritis Rheum 32:544–551
15. Akhter E, Burlingame RW, Seaman AL, Magder L, Petri M (2011) Anti-C1q antibod-

ies have higher correlation with flares of lupus nephritis than other serum markers. Lupus 20:1267–1274

16. Trouw LA, Groeneveld TW, Seelen MA, Duijs JM, Bajema IM, Prins FA et al (2004) Anti-C1q autoantibodies deposit in glomeruli but are only pathogenic in combination with glomerular C1q-containing immune complexes. J Clin Invest 114:679–688
17. Levinson SS, Goldman JO (1987) Evaluation of anti-C1q capture assay for detecting circulating immune complexes and comparison with polyethylene glycol-immunoglobulin G, C1q-binding, and Raji cell methods. J Clin Microbiol 25:1567–1569
18. Mahler M, Van Schaarenburg RA, Trouw LA (2013) Anti-C1q autoantibodies, novel tests, and clinical consequences. Front Immunol 4:117

Chapter 5

Methods for Measuring Antibody-Dependent Cell-Mediated Cytotoxicity In Vitro

Aaron S. Miller, Max L. Tejada, and Hélène Gazzano-Santoro

Abstract

Antibody-dependent cell-mediated cytotoxicity (ADCC) is a relevant characteristic to measure for a number of therapeutic monoclonal antibodies (mAbs) under development. ADCC is a mechanism by which antibody-opsonized, infected, or cancerous cells are destroyed by FcγRIII (CD16)-expressing effector cells. Here we describe three methods that can be used to quantify the ADCC activity of mAbs by measuring distinct aspects of the ADCC mechanism.

Key words Cell death, Fc receptors, Natural killer cells, Interferon gamma, Tumor necrosis factor

1 Introduction

Antibody-dependent cell-mediated cytotoxicity (ADCC) is a part of the innate immune system through which activated effector cells destroy infected or cancerous cells [1]. ADCC is initiated when opsonized target cells are recognized by natural killer (NK) cells. Antibodies bind to a surface antigen on the target cell and then the Fc domain of the antibodies binds to FcγRIIIa (CD16) on the surface of the NK cell [2]. Coupling of the target cell to NK cell initiates FcγRIII signaling which triggers the release of perforin and granzyme inducing cell lysis and apoptosis in target cells, respectively [3]. The concurrent release of cytokines including IFNγ and TNFα further activates the immune response. Many therapeutic monoclonal antibodies (mAbs) include ADCC as part of their mechanism of action (MoA) [4, 5]. As such, it is essential to measure ADCC activity as part of mAb development.

Here we describe three different methods to quantify the ADCC activity for a mAb of interest by measuring distinct aspects of the ADCC mechanism. Each of these methods has previously been shown to be sensitive to fucose levels of the mAb and is able to detect degradation of the antibody induced by exposure to

Paul Eggleton and Frank J. Ward (eds.), *Systemic Lupus Erythematosus: Methods and Protocols*, Methods in Molecular Biology, vol. 1134, DOI 10.1007/978-1-4939-0326-9_5,

stressed conditions [6–8]. These methods are presented as examples and should be broadly applicable to all mAbs where ADCC is involved in the MoA. However, the assay for each mAb will require empirical optimization of critical parameters including but not limited to reagent and cell concentrations, choice of FcγRIII polymorphism, target-to-effector cell ratio, and incubation times. First, a method is described that reflects the initial step in the initiation of ADCC. This cell-free, ELISA-based method measures the ability of a therapeutic mAb to bridge an antigen coated to the surface of an ELISA plate to the soluble, extracellular domain of FcγRIIIa. Next is a method that measures the activation of NK cells by monitoring the release of IFNγ and TNFα. The final method measures cytotoxicity of the target cells, the ultimate biological output of ADCC.

2 Materials

2.1 ELISA Components

1. 96-well high-binding polystyrene microtiter plates Nunc (Rochester, NY).
2. Target antigen (*see* **Note 1**).
3. Wash Buffer: 10 mM sodium phosphate, 0.15 M NaCl, 0.05 % polysorbate 20, pH 7.5.
4. Assay Diluent: 10 mM sodium phosphate, 0.15 M NaCl, 0.5 % v/v bovine serum albumin, 0.05 % v/v polysorbate 20.
5. FcγRIII-GST (*see* **Note 2**).
6. Anti-GST-HRP (Rockland Immunochemicals Inc., Gilbertsville, PA).
7. SureBlue Reserve™ TMB Microwell Peroxidase Substrate (Gaithersburg, MD).
8. 0.6 M H_2SO_4.

2.2 Cytokine Release Method Components

1. Growth medium (*see* **Note 3**).
2. Target cells (*see* **Note 4**).
3. NK cells (*see* **Note 5**).
4. TNF-alpha or IFN-gamma 96-well MSD plates (Meso Scale Discovery, Gaithersburg, MD).
5. Ruthenium-tagged anti-human IFNγ and anti-human TNFα (Meso Scale Discovery, Gaithersburg, MD).
6. 2× Read Buffer T with surfactant (Meso Scale Discovery, Gaithersburg, MD).

2.3 NK Cell-Based Method Components

1. Growth medium (*see* **Note 3**).
2. Target cells (*see* **Note 4**).

3. NK cells (*see* **Note 5**).
4. DELFIA BATDA labeling reagent (PerkinElmer, Waltham, MA).
5. 96-well U-bottom plate (BD Falcon, Franklin Lakes, NJ).
6. OptiPlate-96 white (PerkinElmer, Waltham, MA).
7. DELFIA europium solution (PerkinElmer, Waltham, MA).
8. DELFIA lysis buffer (PerkinElmer, Waltham, MA).

3 Methods

3.1 ADCC Bridging Method

1. Coat 96-well plates overnight with 100 μL per well target antigen diluted to 1 μg/mL (*see* **Note 6**).
2. Thoroughly wash plates with Wash Buffer and blot plates on paper towel to dry.
3. Block plate by adding 200 μL Assay Diluent to each well and incubate in a 25 °C plate shaker for 1–2 h.
4. During plate blocking, dilute reference and sample antibodies in Assay Diluent.
5. Thoroughly wash plates with Wash Buffer and blot plates on paper towel to dry.
6. Add 100 μL of antibody dilutions per well and add 100 μL Assay Diluent to any unused wells.
7. Incubate plates in a 25 °C plate shaker for 1 h.
8. During the antibody incubation, dilute FcγRIII-GST to desired concentration in Assay Diluent (*see* **Note 2**).
9. Thoroughly wash plates with Wash Buffer and blot plates on paper towel to dry.
10. Add 100 μL of FcγRIII-GST solution to each well and incubate in a 25 °C plate shaker for 1 h.
11. Thoroughly wash plates with Wash Buffer and blot plates on paper towel to dry.
12. During FcγRIII-GST incubation, dilute anti-GST-HRP to desired concentration in Assay Diluent (*see* **Note 7**).
13. Thoroughly wash plates with Wash Buffer and blot plates on paper towel to dry.
14. Add 100 μL of FcγRIII-GST solution to each well and incubate in a 25 °C plate shaker for 1 h.
15. Thoroughly wash plates with Wash Buffer and blot plates on paper towel to dry.
16. Add 100 μL TMB solution to each well and incubate until a gradient is visible across the antibody concentrations, approximately 10 min (*see* **Note 7**).

17. Add 100 μL 0.6 M H_2SO_4 to each well and mix the plate on a plate shaker for 1–2 min.
18. Measure optical density (OD) at 450 nm on a 96-well plate reader and plot each value against antibody concentration.

3.2 Cytokine Release Method

1. Dilute reference and sample antibodies in growth medium.
2. Harvest target cells by centrifugation, resuspend in growth medium, and determine cell viability and concentration.
3. Harvest NK92 cells by centrifugation, resuspend in growth medium, and determine cell viability and concentration.
4. Dilute target cells and NK cells to 4× the desired final concentration and then mix the cell suspensions together in a 1 to 1 volume ratio (*see* **Note 8**).
5. Add 100 μL of the NK92/target cell suspension mixture to the MSD plate.
6. Add 100 μL of the reference and sample antibodies to their corresponding wells in the MSD plate.
7. Incubate the MSD plate for 2 h on an orbital shaker in a humidified CO_2 incubator at 37 °C (*see* **Note 9**).
8. Following the incubation, thoroughly wash plates with Wash Buffer and blot plates on paper towel to dry.
9. Add 50 μL per well mixture of ruthenium-tagged anti-human IFNγ and anti-human TNFα and incubate for 1 h at room temperature on an orbital shaker.
10. Thoroughly wash plates with Wash Buffer and blot plates on paper towel to dry.
11. Add 150 μL per well MSD 2× Read Buffer T with surfactant.
12. Measure electrochemiluminescent signal for IFNγ and TNFα using the MSD Sector Imager 6000 plate reader and plot each value against antibody concentration.

3.3 NK-Based ADCC Method

1. Dilute reference and sample antibodies in growth medium (*see* **Note 3**).
2. Harvest target cells by centrifugation, resuspend in growth medium, and determine cell viability and concentration.
3. Label the target cells at 1.0×10^6 cells/mL by adding 2 μL BATDA per mL of cell suspension. Mix thoroughly and incubate for 25 min in a humidified CO_2 incubator at 37 °C (*see* **Note 10**).
4. Wash labeled target cells by centrifuging and resuspending in PBS. Repeat twice for a total of 3 washes (*see* **Note 11**).
5. After final wash, resuspend labeled target cells in growth medium and determine cell viability and concentration.

6. Dilute labeled target cells to 4× the desired final concentration (*see* **Note 8**).
7. Harvest NK92 cells by centrifugation, resuspend in growth medium, and determine cell viability and concentration.
8. Dilute NK92 cells and target cells to 4× the desired final concentration and then mix the cell suspensions together in a 1 to 1 volume ratio (*see* **Note 8**).
9. Add 100 μL of the NK92/target cell suspension mixture to a 96-well U-bottom plate.
10. Add 100 μL of the reference and sample antibodies to their corresponding wells in the 96-well U-bottom plate.
11. Prepare controls:
    (a) Background Control: Add 150 μL growth medium per well. Centrifuge an aliquot of labeled target cells and add 50 μL of the supernatant per well.
    (b) Spontaneous Release Control: Add 150 μL growth medium per well. Add 50 μL of the labeled target cells per well.
    (c) Maximum Release Control: Add 130 μL growth medium per well. Add 50 μL of the labeled target cells per well. Add 20 μL lysis buffer per well.
    (d) Spontaneous Release with NK Control: Add 100 μL growth medium per well. Add 100 μL NK92/target cell mixture per well (*see* **Note 12**).
12. Incubate plates for 2 h in a humidified CO_2 incubator at 37 °C (*see* **Note 9**).
13. Following the incubation, pellet the cells by centrifuging plates using a swinging bucket plate rotor.
14. Transfer 20 μL of the supernatant from each well to the corresponding well of a white 96-well plate.
15. Add 200 μL europium solution to each well and incubate for 15 min and mix on a plate shaker set at 100 rpm.
16. Measure time-resolved fluorescence by exciting at 345 nm and reading emission at 615 nm with a 50 μs delay and a 1 ms integration time.
17. Using the measured value for Specific Release for each well, calculate %Specific Toxicity (%ST) for each well according to the formula:

$$\%ST = \frac{(\textit{Specific Release} - \textit{Background}) - (\textit{Spontaneous Release} - \textit{Background})}{(\textit{Maximum Release} - \textit{Background}) - (\textit{Spontaneous Release} - \textit{Background})} \times 100$$

18. Plot each value for %ST against the antibody concentration.

4 Notes

1. Target antigen will depend on the antibody being measured. Source of the antigen may be peptides, proteins, cell lysates, live cells, or fixed cells.
2. In Miller et al. a recombinant FcγRIII-GST fusion protein that was prepared in-house was used [6], though various constructs of FcγRIII are available commercially (Peprotech, Rocky Hill, NJ and Abcam, Cambridge, MA). Selection of polymorphism used (F158 or V158) and receptor concentration must be optimized empirically. The goal should be to maximize sensitivity of the assay to differences in fucose levels of the antibody, as in Miller et al. [6].
3. The growth medium components will depend on the specific target cell line used. Substitute FBS with heat-inactivated FBS to avoid lysis of target cells by complement. For WIL2-S cells we use in [6–8], the growth medium was as follows: RPMI 1640, 10 % heat-inactivated FBS, 2 mM L-glutamine, and 20 mM HEPES, pH 7.2 (Gibco).
4. Selection of target cells will depend on antigen expression levels. Generally, higher expression of antigen generates higher levels of cytotoxicity.
5. NK92 cells engineered to stably express either FcγRIII F158 or V158 were used in Miller et al., Schnueringer et al., and Tejada et al. [6–8], though these cells are not publicly available. However, NK cell lines may also be obtained from other sources [9, 10]. Donor peripheral blood mononuclear cells (PBMCs) may also be used as in Schnueringer et al. and Tejada et al. [7, 8], though the engineered NK cell lines have the advantage of being less prone to donor-to-donor and day-to-day variability.
6. For peptides and proteins, 1 μg/mL usually provides sufficient signal and reproducibility.
7. The TMB incubation time will increase with increasing dilution of anti-GST-HRP. Further the anti-GST-HRP concentration and TMB incubation time will also depend on antigen density. We typically target approximately 10 min for improved reproducibility between plates and vary anti-GST-HRP concentration accordingly.
8. Target and effector cell concentration and the target-to-effector cell ratio must be optimized empirically in order to optimize signal to background. For engineered NK92 cell lines, this ratio ranges from 2:1 to 5:1, while PBMCs typically are 25:1 to 50:1 due to the inherent heterogeneity of PBMC preparations.
9. Assay incubation time must be determined empirically to attain optimal signal to background. Typical incubation times range from 2 to 4 h depending on antibody and cell line.

10. BATDA concentration may be increased to 7 μL BATDA per mL of cell suspension to achieve higher signal. The cell labeling incubation step is carried out in a 50 mL conical tube with the cap sitting loosely on the tube to insure sufficient exposure to CO_2.
11. It may be necessary to add 5 mM sulfinpyrazone (Sigma-Aldrich, St. Louis, MO) to the PBS washes in order to increase the intracellular retention of BATDA.
12. Spontaneous Release with NK Control is not used in the calculation of Specific Toxicity. Nevertheless, it is an important control and its value should be similar to the value for Spontaneous Release.

References

1. Janeway C (2005) Immunobiology: the immune system in health and disease, 6th edn. Garland Science, New York
2. Shields RL, Namenuk AK, Hong K, Meng YG, Rae J, Briggs J, Xie D, Lai J, Stadlen A, Li B, Fox JA, Presta LG (2001) High resolution mapping of the binding site on human IgG1 for Fc gamma RI, Fc gamma RII, Fc gamma RIII, and FcRn and design of IgG1 variants with improved binding to the Fc gamma R. J Biol Chem 276:6591–6604
3. Bryceson YT, March ME, Ljunggren HG, Long EO (2006) Synergy among receptors on resting NK cells for the activation of natural cytotoxicity and cytokine secretion. Blood 107:159–166
4. Clynes RA, Towers TL, Presta LG, Ravetch JV (2000) Inhibitory Fc receptors modulate in vivo cytotoxicity against tumor targets. Nat Med 6:443–446
5. Dall'Ozzo S, Tartas S, Paintaud G, Cartron G, Colombat P, Bardos P, Watier H, Thibault G (2004) Rituximab-dependent cytotoxicity by natural killer cells: influence of FCGR3A polymorphism on the concentration-effect relationship. Cancer Res 64:4664–4669
6. Miller AS, Tejada ML, Gazzano-Santoro H (2012) Development of an ELISA based bridging assay as a surrogate measure of ADCC. J Immunol Methods 385:45–50
7. Schnueriger A, Grau R, Sondermann P, Schreitmueller T, Marti S, Zocher M (2011) Development of a quantitative, cell-line based assay to measure ADCC activity mediated by therapeutic antibodies. Mol Immunol 48: 1512–1517
8. Tejada ML, Jia X, Gazzano-Santoro H (2013) Using cytokine release as a surrogate measure of antibody dependent cell-mediated cytotoxicity. mAbs (manuscript submitted for review)
9. Gong JH, Maki G, Klingemann HG (1994) Characterization of a human cell line (NK-92) with phenotypical and functional characteristics of activated natural killer cells. Leukemia 8:652–658
10. Kornbluth J, Flomenberg N, Dupont B (1982) Cell surface phenotype of a cloned line of human natural killer cells. J Immunol 129:2831–2837

Chapter 6

Recombinant Antibody Microarray for Profiling the Serum Proteome of SLE

Carl A.K. Borrebaeck, Gunnar Sturfelt, and Christer Wingren

Abstract

Systemic lupus erythematosus (SLE) is a severe autoimmune connective tissue disease. Our current knowledge about the serum proteome, or serum biomarker panels, reflecting disease and disease status is still very limited. Affinity proteomics, represented by recombinant antibody arrays, is a novel, multiplex technology for high-throughput protein expression profiling of crude serum proteomes in a highly specific, sensitive, and miniaturized manner. The antibodies are deposited one by one in an ordered pattern, an array, onto a solid support. Next, the sample is added, and any specifically bound proteins are detected and quantified. The binding pattern is then converted into a relative protein expression map, or protein map, deciphering the composition of the sample at the molecular level. The methodology provides unique opportunities for delineating serum biomarkers reflecting SLE, thus paving the way for improved diagnosis, classification, and prognosis.

Key words Antibody microarray, Protein expression profiling, SLE, Biomarkers, Diagnosis, Prognosis, Classification

1 Introduction

Systemic lupus erythematosus (SLE) is a severe, chronic autoimmune connective tissue disease with a prevalence of 40–200 cases per 100,000 persons [1]. Despite major efforts, SLE remains a poorly understood disease with unknown etiology and complex pathogenesis [1, 2]. The course of this multifaceted disease is unpredictable, with periods of flares (active disease), alternating with remission (inactive disease), and its symptoms vary so much it often mimics or is mistaken for other illnesses. In fact, SLE is often called "the invisible disease." Thus, further studies delineating SLE and revealing the underlying disease biology at the molecular level would be of great clinical importance [1, 2].

Our current knowledge about the serum proteome reflecting SLE is still limited and mainly restricted to single laboratory variables [1–4]. The quest of defining disease-associated serum

Paul Eggleton and Frank J. Ward (eds.), *Systemic Lupus Erythematosus: Methods and Protocols*, Methods in Molecular Biology, vol. 1134, DOI 10.1007/978-1-4939-0326-9_6, © Springer Science+Business Media New York 2014

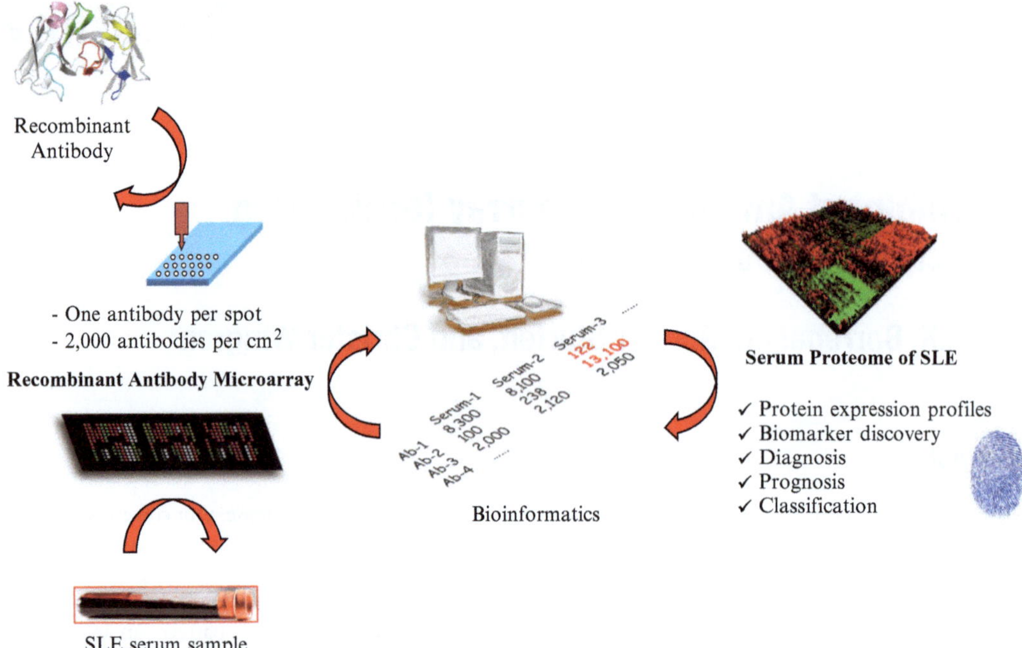

Fig. 1 Schematic illustration of serum proteome profiling of SLE patients using recombinant antibody microarrays

biomarkers for most diseases, including SLE, has, however, turned out to be very challenging due to technical limitations [5]. In this context, antibody-based microarrays are among the new class of promising proteomic technologies that hold great promise in biomedicine (Fig. 1) [6–12]. Recent efforts have outlined the potential and applicability of antibody-based microarrays for serum protein (proteome) profiling of SLE [13, 14].

The antibody microarray methodology can be used for high-throughput protein expression profiling of crude, non-fractionated samples, such as serum, targeting both high- and low-abundant analytes in a multiplex fashion [6, 7, 9]. The concept of antibody arrays is based on printing minute amounts of numerous (a few to several thousands) antibodies with the desired specificities one by one in discrete positions in an ordered pattern, an array (<1 cm^2 in size), onto a solid support (Fig. 1). The arrayed antibodies will then act as specific catcher probes for the target protein analytes. These miniaturized arrays are then incubated with μL scale of crude, non-fractionated serum. Next, specifically bound analytes are detected and quantified, mainly using fluorescence as mode of detection [15]. The complete assay is run within less than 4 h, where after the microarray images are transformed into protein expression profiles, or protein maps, revealing the detailed composition of the sample. Depending on the application at hand, different bioinformatic strategies can be applied [16, 17] to further explore the wealth of data generated, e.g., pinpointing differentially expressed protein analytes between, e.g., SLE patients and healthy controls [13, 14]. In this protocol, we will describe the generation and use of recombinant antibody microarrays for protein expression profiling of SLE serum samples.

2 Materials

2.1 Preparation of Antibodies

1. Use well-characterized recombinant antibodies, e.g., single-chain fragment variable (scFv) antibodies, with validated on-chip performances, as specific catcher probes on the arrays [16, 18] (*see* **Note 1**).
2. PBS stock solution: 140 mM NaCl, 2.7 mM KCl, and 10 mM sodium phosphate buffer, pH 7.4.

2.2 Clinical Sample Preparation

1. Collect the serum samples using a standardized protocol and store them as aliquots at −20 °C or −80 °C prior to use (*see* **Note 2**).
2. PBS stock solution.
3. Micro bicinchoninic acid (BCA™) Protein Assay Kit (Pierce, Rockford, IL, USA).

2.3 Labeling of Serum Samples

1. EZ-Link Sulfo-NHS-LC-Biotin (Pierce) [15] (*see* **Note 3**).
2. PBS stock solution.
3. 3.5 kDa molecular weight cutoff dialysis units (Thermo Scientific, Rockford, IL, USA).

2.4 Printing of Antibody Microarrays

1. Printing buffer: PBS stock solution.
2. Array support: polymer MaxiSorp microarray slides (NUNC, Roskilde, Denmark) (*see* **Note 4**).
3. Protein printer: sciFLEXARRAYER 11 (Scienion, Berlin, Germany) (*see* **Note 5**).
4. Positive control: biotinylated bovine serum albumin (BSA) (Sigma) (*see* **Note 6**).
5. Negative control: antibody (protein) or PBS stock solution (*see* **Note 7**).
6. Hydrophobic pen (DakoCytomation Pen, DakoCytomation, Glostrup, Denmark).
7. Nexterion IC 16 incubation chamber with 16-well silicone superstructure (Schott-Nexterion, Mainz, Germany).

2.5 Antibody Microarray Assay

1. Blocking buffer: 1 % (w/v) fat-free milk powder and 1 % (v/v) Tween-20 in PBS (PBS-MT).
2. Washing buffer: 0.05 % (v/v) Tween-20 in PBS (PBS-T).

3. Sample buffer: PBS-MT.
4. Alexa647-conjugated streptavidin (Invitrogen, Carlsbad, CA, USA).
5. Incubation chamber (box with tight lid and a moist Wettex cloth).
6. Nitrogen gas.

2.6 Data Analysis

1. Confocal fluorescence slide scanner (ScanArray Express scanner, PerkinElmer Life Sciences) (*see* **Note 8**).
2. ScanArray Express software v4.0 (PerkinElmer Life & Analytical Sciences, Wellesley, MA, USA) (*see* **Note 9**).
3. Statistical computing environment R.
4. Additional high-end software(s) for data analysis, e.g., Qlucore Omics Explorer (Qlucore, Lund, Sweden).

3 Methods

3.1 Preparation of Antibodies

1. Select the range of proteins (e.g., key immunoregulatory analytes) to be targeted by your multiplexed recombinant antibody array setup [6, 17, 18] (*see* **Note 1**).
2. Use the antibodies fresh or longtime store the antibody stock solutions at 4 °C or −20 °C based on the recommendations provided (tested) for each antibody preparation (*see* **Note 10**).
3. Use only well-characterized (e.g., specificity and affinity) antibodies as specific catcher probes. The recombinant antibodies can be generated through, e.g., stringent selections from large human recombinant scFv phage display libraries [19] (*see* **Note 1**).
4. Use only antibodies with validated on-chip array performances (e.g., specificity, stability, and functionality) (*see* **Note 1**).
5. Dilute the antibodies to 0.1 mg/ml in PBS (printing buffer) (just prior to array production) (*see* **Note 11**).

3.2 Clinical Sample Preparation

1. Collect the clinical serum samples using a standardized protocol (*see* **Note 2**).
2. Characterize (e.g., diagnose, phenotype, disease activity (SLEDAI-2K), and renal involvement) each individual sample (patient) using current orthogonal clinical methodologies to enable a correlation between the observed protein expression profiles generated using the antibody arrays and clinical/biological features for the SLE patients (*see* **Note 2**).
3. Longtime store the serum samples as aliquots at −20 °C or −80 °C (thaw each aliquot only once) (*see* **Note 2**).
4. Thaw the samples on ice, and centrifuge at 16,000 × *g* for 20 min at 4 °C.

5. If so required, determine the total protein concentration in the samples using a micro BCA Protein Assay Kit.
6. Dilute the sample to 2 mg/ml in PBS (45× dilution assuming a serum protein concentration of 90 mg/ml).
7. Mix the serum with EZ-Link Sulfo-NHS-LC-Biotin to a final concentration of 0.6 mM, and incubate on ice for 2 h (*see* **Note 12**).
8. Remove any free biotin by extensive dialysis against PBS for 72 h at 4 °C, using 3.5 kDa molecular weight cutoff dialysis units.
9. Aliquot the samples, and store them at −20 °C prior to use.

3.3 Printing of Antibody Microarrays

1. Centrifuge the antibodies and controls to be arrayed in order to remove any precipiates, etc.
2. Dilute the antibodies (0.1 mg/ml) (*see* **Note 11**) and the positive control (10 μg/ml) (*see* **Note 13**) in spotting buffer (i.e., PBS) (*see* **Note 14**).
3. Design the array print layout (*see* **Note 15**).
4. Print the arrays using a protein printer (*see* **Note 5**).
5. Use the slides directly or store them at RT overnight (*see* **Note 16**).
6. Preferentially, print the arrays in a room with controlled temperature and humidity.

3.4 Antibody Microarray Assay

All incubation and washing steps are performed at RT with gentle shaking. A humidity chamber, generated by placing a moist Wettex cloth in an ordinary box with a tight lid, can be used in order to make sure that the arrays do not dry out during the assay.

1. Create individual sub-arrays either by mounting the slide in a multi-well incubation chamber (e.g., 16 sub-arrays/slide) or by manually drawing a hydrophobic barrier around each sub-array using a hydrophobic pen. The steps below assume that a 16-well incubation chamber is used, representing the preferred approach.
2. The individual sub-arrays are blocked with 150 μL blocking buffer for 1 h.
3. Wash the arrays with 4 × 150 μL washing buffer.
4. Add 100 μL labeled serum sample (diluted 10 times in sample buffer, thus resulting in a final concentration of about 0.2 mg/ml) and incubate for 1 h (or 2 h) (*see* **Note 17**).
5. Wash the arrays with 4 × 150 μL washing buffer.
6. Add 100 μL 1 μg/ml Alexa647-conjugated streptavidin and incubate for 1 h.

7. Wash the arrays with 4 × 150 μL washing buffer.
8. Dismount the chip holder, and immerse the entire chip in distilled water, whereafter the slides are directly dried under a stream of nitrogen gas.
9. Store the slides in the dark at RT prior to scanning (if possible scan immediately).

3.5 Data Analysis

1. Slides are scanned dry with the confocal ScanArray Express scanner or equivalent (scan settings 5 or 10 μm resolution, laser power 90 (fixed), and a PMT gain of 50 or higher) (*see* **Note 18**).
2. Image analysis (quantification) can be performed using the ScanArray Express software v4.0 using the fixed circle method. Use only non-saturated spots (*see* **Note 18**).
3. Subtract the local background, and to compensate for any possible local defects, the highest and lowest replicate values are automatically removed, and each data point represents the mean (or median) value of the remaining data points (*see* **Note 19**).
4. Perform chip-to-chip normalization to eliminate any technical variations (e.g., day-to-day variations). Various approaches are at hand, but we have often used a semi-global normalization approach [14], conceptually similar to the normalization developed for DNA microarrays (*see* **Note 20**). Calculate and rank the coefficient of variation (CV) for each analyte. Fifteen percent of the analytes that display the lowest CV values over all samples are then identified and used to calculate a chip-to-chip normalization factor. The normalization factor N_i is calculated by the formula $N_i = S_i/\mu$, where S_i is the sum of the signal intensities for the selected analytes for each sample and μ is the sum of the signal intensities for the selected analytes averaged over all samples. Each data set generated from one sample is divided with the normalization factor N_i.
5. For the intensities, use log2 values.
6. The signal intensity values can be seen as detailed protein expression profile, or protein maps, revealing which proteins are present and at what relative levels in each serum sample. Set adequate cutoff values using the negative control(s) to finalize the protein expression profile in each individual sample. Hence, this profile represents the serum proteome map of the sample, and the resolution (detailed information) of this map is directly dependent on the number of antibodies and their range of specificities included on the microarray.
7. Comparison of protein expression profiles for different sample cohorts, e.g., healthy versus SLE or active SLE versus non-active SLE, can be performed using statistical computing environment R (*see* **Note 21**). Differentially expressed analytes

($p<0.05$) can be delineated using Wilcoxon signed-rank test (assuming non-normally distributed data) or Student's *t*-test (assuming normally distributed data, which must be verified). The ability to classify two groups can be estimated using support vector machine (SVM) in R and be described by a receiver operating characteristic curve (ROC). The data can also be visualized and analyzed using principle component analysis in Qlucore Omics Explorer (*see* **Note 21**). Evaluate the protein expression maps in relation to the clinical parameters (e.g., degree of disease activity or renal involvement) of relevant patient cohorts in order to decipher any biomarker or more likely panels of biomarkers reflecting biologically relevant properties (e.g., disease activity or renal involvement) of the samples. Stringent data analysis approaches, e.g., dividing the data set into a training set (2/3 of all samples) and a test set (1/3 of the samples), should preferentially be adopted. Candidate biomarker signatures must be pre-validated and validated using novel-independent sample cohorts and/or by using orthogonal methods (e.g., ELISA and mass spectrometry).

4 Notes

1. Recombinant scFv antibody fragments, selected from large phage display libraries, have predominantly been used as probes for recombinant antibody-based micro- and nano-arrays. The specificity (and affinity) should be pre-validated prior to use. Most importantly, the on-chip performances (e.g., stability and functionality) of the antibodies should also be (extensively) validated prior to use [18, 20]. The performance of arrayed antibodies has been shown to vary significantly, simply reflecting the facts that the antibodies are subjected to harsh conditions when they are deposited onto a solid support and stored in a dried-out condition. This could potentially result in denaturing of the antibody molecules and subsequently loss of functionality, why recombinant antibodies, microarray adapted by molecular design to withstand such conditions, represent the optimal choice of probes [18]. Antibody microarrays based on a sandwich approach could also be adopted, but then two specific antibodies (catcher antibody and detector antibody) must be generated per target analyte, which might cause logistical issues. The number of antibodies (<2,000 antibodies/cm^2 [6]) and their range of specificities determine the resolution at which the serum proteome can be described, i.e., the resolution can be increased by including more antibodies with a wider range of specificities. The range of specificities should be selected for the application at hand. We have often used arrays targeting immunoregulatory analytes, taking advantage of the immune system

as an early sensor for disease (i.e., immunosignaturing) [14, 21, 22]; for review *see* refs. 6, 12.

2. The serum samples should be collected using a standardized protocol, in order to make sure that the integrity of the sample (proteins) is conserved. Next, the sample should be aliquoted and rapidly frozen at −20 °C or −80 °C, and the thawing-freezing cycle of each vial should be kept at a minimum (i.e., only thaw each vial one time). The collection protocol at hand will reflect/depend on the organization responsible for collecting and storing the sample.
3. The sample can be labeled using a wide range of reagents, ranging from direct labeling with a fluorescent dye (e.g., Alexa-647) to indirect labeling with, e.g., biotin and subsequent visualization using fluorescently labeled streptavidin. We have based our approach on biotinylation of the serum samples [15, 23]. The labeling protocol depends on the particular labeling reagent. Further, additional clinical and laboratory parameters should be determined and collected for each sample, which will enable the observed protein expression profiles to be correlated with known clinical/biological properties of the samples/patients.
4. Many different surfaces can be used as planar, solid supports for antibody microarrays, and the precise choice will mainly depend on (1) how well the slide can be blocked for nonspecific background binding and (2) biocompatibility (i.e., functionality of arrayed probes). We have mainly used black polymer MaxiSorp slides from Nunc as support (displaying low nonspecific background binding and high biocompatibility) [23]. The microarray assay protocol, ranging from the amount of antibody deposited to choice of buffers (e.g., blocking buffer), depends on the particular solid support.
5. Different printers can be used for the preparation of antibody microarrays. We have frequently used sciFLEXARRAYER 11 (Scienion, Berlin, Germany) which deposits antibodies in the 300 pL scale using inkjet technology (i.e., noncontact printer). The preparation protocol depends on the particular spotter.
6. Different reagents (proteins or dyes) can be used as positive control. We have often used biotinylated BSA as positive control.
7. Different reagents can be used as negative control(s), including an antibody directed against an antigen (analyte) not present in the sample (control antibody) (representing the preferred choice), a completely different protein, or simply spotting buffer (PBS). We have mainly used a control antibody and/or spotting buffer as negative control.
8. Different scanners can be used for scanning the slides. We have predominantly used the confocal ScanArray Express scanner. The scanner setting depends on the particular scanner.

9. Different software can be used for detecting and quantifying each individual spot. We have mainly used the ScanArray Express software v4.0. The settings depend on the particular software and spot intensity.
10. The storage condition depends on the particular recombinant antibody (and format) at hand. While some should be used fresh, some can be stored frozen in a certain buffer, while others are preferentially stored at 4 °C. This should to be tested and evaluated for each antibody in order to ensure high functionality.
11. The spotting concentration depends on the antibody and solid support at hand. This will have to be tested and evaluated for each individual antibody and surface. We have frequently used an antibody (scFv) concentration of 0.1 mg/ml as starting concentration. A too low concentration will result in partial spots, while too high concentration will result in blurry spots. Dilute the antibodies just prior to use, i.e., store them at as high concentration as possible.
12. This is a key feature, as a too high molar ratio of biotin to protein can result in overlabeling and thereby reduced immunoreactivity due to epitope masking, and a too low molar ratio will give very weak signals in particular for low-abundant analytes. We have frequently used a molar ratio of biotin to protein of 15:1, assuming an average molecular weight of serum proteins of 50 kDa [23, 24].
13. The concentration of the positive control depends on the particular positive control.
14. The printing buffer could be spiked with a fluorescently labeled (a different dye than the one used to visualize binding of sample) protein, e.g., cadherin, which then could be used as a positive control for printing of antibodies in each individual position.
15. The array print layout depends on several factors, such as the size and number of sub-arrays, and application. The array layout should include the antibody probes, positive and negative controls, deposited with an adequate number of replica spots (≥3). We have frequently used five to eight replicate spots of each individual antibody/control. If possible, the replicate spots should be spread across the entire array. In order to facilitate the subsequent spot finding and quantification process, the positive control should be included at regular intervals, e.g., every 20th row. If multi-well incubation chamber is used, up to 16 sub-arrays/slide could be generated. If the sub-arrays are created using a hydrophobic pen, two to eight sub-arrays per slide could normally be generated.

16. For how long printed arrays can be stored depends on the functional on-chip stability of the arrayed antibodies. We have normally used the slide the day after production in order to standardize and eliminate (minimize) any impact of storage time on the performances of the antibody arrays. The storage conditions depend on the particular combination of antibodies and solid support. We have normally stored our slide in the dark at RT.
17. The concentration of serum sample depends on several factors, such as concentration of the target analytes, choice of labeling reagent, solid support, and blocking buffer. The signal-to-noise ratios should be optimized for each setup. We have mainly used a concentration of 0.2 mg/ml directly biotinylated non-fractionated serum.
18. The scanner settings depend on the observed signal intensity, reflecting several factors, such as concentration of the target analyte and how well the support can be blocked for nonspecific background binding. Non-saturated spots only should be used. We usually scan the slide at two or more predefined scanner settings, e.g., a laser power of 90 combined with different PMT gain settings. The quenching effects need to be evaluated for each setup at hand in order to eliminate (minimize) any effects.
19. The spot quality is essential for the subsequent array data analysis. In order to facilitate the quality control, the replica spots with the highest and lowest signal intensities are often automatically removed in order to compensate for any technical issues (e.g., surface imperfections and/or dust), and a mean (median) value of the remaining replicates is then used. We have often generated eight replicate spots, automatically removed the two highest and two lowest signal intensities, and then reported the mean (median) value of the four remaining spots.
20. The array data should be normalized in order to enable a comparison of data generated on different sub-arrays, slides, and/or days. A range of different normalization procedures can be used, and the choice needs to be evaluated for the application/array setup at hand. We have frequently used the semi-global CV normalization process described here.
21. Different statistical software can be used to (1) identify any differentially expressed ($p < 0.05$) analytes between two or more sample cohorts and (2) determine how well two or more sample cohorts can be differentiated or classified. We have mainly used statistical computing environment R for delineating differentially expressed analytes and for determining how well two groups can be classified (using support vector

machine, a supervised learning method in R). The software settings depend on the particular question and data set. The data can also be visualized and analyzed using principle component analysis in Qlucore Omics Explorer. This software can also be used if three or more groups are to be compared.

Acknowledgements

This work was supported by grants from the Swedish National Science Council (VR-NT and VR-M), the SSF Strategic Center for Translational Cancer Research (CREATE Health), and Vinnova.

References

1. Rahman A, Isenberg DA (2008) Systemic lupus erythematosus. N Engl J Med 358: 929–939
2. D'Cruz DP, Khamashta MA, Hughes GR (2007) Systemic lupus erythematosus. Lancet 369:587–596
3. Liu CC, Ahearn JM (2009) The search for lupus biomarkers. Best Pract Res 23:507–523
4. Rovin BH, Zhang X (2009) Biomarkers for lupus nephritis: the quest continues. Clin J Am Soc Nephrol 4:1858–1865
5. Hanash S (2003) Disease proteomics. Nature 422:226–232
6. Borrebaeck CAK, Wingren C (2009) Design of high-density antibody microarrays for disease proteomics: key technological issues. J Proteomics 72:928–935
7. Haab BB (2006) Applications of antibody array platforms. Curr Opin Biotechnol 17:415–421
8. Kingsmore SF (2006) Multiplexed protein measurement: technologies and applications of protein and antibody arrays. Nat Rev 5: 310–320
9. Sanchez-Carbayo M (2011) Antibody microarrays as tools for biomarker discovery. Methods Mol Biol 785:159–182
10. Wingren C, Borrebaeck CAK (2006) Antibody microarrays: current status and key technological advances. OMICS 10:411–427
11. Wingren C, Borrebaeck CAK (2007) Progress in miniaturization of protein arrays—a step closer to high-density nanoarrays. Drug Discov Today 12:813–819
12. Wingren C, Borrebaeck CAK (2009) Antibody-based microarrays. Methods Mol Biol 509: 57–84
13. Bauer JW, Baechler EC, Petri M, Batliwalla FM, Crawford D, Ortmann WA, Espe KJ, Li W, Patel DD, Gregersen PK, Behrens TW (2006) Elevated serum levels of interferon-regulated chemokines are biomarkers for active human systemic lupus erythematosus. PLoS Med 3:e491
14. Carlsson A, Wuttge DM, Ingvarsson J, Bengtsson AA, Sturfelt G, Borrebaeck CAK, Wingren C (2011) Serum protein profiling of systemic lupus erythematosus and systemic sclerosis using recombinant antibody microarrays. Mol Cell Proteomics 10(M110):005033
15. Wingren C, Borrebaeck CAK (2008) Antibody microarray analysis of directly labelled complex proteomes. Curr Opin Biotechnol 19:55–61
16. Borrebaeck CAK, Wingren C (2007) High-throughput proteomics using antibody microarrays: an update. Expert Rev Mol Diagn 7: 673–686
17. Borrebaeck CAK, Wingren C (2009) Transferring proteomic discoveries into clinical practice. Expert Rev Proteomics 6:11–13
18. Borrebaeck CAK, Wingren C (2011) Recombinant antibodies for the generation of antibody arrays. Methods Mol Biol 785: 247–262
19. Soderlind E, Strandberg L, Jirholt P, Kobayashi N, Alexeiva V, Aberg AM, Nilsson A, Jansson B, Ohlin M, Wingren C, Danielsson L, Carlsson R, Borrebaeck CA (2000) Recombining germline-derived CDR sequences for creating diverse single-framework antibody libraries. Nat Biotechnol 18:852–856
20. Haab BB, Dunham MJ, Brown PO (2001) Protein microarrays for highly parallel detection and quantitation of specific proteins and antibodies in complex solutions. Genome Biol 2:RESEARCH0004
21. Carlsson A, Wingren C, Kristensson M, Rose C, Ferno M, Olsson H, Jernstrom H, Ek S,

Gustavsson E, Ingvar C, Ohlsson M, Peterson C, Borrebaeck CAK (2011) Molecular serum portraits in patients with primary breast cancer predict the development of distant metastases. Proc Natl Acad Sci U S A 108:14252–14257

22. Sandstrom A, Andersson R, Segersvard R, Lohr M, Borrebaeck CAK, Wingren C (2012) Serum proteome profiling of pancreatitis using recombinant antibody microarrays reveals disease-associated biomarker signatures. Proteomics Clin Appl 6:486–496

23. Wingren C, Ingvarsson J, Dexlin L, Szul D, Borrebaeck CAK (2007) Design of recombinant antibody microarrays for complex proteome analysis: choice of sample labeling-tag and solid support. Proteomics 7:3055–3065

24. Ingvarsson J, Larsson A, Sjoholm AG, Truedsson L, Jansson B, Borrebaeck CAK, Wingren C (2007) Design of recombinant antibody microarrays for serum protein profiling: targeting of complement proteins. J Proteome Res 6:3527–3536

Chapter 7

Bifunctional Antibody Fragment-Based Fusion Proteins for the Targeted Elimination of Pathogenic T-Cell Subsets

Wijnand Helfrich and Edwin Bremer

Abstract

Pathogenic effector T cells are key contributors to autoimmune diseases such as systemic lupus erythematosus (SLE). General inhibition of T cells using, e.g., methotrexate, prednisolone, or TNF blockers, has prominent therapeutic effects frequently at the cost of severe long-term side effects and toxicity. Therefore, targeted strategies that can selectively inhibit or eliminate pathogenic T cells are sought after as a new approach to safely block perpetual inflammatory T-cell responses and inhibit concomitant progressive tissue destruction. Of particular interest in this respect is the use of the so-called single-chain fragments of variable region (scFv) antibody fragments for the targeted reactivation of Fas-dependent activation-induced cell death (AICD). Recently, we demonstrated that a recombinant fusion protein comprising a T-cell-targeted anti-CD7 scFv antibody fragment genetically fused to soluble FasL (sFasL) can eliminate synovial fluid T cells in the absence of activity toward resting peripheral blood cells. Here, we describe a detailed protocol for construction and preclinical evaluation of such scFv:FasL fusion proteins that may be used to selectively eliminate pathogenic immune cells.

Key words Autoimmune, T cell, FasL, Antibody fragment, Apoptosis

1 Introduction

Clonally expanded T helper I (T_{HI}) cells and, as recent studies highlight, T helper 17 (T_{H17}) cells appear to be key components in the perpetual inflammatory responses in autoimmune diseases such as systemic lupus erythematosus (SLE) and rheumatoid arthritis (RA) [1–3]. Therefore, selective inhibition or elimination of these pathogenic T-cell subsets is actively being pursued as a potential therapeutic strategy. Unfortunately, early clinical trials evaluating the efficacy of CD4- and CD7-targeted depletion of T cells showed no clinical improvement [4–6]. Therefore, other approaches were developed that involved the use of targeted protein drugs designed to prevent antigen-presenting cells (APCs) from delivering costimulatory signals to T cells. In the absence of appropriate complementary costimulatory signals, T cells become largely inactivated

Paul Eggleton and Frank J. Ward (eds.), *Systemic Lupus Erythematosus: Methods and Protocols*, Methods in Molecular Biology, vol. 1134, DOI 10.1007/978-1-4939-0326-9_7, © Springer Science+Business Media New York 2014

in a process known as anergy. A prominent example is fusion protein Abatacept (also known as Orencia) in which the extracellular domain of CTLA-4 is genetically fused to the Fc domain of human IgG1 [7]. Abatacept selectively inhibits the costimulation of T cells by blocking CD80 (B7-1) and to a lesser extent to CD86 (B7-2). Abatacept is licensed in the USA for the treatment of RA after failure to respond to anti-TNFα therapy and has been shown to yield durable responses of up to 1 year [7].

Recently, selective depletion of T_{H1} and T_{H17} subsets was shown feasible in preventive and therapeutic models of collagen-induced arthritis (CIA) by exploiting an antibody that blocks the biological activity of the cytokine lymphotoxin-alpha (LTα) [8]. LTα is a member of the tumor necrosis factor family and is secreted primarily by activated T_{H1} and B lymphocytes and natural killer (NK) cells. LTα forms heterotrimers with lymphotoxin-β by which it is anchored to the cell surface. LTα mediates various pro-inflammatory, immunostimulatory, and antiviral responses. Currently, various strategies are under development that aim to selectively interfere with LTα activation and its binding to various receptors.

An alternative approach, which is the topic of the current method, is aimed at the removal of pathogenic T cells by the targeted reactivation of the elimination pathway that normally ensures T-cell removal during the resolution phase of the immune response. The resolution of a T-cell immune response is regulated by a process dubbed activation-induced cell death (AICD) [9, 10]. AICD is reciprocally executed via interaction of the TNF-ligand FasL with its cognate agonistic TNF-receptor Fas between neighboring T cells. FasL is a prominent member of the TNF-ligand family. We and others have previously shown that such TNF ligands are particularly amenable for use as therapeutic payload in antibody-based therapy [11].

Although TNF ligands such as FasL are expressed as type II transmembrane proteins, most ligands are also proteolytically processed into soluble trimeric ligands (Fig. 1a). Many of these soluble TNF ligands have a significantly reduced signaling activity compared to their transmembrane counterparts. Indeed, soluble FasL (sFasL) has all but lost the capacity to activate Fas and has been shown to competitively inhibit Fas activation by membrane FasL [12]. Nevertheless, the soluble trimeric ligand typically still binds to the receptor. This soluble ligand requires secondary cross-linking to achieve receptor activation, a process reminiscent of TNFR activation after being cross-linked by its transmembrane counterpart. The cross-linking requirements of Fas by FasL are illustrated in Fig. 1b. This general feature of the TNF superfamily has formed the basis for their incorporation into antibody-based targeted therapies (*see* Fig. 1b) [11]. In brief, a soluble TNF ligand is genetically fused to a tumor-directed antibody fragment,

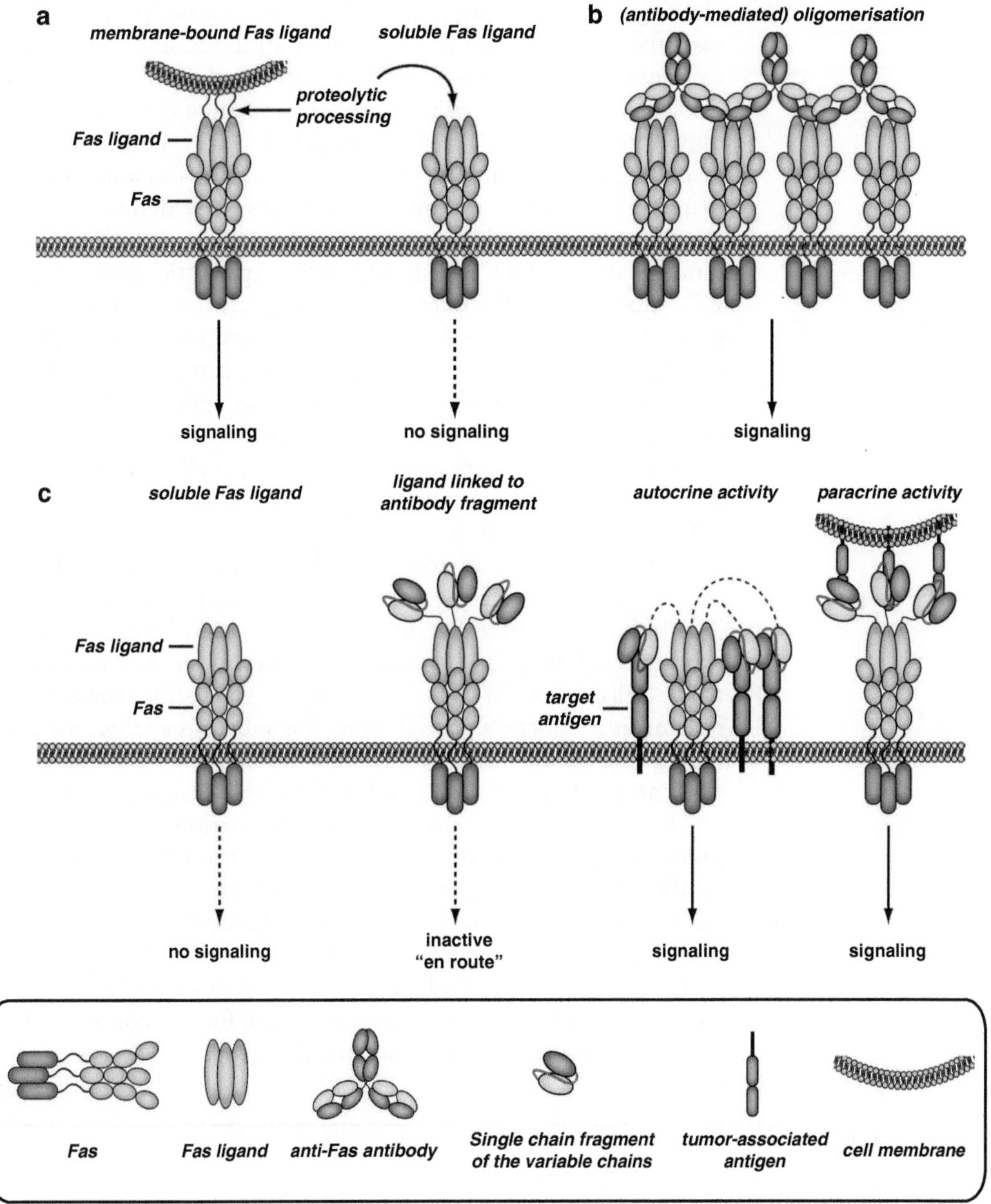

Fig. 1 FasL/Fas signaling characteristics. (**a**) FasL is typically produced as a type II transmembrane protein, but the extracellular domain can also be proteolytically cleaved by proteases into a soluble form (sFasL). Soluble FasL has lost Fas receptor-activating activity. However, this activity can be restored by secondary cross-linking. (**b**) The cross-linking requirement of sFasL makes its inclusion into an antibody fragment approach attractive. In brief, such a sFasl fusion protein comprises a scFv antibody fragment genetically fused to the sFasL. This scFv:sFasL fusion protein is essentially inactive en route. However, upon target binding of the scFv antibody fragment, domain sFasL is converted into signaling competent membrane-like Fas. (**c**) On the same cell (autocrine) or on neighboring cells (paracrine)

yielding a soluble-targeted TNF ligand fusion protein that is essentially inactive “en route.” Upon antibody fragment binding to the target cell, this ligand is converted into a membrane-associated and fully signaling competent form of the TNF ligand as illustrated in Fig. 1c for T-cell-targeted sFasL. Thus, such scFv-targeted FasL fusion proteins can be considered as a form of pro-drug. The feasibility of this approach has been demonstrated for the Fas-mediated elimination of cancer cells, with CD7-specific binding of scFvCD7:sFasL triggering apoptotic elimination of CD7-positive T-cell leukemic cells [13]. Of note, scFvCD7:FasL proved inactive toward normal CD7-positive cells, including resting T cell and NK cells. In contrast, activated T cells were highly sensitive to apoptotic elimination by scFvCD7:FasL, probably due to the intrinsic increase in sensitivity to AICD occurring in T cells at later activation stages. In actual fact, this T-cell-restricted activity profile also enabled the selective elimination of pathogenic synovial fluid T cells [14].

Of note, we and others have recently reported on a subset of T cells that expresses the B-cell antigen CD20 [15–17]. This subset of T cells was detected in RA and in the brain of MS patients and was characterized by a T_{H17} phenotype, whereas in healthy controls these cells were of T_{H1} phenotype. This shift toward pro-inflammatory phenotype highlights this subset as a target for elimination. In line with this, we have shown that such CD20-positive T cells can be eliminated by an scFvCD20:FasL fusion protein [18].

Here, we provide a protocol for construction, production, and preclinical evaluation of such scFv-based fusion protein. Of note, to allow for rapid evaluation of candidate therapeutic proteins, we have generated a versatile expression platform that enables easy exchange of scFv domains and effector domains [19]. Thus, the construction of scFv:sFasL fusion proteins described here is used to exemplify a widely applicable procedure for the construction of therapeutic proteins with bifunctional activity.

2 Materials

2.1 Components for Construction of Eukaryotic Expression Plasmids Encoding T-Cell Targeting scFv:FasL Fusion Proteins

1. A DNA fragment encoding an appropriate T-cell targeting scFv antibody fragment (*see* **Note 1**). A DNA fragment encoding the extracellular domain of human FasL. In short, full-length cDNA encoding human FasL (NCBI Reference Sequence: NM_000639.1) is used as template and subjected to a standard PCR reaction using primers T1, 5′-ATCCTCGAGT CTAGTGGGAGCGGATCTACCAGCCAGATGCACA CA-3′ (XhoI site is underlined) and T2, 5′-CCCAAGCTTTGC TTCTCTTAGAGCTT ATATAAG-3′ (HindIII site is underlined). The XhoI and HindIII sites are incorporated for cloning purposes (*see* Fig. 2).

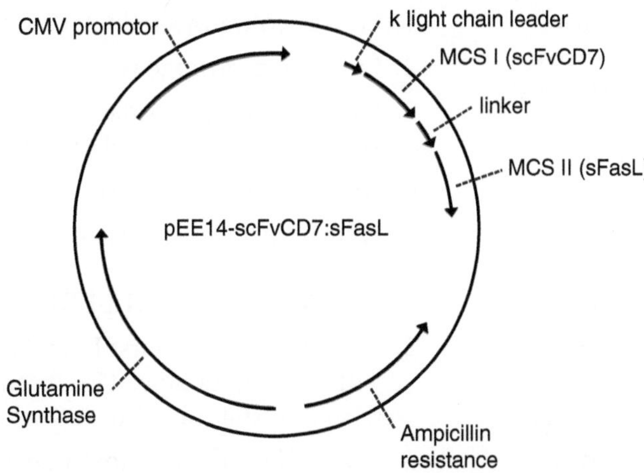

Fig. 2 Vector map of eukaryotic expression vector for production of scFv:FasL

2. An appropriate eukaryotic expression plasmid with suitable multiple cloning sites, e.g., our in-house customized version of the pEE14 plasmid (*see* Fig. 2). In short, we adapted plasmid pEE14 for the rapid construction, evaluation, and stable expression of scFv:sFasL fusion proteins in CHO-K1 cells. Important features of this vector are a murine kappa light-chain leader peptide (*see* **Note 2**) encoded upstream of two multiple cloning sites (MCSs) that are separated by a 26-residue in-frame linker sequence (*see* **Note 3**), and the glutamine synthetase selectable marker mini gene driven by the SV40 late promoter. The vector exploits the strong cytomegalovirus (CMV) promoter to drive recombinant protein expression.
3. Standard reagents for DNA manipulation, plasmid construction, production, and purification.

2.2 Components for Transient Expression in CHO-K1 Cells

1. pEE14 expression plasmid encoding the scFv:FasL fusion protein of interest.
2. CHO-K1 cells (ATCC, Rockville, MD, USA). Of note, CHO-K1 cells have been used for industrial scale and clinical grade production of numerous therapeutic proteins. Lab scale production of scFv-based proteins using the pEE14 expression plasmid platform and CHO-K1 expression cells may help to accelerate future large-scale production.
3. Glasgow's Modified Eagle Medium (GMEM) (Lonza).
4. Fetal bovine serum (Sigma-Aldrich Chemie, Zwijndrecht, the Netherlands).
5. Fugene-6 transfection reagent (Promega).
6. 6-well plates (NUNC).

2.2.1 Analysis of Transfection Efficiency by Immunocytochemistry

1. Harvested transfected CHO-K1 cells.
2. Cytospin centrifuge (e.g., StatSpin® CytoFuge 12).
3. Horseradish peroxidase (HRPO)-conjugated anti-HA-tag antibody (e.g., 3F10-HRP, Roche).
4. AEC staining procedure.
5. Hematoxylin counterstain.

2.3 Components for Stable Expression in CHO-K1 Cells

2.3.1 Stable Transfection in Adherent CHO-K1 Cells

1. Transfected CHO-K1.pEE14scFv:sFasL cells.
2. GMEM medium (First Link, West Midlands, UK), formulated without L-glutamine. The absence of glutamine is required for the successful use of the GS selection system.
3. Dialyzed fetal calf serum (Sigma-Aldrich Chemie, Zwijndrecht, the Netherlands). No free amino acids (i.e., glutamine), a requirement for successful use of the GS selection system.
4. L-Methionine-sulfoximine (MSX; Sigma) at a stock solution of 100 mM. MSX is a potent inhibitor of glutamine synthetase activity. MSX has widely been used as a selection agent for plasmid integration in Chinese hamster ovary (CHO) and other mammalian cell lines.

2.3.2 Single Cell Cloning of Optimal CHO-K1 Producer Clone

1. Small-scale culture CHO-K1 cells transfected with plasmid pEE14scFv:sFasL.
2. 96-well plates supplemented with 200 μl of GMEM/5 % dFBS/MSX selection medium (leave outer rim of wells in the plate empty to minimize chance of infections upon long-term culture).
3. FACS tubes (4 ml) and snap cap cell strainer 35-μm nylon mesh (BD biosciences).
4. MoFlo high-speed cell sorter (Cytomation).

2.3.3 Production of scFv:FasL with Stably Transfected CHO-K1 Cells

1. Stably transfected polyclonal or monoclonal CHO-K1. pEE14scFv:FasL cells.
2. Fully formulated CHO-S-SFM suspension medium (Gibco).
3. Standard 162-cm^2 culture flasks (or, e.g., roller-bottle suspension culture flasks (Gibco)).

2.4 Components for Affinity Purification on Anti-HA Agarose

1. Supernatant of stably transfected CHO-K1 pEE14scFv:FasL producer cells.
2. Anti-HA mAb 3F10 agarose (Roche).
3. Wash buffer; TBS (0.02 M Tris, 8 % NaCl, pH 7.6).
4. Elution buffer; HA peptide (100 μg/ml HA peptide; Pierce).

5. Storage buffer (Glycerol 50 % in TBS with 0.02 % sodium azide).
6. Slide-a-Lyzer Dialysis cassette 20K MWCO (Pierce).

2.5 Components for Biochemical Characterization

2.5.1 Analytical Gel Filtration and Downstream Analysis

1. Supernatant of CHO-K1.pEE14scFv:FasL cells or solution of affinity tag-purified scFv:FasL.
2. Gel filtration standards (BioRad).
3. HiLoad 16/60 Superdex 200 Prep grade column (GE Healthcare).
4. Akta system + spectrophotometer + fraction collector.
5. FasL enzyme-linked immunosorbent assay (ELISA) (Axxora, San Diego, CA).
6. A reporter cell line, such as the T-cell line Jurkat or the B-cell line Ramos, that is resistant to homogeneous trimeric sFasL preparations, but sensitive to multimeric and aggregated forms of FasL. Such a cell line can be exploited as a biological indicator for the functional detection of the presence of unwanted aggregates in FasL-based fusion protein formulations.

2.6 Components for Functional Characterization

2.6.1 Analysis of Target Antigen-Restricted Binding Activity

1. Isogenic parental target antigen-negative and stable target antigen-positive transfectant cell lines.
2. Competitive target antigen-blocking antibody. Ideally, the antibody is the parental monoclonal antibody from which the scFv has been derived. Alternatively, an in-house minibody can be generated using the scFv or an antibodies that binds to an overlapping epitope may also be used for this purpose.
3. Fluorescently labeled anti-FasL antibody (we typically use PE-conjugated anti-FasL clone NOK-1 from eBioscience).
4. FACS tubes (4 ml).

2.6.2 Target Antigen-Restricted Apoptotic Activity on T-Cell Line and/or Isolated Lymphocytes

1. Target antigen-positive and target antigen-negative isogenic cell line pair.
2. Competitive target antigen-blocking antibody.
3. Lymphoprep™ for density gradient isolation of lymphocytes (Axis-Shield).
4. 48-well plates.
5. Apoptosis assays (DiOC6, Annexin-V/PI).
6. 4-ml FACS tubes.
7. Appropriate fluorescently conjugated primary T-cell surface antibodies (e.g., CD3/CD4/CD8) for immune phenotyping.
8. Flow cytometer; benchtop Accuri flow cytometer (BD) for 4-color flow cytometry or LSR-II (BD) for multicolor flow cytometry.

3 Methods

3.1 Construction of Eukaryotic Expression Plasmids Encoding scFv:sFasL Fusion Proteins

1. Construct an expression cassette (or order a synthetic gene) encoding a protein of interest with the following general features: leader sequence HA-tag–scFv–linker–sFasL domain (*see* **Notes 1** and **2**; Fig. 2). In the case of scFvCD7:sFasL, a 745-bp DNA fragment encoding anti-CD7 antibody fragment scFv3A1F is excised from Phagemid pCANTAB pCANTAB5E/scFv3A1F using restriction enzymes SfiI and NotI. PCR-produced sFasL encoding DNA is digested using restriction enzymes XhoI and HindIII. The resulting DNA fragments should be isolated after separation using standard agarose gel electrophoresis separation and subsequent gel extraction.
2. Subclone the expression cassette in a eukaryotic expression plasmid, e.g., pEE14, or comparable eukaryotic expression plasmid. For scFvCD7:sFasL, the scFv3A1F antibody fragment is directionally inserted using the unique SfiI and NotI restriction enzyme sites. In the second MCS, the extracellular domain of human sFasL is directionally inserted using restriction enzymes XhoI and HindIII. The sFasL domain must contain the trimerization domain to allow receptor binding.

3.1.1 Transient Expression of scFv:sFasL in CHO-K1 Cells

1. Culture CHO-K1 cells in standard culture flasks in GMEM/5 % v/v FBS (to 70–80 % confluency).
2. Harvest cells by trypsin digestion and plate in 6-well plates at a concentration of 1×10^5/well in GMEM/5 % FBS.
3. Next day check whether confluency is ~70–80 %, then transfect using FuGENE transfection reagent (or alternate transfection method) according to manufacturer's instructions.
4. After 3 days, collect cell culture supernatant and verify for the presence of functional scFv:sFasL fusion protein (*see* Subheading 3.4) and determine its concentration using FasL ELISA (*see* Subheading 3.3.1). Harvest cells to determine transfection percentage by standard immunocytochemistry (*see* Subheading 3.1.2).

3.1.2 Analysis of Transfection Efficiency by Immunocytochemistry

1. Pellet harvested cells and resuspend at 1×10^6 cells/ml in PBS.
2. Spot cells on microscope glass slides using Cytospin centrifuge.
3. Dry microscope slides for 30 min using blow-dryer.
4. Fixate cells for 10 min using pure acetone (acetone used for this purpose can be reused up to ten times) and dry microscope slides (*see* **Note 4**).
5. Use a Pap Pen slide marker to circle a thin filmlike barrier around the spotted cells to hold antibody solutions within the designated area.

6. Add HRP-conjugated anti-HA antibody at a concentration of 1 μg/ml and use a minimum of 50 μl/slide.
7. Incubate for 45 min at room temperature in a humidified environment to prevent evaporation, which may result in a precipitation of antibodies.
8. Wash twice with excess PBS.
9. Perform AEC staining according to standard protocol and counterstain with hematoxylin.
10. Microscopically analyze the staining results and quantify percentage of transfected cells by enumeration.

3.1.3 Stable Expression of scFv:sFasL in CHO-K1 Cells

1. After verifying transfection efficiency, wash remaining transfected wells with prewarmed PBS.
2. Add 2 ml of GS selection medium (GMEM/5 % dFBS) to the well.
3. Add MSX to select for cells containing exogenously overexpressed glutamine synthetase gene as present in the backbone of the pEE14 plasmid. The typical effective selection range is 50–150 μM MSX.
4. After ~3 weeks selected clones can be visually detected. Subsequently, harvest clonally expanded cells and seed at 3×10^5 cells/well in a 6-well plate or 25-cm^2 culture flask.
5. Use a small aliquot of cells to verify the percentage of stably selected CHO-K1 producer cells using immunocytochemistry (*see* Subheading 3.1.2).
6. Verify the presence of functional scFv:sFasL fusion protein in the supernatant (*see* Subheading 3.4) and determine concentration using FasL ELISA (*see* Subheading 3.3.1).
7. Store the polyclonal CHO-K1 pEE14scFv:sFasL producing cell population in liquid nitrogen. Typical productivity of such stably transfected polyclonal producer cells ranges from 1 to 10 μg/ml.

3.1.4 Isolation of Single Cell Clones of CHO-K1 pEE14scFv:sFasL

1. Harvest polyclonal CHO-K1 pEE14scFv:sFasL producer cell line by trypsin digestion, resuspend in complete selection medium at 1×10^6 cells/ml.
2. For high-speed sorting, use round-bottom tubes with snap cap cell strainer (35-μm nylon mesh) to remove aggregated cells from cell suspension.
3. Add cells to sterile 4-ml FACS tube and use high-speed cell sorter to inject a single cell/well to 96-well plates (use approx. 10–15 plates).
4. Incubate for 3–4 weeks and continually monitor for signs of infection.
5. Upon visual discoloration of medium and microscopic confirmation of clonal outgrowth; trypsin digest individual wells and replate in 24-well plates.

6. Check the various producer cell clones for activity using, e.g., apoptosis assay on Jurkat T cells to identify highest producers.
7. Freeze aliquot of high producers, check for transfection efficiency by immunocytochemistry, and proceed to large-scale production with selected clone.

3.1.5 Large-Scale Production of scFv:FasL

1. Culture CHO-K1 producer cell clone in 162-cm^2 culture flasks in GMEM/5 % v/v FBS in the presence of the appropriate concentration of MSX.
2. After sufficient expansion (for 300 ml ~10 culture flasks are needed), wash cells with PBS and replace medium with CHO-S-SFMII complete medium.
3. After 1 week of culture, harvest the supernatant and remove detached cells and cell debris by centrifugation (1,000×*g*, 15 min). Check the cleared supernatant for functional scFv:FasL fusion protein as described in Subheading 3.4.
4. Store cleared supernatant for purification at −20 °C.

3.2 Purification of scFv:FasL Using Anti-HA Affinity Chromatography

1. Pack an anti-HA agarose column with a minimum bed volume of 200 μl (minimal bed height 3× diameter).
2. Allow resin to settle and connect to standard peristaltic pump. Be sure to position plunger as close to the resin bed as possible and to avoid any air bubbles in the system. Connect spectrophotometer for monitoring elution of bound protein by OD280. Flow rate for the column should be set at 1 ml/min.
3. Equilibrate the column with ten column volumes of wash buffer.
4. Load scFv:sFasL fusion protein-containing cell culture supernatant (before loading add NaCl to a final concentration 150 mM).
5. Wash the column with 15–20 column volumes of wash buffer.
6. Elute bound protein with HA peptide containing elution buffer.
7. Dialyze the elution fractions containing scFv:sFasL using 20K MWCO Slide-a-Lyzer dialysis cassette to remove free HA peptide.
8. Determine the concentration of purified scFv:sFasL using a commercially available FasL ELISA (*see* Subheading 3.3.2 and **Note 5**).
9. Regenerate column by acid wash with glycine buffer (0.1 M glycine HCl, pH 3.5) to ensure complete elution of all HA-tag bound material.
10. Immediately re-equilibrate column at neutral pH.
11. Store the column in TBS/50 % glycerol supplemented with 0.02 % NaN_3.

3.3 Biochemical Characterization

3.3.1 Gel Filtration Analysis

1. Equilibrate the HiLoad 16/60 Superdex 200 Prep grade gel filtration column (separation range 10^4–10^6 Da) with 5 bed volumes of PBS. The column should be connected to a non-pulsed pump to ensure equal flow.
2. Calibrate column using a mix of standard proteins (we typically use the gel filtration standard provided by BioRad, which provides a range from ~1.35 to 670 kDa. A range covering with a monomeric size of scFv:FasL of ~58 kDa, a trimeric size of ~160 kDa and possible aggregates).
3. Load the column with 5 ml of scFv:sFasL fusion protein using the flow rate recommended for the gel filtration column and collect 1 ml samples of flow through. Hereto, we use an automated sample collector connected to the AKTA system.
4. Use a system with an in-line connected spectrophotometer to monitor protein elution at OD280.
5. Wash column with 5 bed volumes of PBS and store the column in 20 % ethanol for future use.

3.3.2 Solution Behavior Analysis of scFv:sFasL

1. Determine the presence of FasL in all of the fractions obtained after gel filtration using a standard commercially available FasL catching type ELISA. In brief, add undiluted and 1:10 diluted fractions to the ELISA plate and use biotin-conjugated anti-FasL antibody and HRPO-conjugated streptavidin to determine which fractions contain FasL. Typically, scFv:sFasL should be present in fractions corresponding to a MW of 160 kDa (the size of trimeric scFv:sFasL) (*see* **Note 7**). For publication describing exemplary results using scFv:sTRAIL, *see* ref. 20.
2. Check all isolated fractions for the presence of FasL-mediated apoptotic activity using the sensitive target antigen-negative/antigen-positive isogenic reporter cell line pair. Of note, properly folded homotrimeric scFv:FasL will be of ~160 kDa size and will trigger apoptosis in the appropriate target antigen-positive line only. Off-target/aggregated activity can be identified using the target antigen-negative reporter line, which will only be sensitive to aggregated FasL (*see* **Note 6**).

3.4 Characterization of Biological Activity

3.4.1 Target Antigen-Restricted Binding by scFv:FasL

1. Prepare target antigen-positive and target antigen-negative cell lines in 4-ml FACS tubes at 1×10^6/ml.
2. Add scFv:sFasL fusion protein and incubate for 1.5 h at 0 °C. Note: for the TAA-positive cells also add a condition in which cells were preincubated for 45 min at 0 °C with target antigen-blocking monoclonal antibody. Hereto, an in-house constructed minibody of the scFv contained in the fusion protein, or the parental antibody, can be used.
3. Collect cells ($1,000 \times g$/5 min) and wash twice with 4 ml PBS.

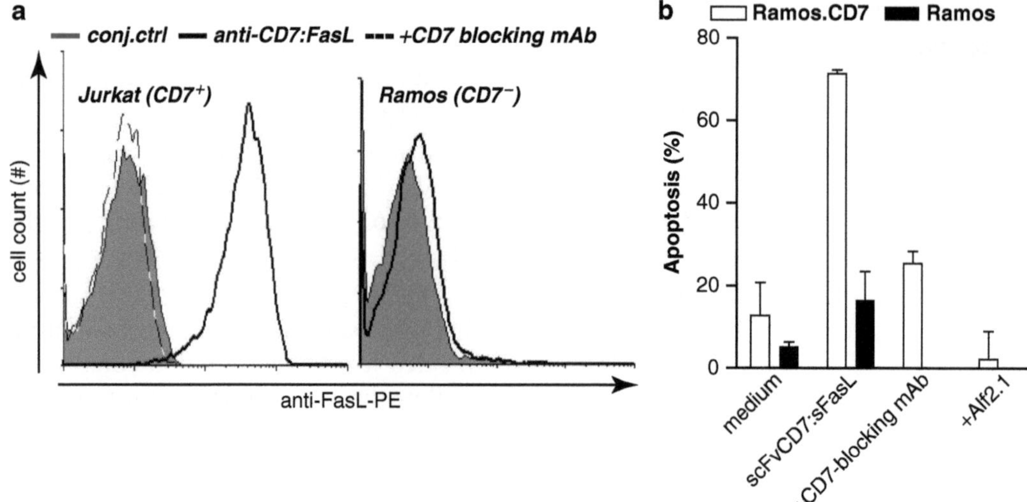

Fig. 3 Target antigen-restricted binding and apoptosis induction. (**a**) Flow cytometric binding analysis of anti-CD7:sFasL on CD7-positive Jurkat cells and CD7-negative Ramos cells. On Jurkat cells, CD7-specific binding is also competitively inhibited by preincubation with CD7-blocking monoclonal antibody TH69. (**b**) Analysis of CD7-restricted induction of apoptosis on Ramos (CD7-negative) and CD7-transfected Ramos cells (Ramos.CD7). Cells were incubated for 24 h with anti-CD7:sFasL and analyzed for apoptosis by loss of mitochondrial membrane potential. For Ramos.CD7, cells were additionally co-treated with CD7-blocking mAb TH69 and FasL-neutralizing mAb Alf2.1

4. Incubate cells with fluorescently conjugated anti-FasL mAb for 45 min at 0 °C.
5. Collect cells (1,000 × *g*/5 min) and wash twice with 4 ml PBS.
6. Analyze cell surface staining by flow cytometry (*see* Fig. 3a).

3.4.2 Target Antigen-Restricted Activity by scFv:sFasL

1. Seed target antigen-positive and target antigen-negative T-cell line or primary T cells in 96-well round-bottom tissue culture plates at 40×10^3 cells/well.
2. Incubate cells with serial dilutions of scFv:sFasL. Note: for the target antigen-positive cell line, also add conditions in which cells were preincubated for 30 min with molar excess of epitope-competing target antigen-blocking antibody.
3. Incubate for 24 h and analyze for cell death induction using standard apoptosis assays, such as Annexin-V/PI according to manufacturer's instruction.
4. Analyze induction of cell death using flow cytometer (*see* Fig. 3b for representative data).

3.4.3 Target Antigen-Restricted Activity on Isolated Lymphocytes

1. After obtaining ethical approval and informed consent, isolate mononuclear cells from heparinized blood of healthy volunteers and/or patients using standard density gradient procedures (Axis).

2. Treat isolated mononuclear for 24 h with the scFv:FasL fusion protein. Also include control conditions in which cells have been preincubated with epitope-competing target antigen-blocking or FasL-neutralizing mAb ALF2.1 (1 μg/ml). As a positive control for FasL sensitivity, including a condition with a FLAG-tagged sFasL preparation secondarily cross-linked by anti-Flag mAb M2.
3. Assess apoptosis by Annexin-V-FITC staining (Immunotools, Germany) and combine with multicolor flow cytometric immunophenotyping to determine specific subpopulations eliminated by scFv:FasL fusion protein. For illustrative flow cytometry stainings *see* [14].

4 Notes

1. As an alternative to the generation of an scFv antibody fragment, the extracellular domain of a natural ligand that binds with high affinity to its corresponding counterpart on T cells may be used. For instance, our studies have shown that K12, the high-affinity ligand for CD7, is equally effective as an anti-CD7 scFv antibody fragment in the targeted delivery of sFasL or sTRAIL to CD7 on T cells [14, 21]. We strongly recommend that fusion proteins of either composition should be subjected to an early-on detailed assessment of solution behavior, stability, and yield of homotrimeric fusion protein.
2. We used a murine kappa light-chain leader peptide to direct produced scFvCD7: sFasL through the endoplasmic reticulum (ER) and Golgi complex, thus taking advantage of the associated stringent quality control mechanisms that facilitates secretion of correctly folded and non-aggregated scFvCD7:sFasL into the culture medium.
3. The various domains are separated by a glycine-serine rich 21 amino acid linkers to ensure flexibility of the respective domains. Different linker lengths may be explored in case of suboptimal activity.
4. If **steps 3** and **4** are not performed sufficiently long, cells will detach upon immunocytochemistry procedure.
5. The concentration of an scFv:FasL fusion protein should be determined by various methods, the outcome of which should correspond closely. Although ELISA is the most sensitive, the genetic fusion of an scFv antibody fragment to FasL may influence the sensitivity of the respective ELISA. However, our experience suggests that the FasL ELISA data closely correspond to other methods of scFv:FasL determination.

6. If significant amount of aggregates are detected, use preparative gel filtration to isolate trimeric and properly folded scFv:FasL. Reevaluate this scFv:FasL preparation for aggregates after (extended) storage to ensure stability of the isolated protein. In the case of continuous aggregate formation, it may be that the selected scFv has a tendency to aggregate or to interfere with proper trimerization of FasL. Therefore, exchange the scFv for an alternate scFv or targeting domain (e.g., the high-affinity CD7-ligand K12 as used by us) and reanalyze for stability.
7. It cannot be ruled out that a FasL ELISA fails to recognize a corresponding scFv:sFasL fusion protein or detects it with lower efficacy due to steric hindrance related to the scFv domain. It is therefore prudent to confirm the ELISA results using alternate methods.

References

1. Lubberts E, Koenders MI, van den Berg WB (2005) The role of T-cell interleukin-17 in conducting destructive arthritis: lessons from animal models. Arthritis Res Ther 7:29–37
2. Lubberts E (2010) Th17 cytokines and arthritis. Semin Immunopathol 32:43–53
3. Shah K, Lee WW, Lee SH et al (2010) Dysregulated balance of Th17 and Th1 cells in systemic lupus erythematosus. Arthritis Res Ther 12:R53
4. Moreland LW, Pratt PW, Mayes MD et al (1995) Double-blind, placebo-controlled multicenter trial using chimeric monoclonal anti-CD4 antibody, cM-T412, in rheumatoid arthritis patients receiving concomitant methotrexate. Arthritis Rheum 38:1581–1588
5. Choy EH, Chikanza IC, Kingsley GH, Corrigall V, Panayi GS (1992) Treatment of rheumatoid arthritis with single dose or weekly pulses of chimeric anti-CD4 monoclonal antibody. Scand J Immunol 36:291–298
6. Kirkham BW, Thien F, Pelton BK et al (1992) Chimeric CD7 monoclonal antibody therapy in rheumatoid arthritis. J Rheumatol 19: 1348–1352
7. Schiff M, Keiserman M, Codding C et al (2008) Efficacy and safety of abatacept or infliximab vs placebo in ATTEST: a phase III, multi-centre, randomised, double-blind, placebo-controlled study in patients with rheumatoid arthritis and an inadequate response to methotrexate. Ann Rheum Dis 67:1096–1103
8. Chiang EY, Kolumam GA, Yu X et al (2009) Targeted depletion of lymphotoxin-alpha-expressing TH1 and TH17 cells inhibits autoimmune disease. Nat Med 15:766–773
9. Brenner D, Krammer PH, Arnold R (2008) Concepts of activated T cell death. Crit Rev Oncol Hematol 66:52–64
10. Green DR, Droin N, Pinkoski M (2003) Activation-induced cell death in T cells. Immunol Rev 193:70–81
11. de Bruyn M, Bremer E, Helfrich W (2013) Antibody-based fusion proteins to target death receptors in cancer. Cancer Lett 332:175–183
12. Schneider P, Holler N, Bodmer JL et al (1998) Conversion of membrane-bound Fas(CD95) ligand to its soluble form is associated with downregulation of its proapoptotic activity and loss of liver toxicity. J Exp Med 187: 1205–1213
13. Bremer E, ten CB, Samplonius DF, de Leij LF, Helfrich W (2006) CD7-restricted activation of Fas-mediated apoptosis: a novel therapeutic approach for acute T-cell leukemia. Blood 107:2863–2870
14. Bremer E, Abdulahad WH, de BM et al (2011) Selective elimination of pathogenic synovial fluid T-cells from rheumatoid arthritis and juvenile idiopathic arthritis by targeted activation of Fas-apoptotic signaling. Immunol Lett 138:161–168
15. Eggleton P, Bremer E, Tarr JM et al (2011) Frequency of Th17 CD20+ cells in the peripheral blood of rheumatoid arthritis patients is

higher compared to healthy subjects. Arthritis Res Ther 13:R208

16. Sandilands GP, Perry M, Wootton M, Hair J, More IA (1999) B-cell antigens within normal and activated human T cells. Immunology 96:424–433
17. Wilk E, Witte T, Marquardt N et al (2009) Depletion of functionally active CD20+ T cells by rituximab treatment. Arthritis Rheum 60: 3563–3571
18. Holley JE, Bremer E, Kendall AC et al (2013) CD20+ Th17 cells in multiple sclerosis brain may be targeted for apoptosis. Multiple sclerosis and related disorders (in revision)
19. Helfrich W, Haisma HJ, Magdolen V et al (2000) A rapid and versatile method for harnessing scFv antibody fragments with various biological effector functions. J Immunol Methods 237:131–145
20. Bremer E, Kuijlen J, Samplonius D et al (2004) Target cell-restricted and -enhanced apoptosis induction by a scFv:sTRAIL fusion protein with specificity for the pancarcinoma-associated antigen EGP2. Int J Cancer 109:281–290
21. de Bruyn M, Wei Y, Wiersma VR et al (2011) Cell surface delivery of TRAIL strongly augments the tumoricidal activity of T cells. Clin Cancer Res 17:5626–5637

Chapter 8

TLC Immunostaining for Detection of "Antiphospholipid" Antibodies

Fabrizio Conti, Cristiano Alessandri, Francesca Romana Spinelli, Antonella Capozzi, Francesco Martinelli, Serena Recalchi, Roberta Misasi, Guido Valesini, and Maurizio Sorice

Abstract

Thin-layer chromatography (TLC) is a nonquantitative technique, which has been employed in the detection of antiphospholipid (aPL) antibodies. Antiphospholipid syndrome (APS) is the most frequently acquired thrombophilia, characterized by thrombosis and obstetric manifestations associated to an autoimmune trait, represented by the positivity of antiphospholipid (aPL) antibodies. Immunoassays for anticardiolipin (aCL) and anti-β2 glycoprotein I (aβ2GPI) antibodies and clotting tests for lupus anticoagulant (LA) represent the standard tests for the routine detection of aPL. The term "seronegative APS" has been used to describe patients with clinical manifestation of APS and persistently negative aPL assessed with routine assays. TLC immunostaining is a useful method for the detection of different antigenic targets of "antiphospholipid" antibodies; it is able to identify the reactivity of serum aPL experimented with purified phospholipid molecules with a different exposure compared to ELISA methods. This method seems to be applicable in patients who repeatedly tested negative for the standard aPL, i.e., aCL, aβ2GPI, and LA. Therefore, this technique may be proposed as a second step test for the diagnosis of APS.

Key words Thin-layer chromatography immunostaining, Antiphospholipid antibodies, Antiphospholipid syndrome

1 Introduction

Thin-layer chromatography (TLC) immunostaining is a useful method for detection of antibodies to different antigenic targets of antiphospholipid antibodies (aPL) and anti-glycolipid antibodies [1, 2]. Antiphospholipid syndrome (APS) is an autoimmune disease characterized by arterial and/or venous thrombosis and/or obstetric manifestations (recurrent miscarriages, fetal loss, or preterm delivery) associated with antibodies against phospholipid-protein complexes [3]. APS is the most frequently acquired thrombophilia, which can occur apart or associated with other autoimmune diseases, especially systemic lupus erythematosus (SLE), a chronic

Paul Eggleton and Frank J. Ward (eds.), *Systemic Lupus Erythematosus: Methods and Protocols*, Methods in Molecular Biology, vol. 1134, DOI 10.1007/978-1-4939-0326-9_8,

inflammatory disorder with a multifactorial etiology characterized by the production of a wide range of autoantibodies [4–8]. Classification of APS requires the presence of at least one clinical (thrombosis, pregnancy morbidity) and one laboratory (lupus anticoagulants, anticardiolipin antibodies, anti-β2-glycoprotein I antibodies) criterion; the detection of aPL antibodies must be confirmed on two distinct occasions 12 weeks apart [9]. Routine tests for aPL antibodies detection include clotting test for the assessment of lupus anticoagulant (LA) and the immunoenzymatic assays for anticardiolipin (aCL) and anti-β2 glycoprotein I (aβ2GPI) antibodies. However, for patients with symptoms suggestive of APS and persistent negativity for routinely used tests, the term of "seronegative APS" (SN-APS) has been proposed [10, 11].

In the recent past, the role of different antigenic targets has emerged. In particular, antibodies directed to the lyso(bis)phosphatidic acid (aLBPA) [12] may represent a marker of APS, showing similar sensitivity and specificity compared to aβ2GPI and a strong association with LA positivity [13]. Moreover, antiprothrombin antibodies have been reported as the sole antibodies detected in a few patients with thrombosis and SLE, who were persistently negative for aCL or LA [14]. Antiphosphatidylethanolamine antibodies (aPE) have been detected in 15 % of a cohort of thrombotic patients, mainly in the absence of the other laboratory criteria of APS [15]. Recently, using a proteomic approach, we identified vimentin/cardiolipin as a "new" target of the APS, also detectable in SN-APS patients [16].

A different laboratory technique capable of detecting aPL by immunostaining on thin-layer chromatography (TLC) plates has been proposed. This is a nonquantitative technique able to identify the reactivity of serum aPL experimented with purified phospholipid molecules with a different antigenic exposure compared to ELISA methods [2]. Furthermore, TLC immunostaining allows the investigator to simultaneously identify the reactivity of patient's sera with different purified phospholipids. The method exploits the fact that antigens run on aluminum-backed silica gel mimic the exposure of phospholipids binding to proteins.

Originally employed for the detection of aPL in 1994, TLC immunostaining appears to be less sensitive but more specific than ELISA in both autoimmune and infectious diseases [2]. We have recently used TLC immunostaining for the detection of aPL in a group of patients with a clinical picture suggestive of APS, i.e., vascular thrombosis and/or pregnancy morbidity associated with several non-criteria APS features (i.e., livedo reticularis, thrombocytopenia, cognitive dysfunctions, migraine, seizures) persistently negative for the routinely used aPL, demonstrating a positivity for different antibodies (aCL, aLBPA, and aPE) in up to 60 % of subjects [17]. Moreover, our results suggest the biological activity of these antibodies that are able to trigger a signal transduction pathway(s) in endothelial cells with consequent proinflammatory and procoagulant effects in vitro [17]. The most relevant finding of this study is that TLC immunostaining could potentially identify the presence of aPL in patients with clinical features suggestive of APS not ascertained by traditional tests for aPL and such identification could have a major impact on the prognosis and the therapeutic approach. Thus, after the detection of aPL by TLC immunostaining in patients with clinical features of SN-APS, our policy is to treat these patients in the same way as those with APS are usually treated. To date, TLC immunostaining appears not to be suitable for screening purpose, but might represent a rescue test for those patients who present clinical signs of APS but tested repeatedly negative for conventional aPL.

2 Materials

Prepare all solutions using ultrapure water (prepared by purifying deionized water to attain a sensitivity of 18 MΩ cm at 25 °C) and analytical grade reagents.

1. *Phospholipid antigens*: cardiolipin (CL) (from bovine heart), lyso(bis)phosphatidic acid (LBPA), phosphatidylcholine (PC), phosphatidylethanolamine (PE), phosphatidylserine (PS), and phosphatidylinositol (PI) (Sigma Chem Co, St Louis, USA).
2. *Plates*: aluminum-backed silica gel 60 (20×20 cm) high-performance thin-layer chromatography (HPTLC) plates (Merck Co, Darmstadt, Germany).
3. *Eluent system*: chloroform/methanol/acetic acid/water.
4. *Soaking solution*: poly(isobutyl methacrylate) beads (Polysciences, Eppelheim, Germany) in hexane (0.5 % w/v).
5. *Washing solution*: commercially prepared PBS, pH 7.4 (*see* **Note 1**).
6. *Blocking solution*: 1 % w/v bovine serum albumin (BSA) in commercially prepared phosphate buffered saline (PBS pH 7.4).
7. *Secondary antibody*: horseradish peroxidase (HRP)-conjugated goat antihuman IgG, IgM, or IgA.
8. *Developing system*: enhanced chemiluminescence (ECL) detection system (Amersham, Buckinghamshire, UK).

3 Methods

All procedures are conducted at room temperature in a fume hood.

3.1 Detection of aPL by TLC Immunostaining

1. *Antigen separation.* Phospholipids (2 μg each in chloroform/methanol, 2:1 v/v) run on aluminum-backed silica gel 60 (20 × 20) high-performance thin-layer chromatography (HPTLC) plates (Merck Co, Darmstadt, Germany); chromatography is performed in chloroform/methanol/acetic acid/water in a volumetric ratio of 100:75:7:4, respectively. The phospholipid run may be checked by staining with iodide vapors for 5 min.
2. *Soaking.* The dried chromatograms are soaked for 90 s in a 0.5 % w/v solution of poly(isobutyl methacrylate) beads (Polysciences, Eppelheim, Germany), dissolved in hexane (86.18 g/mol).
3. *Blocking.* After air-drying for 5 min, the chromatograms are incubated at 20 °C (room temperature) for 1 h with 1 % w/v BSA in PBS to eliminate nonspecific binding (*see* **Note 2**).
4. *Sera reactivity.* After washing (by gentle shaking, three times for 10 min with PBS), the chromatograms are incubated for 1 h at 20 °C with sera, diluted 1:100 in the blocking solution (1 % BSA in PBS).
5. *Detection.* Sera are removed and chromatograms are washed by gentle shaking three times for 10 min with PBS. Bound antibodies are visualized with HRP-conjugated goat antihuman IgG, IgM, or IgA, diluted 1:1,000 in 1 % w/v BSA in PBS, incubated at 20 °C for 1 h (*see* **Notes 3–5**). After washing (by gentle shaking, three times for 10 min with PBS), immunoreactivity is assessed by chemiluminescence reaction, using an ECL detection system in accordance with the manufacturer's instructions.

   As a control for nonspecific reactivity, parallel blots are processed as above, but without serum or without antigen.

4 Notes

1. TLC immunostaining is an easy and suitable method for detection of aPL antibodies (Fig. 1). However, in the execution of the test, some accuracies are very important: temperature has to be maintained in a range between 20 and 25 °C, and chromatograms during washes have to be shaken very gently, in order to avoid the possible silica breakaway from aluminum plates. Moreover, in some cases you may need to employ different eluent system, depending on the characteristics of the (phospho)lipid antigens under test. For example, in order to better separate molecules with similar polarity, the following may be proposed: chloroform/acetone/methanol/acetic acid/water (40:15:13:12:8) (v:v:v:v:v), following preincubation with 1 % potassium oxalate in methanol/water (2:3, v:v) for

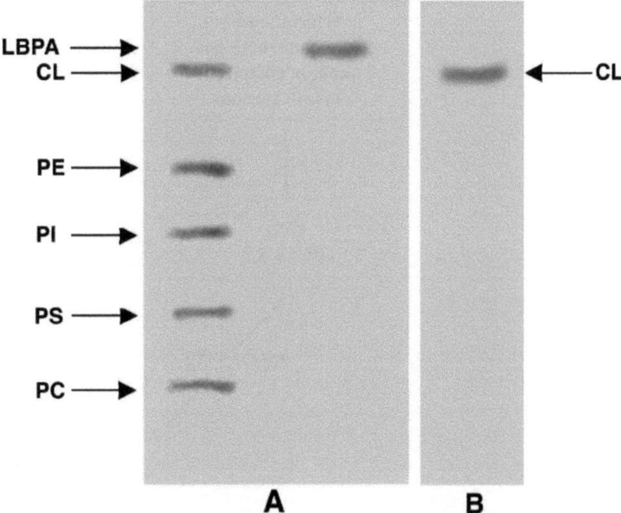

Fig. 1 Representative TLC immunostaining. TLC immunostaining was performed using the following phospholipid antigens: lyso(bis)phosphatidic acid (LBPA), cardiolipin (CL), phosphatidylethanolamine (PE), phosphatidylinositol (PI), phosphatidylserine (PS), and phosphatidylcholine (PC). Lane (**a**), standard phospholipids, stained with iodide vapors; lane (**b**), reactivity of a serum (diluted 1:100 in 1 % BSA in PBS) from an APS patient positive for CL. Bound antibodies were visualized with HRP-conjugated goat antihuman IgG. The reaction was developed using an ECL detection system

1 h at room temperature, drying, and then activation at 100 °C for 5 min [17].

2. Although TLC immunostaining is not quantitative, the use of this technique for detection of aPL allows the simultaneous analysis of reactivity of sera with different phospholipid molecules, thus providing a useful tool for clarifying the immunological specificity of these antibodies in autoimmune or infectious diseases. With this aim, two variations/alternatives to blocking solution are available. The first one, 0.5 % (w/v) gelatin/PBS, works in the absence of protein cofactors and is suitable for detection of aβ2GPI independent antiphospholipid antibodies [18], which are usually detectable in infectious diseases [19]; the second one, 10 % fetal calf serum in PBS, is useful for detection of aPL in the presence of cofactor proteins, mainly aβ2GPI (provided with the medium) [20].

3. In clinical practice it may happen to find patients with clinical signs of APS, who are persistently negative for the routinely used aPL [10, 11]. The main application of this method is the analysis of aPL in patients negative for the laboratory criteria of APS, i.e., aCL, aβ2GPI, and LA. These patients have been recently termed "seronegative APS" [10]. Indeed, we recently

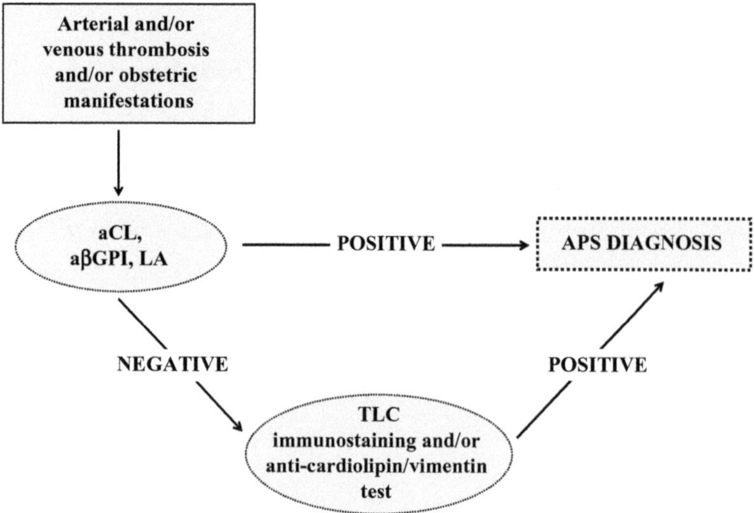

Fig. 2 Algorithm for APS diagnosis. Schematic drawing depicting a proposed algorithm for diagnosis in "seronegative" APS patients. *LA* lupus anticoagulant and the immunoenzymatic assays for *aCL* anticardiolipin antibodies, *aβ2GPI* anti-β2 glycoprotein I antibodies, *TLC* thin-layer chromatography

demonstrated that aPL detected by TLC immunostaining associate with clinical features of APS in these patients [17].

4. As regards the so-called SN-APS patients, the discrepancies between TLC immunostaining and ELISA in detecting aPL may be due to the different antigenic presentation of phospholipids on chromatograms compared to the surface of microtiter wells. Indeed, in TLC immunostaining, the antigen is run on aluminum-backed silica gel plates, and in this way, it may mimic phospholipid exposure after protein binding [17, 19, 21].
5. Thus, although this method has a sensitivity of about 70 %, it represents a rescue test for those patients with clinical features suggestive of APS in which the classical tests for detection aPL result persistently negative. Therefore, it may be proposed, together with anticardiolipin/antivimentin test [16], as a second step test for the diagnosis of "seronegative APS" (Fig. 2).

References

1. Li JL, Matsuda K, Takagi M, Yamamoto N (1997) Detection of serum antibodies against phosphocholine-containing aminoglycoglycerolipids specific to Mycoplasma fermentans in HIV-1 infected individuals. J Immunol Methods 208:103–113
2. Sorice M, Griggi T, Circella A, Garofalo T, d'Agostino F F, Pittoni V et al (1994) Detection of antiphospholipid antibodies by immunostaining on thin layer chromatography plates. J Immunol Methods 173:49–54
3. Hughes GR (1985) The anticardiolipin syndrome. Clin Exp Rheumatol 3:285–286
4. Conti F, Alessandri C, Bompane D, Bombardieri M, Spinelli FR, Rusconi AC, Valesini G (2004) Autoantibody profile in

systemic lupus erythematosus with psychiatric manifestations: a role for anti-endothelial-cell antibodies. Arthritis Res Ther 6:R366–R372

5. Valesini G, Alessandri C, Celestino D, Conti F (2006) Anti-endothelial antibodies and neuropsychiatric systemic lupus erythematosus. Ann N Y Acad Sci 1069:118–128
6. Alessandri C, Barbati C, Vacirca D, Piscopo P, Confaloni A, Sanchez M et al (2012) T lymphocytes from patients with systemic lupus erythematosus are resistant to induction of autophagy. FASEB J 26:4722–4732
7. Colasanti T, Maselli A, Conti F, Sanchez M, Alessandri C, Barbati C et al (2012) Autoantibodies to estrogen receptor α interfere with T lymphocyte homeostasis and are associated with disease activity in systemic lupus erythematosus. Arthritis Rheum 64: 778–787
8. Conti F, Alessandri C, Perricone C, Scrivo R, Rezai S, Ceccarelli F et al (2012) Neurocognitive dysfunction in systemic lupus erythematosus: association with antiphospholipid antibodies, disease activity and chronic damage. PLoS ONE 7(3):e33824
9. Miyakis S, Lockshin MD, Atsumi T, Branch DW, Brey RL, Cervera R et al (2006) International consensus statement on an update of the classification criteria for definite antiphospholipid syndrome (APS). J Thromb Haemost 4:295–306
10. Hughes GR, Khamashta M (2003) Seronegative antiphospholipid syndrome. Ann Rheum Dis 62:1127
11. Rodriguez-Garcia JL, Bertolaccini ML, Cuadrado MJ, Sanna G, Ateka-Barrutia O, Khamashta MA (2012) Clinical manifestations of antiphospholipid syndrome (APS) with and without antiphospholipid antibodies (the so-called "seronegative APS"). Ann Rheum Dis 71:242–244
12. Sorice M, Ferro D, Misasi R, Pittoni V, Longo A, Circella A et al (2002) Evidence for anticoagulant activity and β2-GPI accumulation in late endosomes of endothelial cells induced by anti-LBPA antibodies. Thromb Haemost 87: 735–741
13. Alessandri C, Bombardieri M, Di Prospero L, Conigliaro P, Conti F, Labbadia G et al (2005) Anti-lysobisphosphatidic acid antibodies in patients with antiphospholipid syndrome and systemic lupus erythematosus. Clin Exp Immunol 140:173–180
14. Oku K, Atsumi T, Amengual O, Koike T (2008) Antiprothrombin antibody testing: detection and clinical utility. Semin Thromb Haemost 34:335–339
15. Sanmarco M et al (2007) Antiphosphatidylethanolamine antibodies are associated with an increased odds ratio for thrombosis. A multicenter study with the participation of the European Forum on antiphospholipid antibodies. Thromb Haemost 97:949–954
16. Ortona E, Capozzi A, Colasanti T, Conti F, Alessandri C, Longo A et al (2010) Vimentin/cardiolipin complex as a new antigenic target of the antiphospholipid syndrome. Blood 116: 2960–2967
17. Conti F, Alessandri C, Sorice M, Capozzi A, Longo A, Garofalo T et al (2012) Thin-layer chromatography immunostaining in detecting anti-phospholipid antibodies in seronegative anti-phospholipid syndrome. Clin Exp Immunol 167:429–437
18. Sorice M, Circella A, Griggi T, Garofalo T, Nicodemo G, Pittoni V et al (1996) Anticardiolipin and anti-β2GPI are two distinct populations of autoantibodies. Thromb Haemost 75:303–308
19. Sorice M, Pittoni V, Griggi T, Losardo A, Leri O, Magno MS et al (2000) Specificity of antiphospholipid antibodies in infectious mononucleosis: a role for anti-cofactor protein antibodies. Clin Exp Immunol 120:301–306
20. Alessandri C, Sorice M, Bombardieri M, Conigliaro P, Longo A, Garofalo T et al (2006) Antiphospholipid reactivity against cardiolipin metabolites occurring during endothelial cell apoptosis. Arthritis Res Ther 8:R180–R190
21. Capozzi A, Lococo E, Grasso M, Longo A, Garofalo T, Misasi R, Sorice M (2012) Detection of antiphospholipid antibodies by automated chemiluminescence assay. J Immunol Methods 379:48–52

Chapter 9

Induced Murine Models of Systemic Lupus Erythematosus

Yuan Xu, Leilani Zeumer, Westley H. Reeves, and Laurence Morel

Abstract

Induced mouse models of systemic lupus erythematosus (SLE) have been developed to complement the spontaneous models. This chapter describes the methods used in the pristane-induced model and the chronic graft-versus-host disease (cGVHD) model, both of which have been extensively used. We will also outline the specific mechanisms of systemic autoimmunity that can be best characterized using each of these models.

Key words Pristane, Graft-versus-host disease, Systemic lupus erythematosus, Autoantibodies, Glomerulonephritis, Arthritis, Mice, Murine lupus, Alveolar hemorrhage, Type 1 interferon, Sex difference

1 Introduction

Spontaneous mouse models of SLE have been used extensively over the years (*see* [1] for review). Although these models are diverse and present many advantages, they have also drawbacks, the two major ones being that (1) their clinical manifestations present relatively late in life (5–8 months of age) with a high interindividual variability disease in the time-course and (2) they do not represent some of the phenotypes found across the broad spectrum of SLE clinical manifestations. To overcome these problems, induced models of lupus have been developed and used to offer additional tools either to investigate the cellular mechanisms of the disease or to test the hypothesis that specific genetic variations contribute to the induction of pathogenic systemic autoimmunity. The two major types of induced models that have been used extensively, the pristane-induced model and the chronic graft-versus-host disease (cGVHD) model, will be covered in this chapter.

Paul Eggleton and Frank J. Ward (eds.), *Systemic Lupus Erythematosus: Methods and Protocols*, Methods in Molecular Biology, vol. 1134, DOI 10.1007/978-1-4939-0326-9_9,

2 Materials

2.1 The Pristane-Induced Model

1. *Pristane preparation:* Pristane can be purchased from a number of commercial sources and they appear to give comparable results (*see* **Note 1**). Before injection, filter the pristane through a 0.22 μm syringe-driven filter unit, especially if injecting into C57BL/6 (B6) or C57BL/10 (B10) mice, which are susceptible to alveolar hemorrhage (discussed further below). BALB/c mice are resistant to alveolar hemorrhage and pristane filtration is unnecessary with these mice.

2.2 cGVHD-Induced Model

1. *Splenocyte preparation:* Plan to use one donor mouse per each recipient mouse. Make a sterile single-cell suspension from spleen in cRPMI (RPMI 1640, 5 % fetal bovine serum [FBS], 2-mercaptoethanol, penicillin) and centrifuge at 450 × *g* for 5 min.
2. Discard supernatant and lyse the cell pellet in 5 mL of sterile RBC lysis buffer (1 M Tris, NH_4Cl) at room temperature for 5 min and then add 5 mL cRPMI before centrifuging for 8 min at 450 × *g*.
3. Discard supernatant, add 5 mL cRPMI, and filter the cell suspension through a 30 μm pre-separation filter (Miltenyi Biotec).
4. Count splenocytes. We use a Cellometer Auto 2000 (Nexcelom Bioscience), but any method for counting live cells will work. Then centrifuge the cells for 5 min at 450 × *g*.
5. Discard supernatant and add 5 mL sterile PBS to the cell pellet.
6. Centrifuge at 450 × *g* for 5 min, discard supernatant, and then resuspend the cell pellet in sterile PBS for a final cell suspension of 60–80 × 10^6 cells/200 μL.

3 Methods

Carry out all procedures in accordance with animal husbandry regulations.

3.1 The Pristane-Induced Model

Pristane (tetramethylpentadecane, TMPD) is an isoprenoid alkane found naturally in plants and shark liver [2] and is also a constituent of mineral oil, a by-product of the fractional distillation of petroleum [2]. In 1994, it was found that intraperitoneal (i.p.) administration of pristane could induce lupus-specific IgG autoantibodies against a variety of nuclear antigens including double-stranded (ds) DNA, single-stranded (ss) DNA, chromatin, Sm, RNP, Su, and ribosomal P starting 3 months after treatment of non-autoimmune mice [3, 4]. Experimental lupus induced by pristane mimics several features of human SLE including the production of antinuclear antibodies (ANA), lupus-specific autoantibodies (anti-dsDNA, anti-Sm), and the development of immune-complex-mediated glomerulonephritis and arthritis. Importantly, pristane-induced lupus is associated with the increased expression of a group of genes regulated by type I interferons (IFN-I), e.g., IFNα and IFNβ [5]. This "interferon signature" is found in approximately two thirds of adult lupus patients and nearly all pediatric lupus patients [6]. At present, pristane-induced lupus is the best animal model of SLE associated with the interferon signature [2], making it valuable for understanding the role of IFN-I in SLE. On the other hand, pristane-induced lupus is of limited value for the understanding the role of natural genetic variation in lupus. The discussion below is a practical guide to the application of pristane-induced lupus to study of SLE pathogenesis.

1. *Injection of pristane:* Wearing gloves, take up pristane from the stock container into a syringe through an 18-gauge needle. To induce lupus in mice, administer 0.5 mL of pristane i.p. using a 25-gauge 5/8″ needle and a 3 mL syringe with Luer-Lock top into the mouse's lower abdomen. The Luer-Lock top helps to prevent the needle becoming detached during injection of the viscous oil. Avoid piercing the mouse's organs (bladder or intestines) with the needle. Be careful to inject the oil into the peritoneum and not subcutaneously. In general, the mice should be at least 8–12 weeks of age before injecting with pristane (*see* **Note 2**).
2. After injection, hold the mouse upright to allow the pristane to flow into the lower abdomen for a few seconds prior to withdrawing the needle. This avoids loss of the pristane through the needle hole. Although a small amount of leakage is common, a large leak of oil out of the peritoneum should be considered a "mis-injection," which may lead to failure of the mouse to develop lupus. At the conclusion of the experiment, it is helpful to examine peritoneal fluid for the presence of droplets of the pristane oil. These are less apparent with increasing time after pristane injection.
3. *Use of other alternative oils:* The capacity to induce lupus-like autoimmunity is shared by several hydrocarbons and is not a unique property of pristane [7]. I.p. injections of 0.5 mL of squalene (a metabolite of the cholesterol biosynthetic pathway used as an adjuvant for human vaccines), hexadecane, and incomplete Freund's adjuvant (containing the mineral oil Bayol F) induce a similar spectrum of autoantibodies, but less efficiently than pristane [2, 7, 8]. In contrast, medicinal mineral oil does not induce lupus autoantibodies or glomerulonephritis and can be considered as a control for pristane injection [7, 8].

3.1.1 Evaluation of Early Disease Manifestations (Collection of Cells and Lavage)

The evaluation of the disease includes short-term (2–6 weeks) effects such as peritoneal and systemic inflammatory responses, as well as the initiation of IFN-I and polyclonal immunoglobulin production, which will be covered in this section, and long-term (3–6 months) effects, such as the development of IgG autoantibodies and glomerulonephritis [9, 10], which will be covered in the next section. Within 2 weeks of injecting pristane, the peritoneum is infiltrated by neutrophils, Ly6C^{hi} monocytes, dendritic cells, and T cells [10]. In contrast, resident B cells, in particular the B-1 subset, become depleted [11]. These cells are the source of cytokines secreted into the peritoneal cavity: The neutrophils produce TNFα, Ly6C^{hi} monocytes and plasmacytoid dendritic cells (pDC) produce IFNα and IFNβ, and myeloid dendritic cells (mDC) produce IL-12. The infiltrating cells as well as the cytokines they produce can be evaluated by peritoneal lavage.

1. Method for collecting peritoneal cells and secreted cytokines by lavage: Use an 18-gauge needle attached to a 5 mL syringe to draw up 5 mL of sterile PBS into the syringe.
2. Euthanize the mouse and clean the fur by spraying with 70 % ethanol. Lay the mouse on its back and grab the skin with forceps. Nick the skin with scissors (sterilized in 70 % v/v ethanol) and expose the muscle layer. Avoid puncturing the muscular layer to prevent leakage of peritoneal exudate. Inject 5 mL sterile PBS into the peritoneal cavity and gently shake the mouse to resuspend the peritoneal exudate cells in the PBS. Collect the fluid while moving the tip of the needle gently to avoid clogging by fat or internal organs. Collect as much fluid as possible and deposit into sterile plastic centrifuge tubes kept on ice. Inject some air and collect the remaining fluid.
3. Centrifuge the cell suspensions at $450 \times g$ for 10 min. There should be three layers in the tubes after centrifugation from top to bottom: pristane, an aqueous layer, and the cell pellet. Carefully aspirate the pristane layer. Store the peritoneal fluid (aqueous layer) in small aliquots at −80 °C as soon as possible for cytokine ELISA (avoid repeated freeze-thaw cycles).
4. Collect the peritoneal cavity cell pellet. Aspirate off any remaining fluid from the cell pellet (*see* **Note 3**). Wash the cells in sterile PBS and spin down before counting. The resulting cells can be used for phenotype and gene expression analysis.
5. Resuspend the cell pellet in 5 mL PBS, count peritoneal cells with a hemocytometer (or other appropriate devices), and calculate the total peritoneal cell number.
6. For gene expression analysis, resuspend 10^6 peritoneal cells in 1 mL TRIzol reagent (Invitrogen, Carlsbad, CA) for isolating RNA. Synthesize cDNA using the Superscript II

First-Strand Synthesis kit (Invitrogen) according to the manufacturer's protocol.

7. For phenotype analysis, aliquot 10,000–50,000 cells (about 100–200 μL of resuspended cells) for each flow cytometry panel.

3.1.2 Analysis of the Peritoneal Exudate and Lipogranuloma Cells by Flow Cytometry

Before surface staining, peritoneal cells are incubated with anti-mouse CD16/32 (Fc Block, BD Bioscience, San Jose, CA) for 10 min. The cells are then stained with an optimized amount of primary antibody for 30 min at room temperature before washing and resuspending in PBS supplemented with 0.1 % v/v BSA. The following panels of antibodies are used to characterize the indicated cell populations (*see* **Notes 4, 5**).

1. *Myeloid cell panel:* Detect neutrophils and monocytes by staining with the following antibodies: anti-Ly6G-PE, anti-Ly6C-FITC (BD Bioscience), and anti-CD11b-Brilliant Violet (BioLegend, San Diego, CA). Ly6C^{hi} monocytes are present in large numbers only in mice treated with hydrocarbon oils that can stimulate IFN-I production, such as pristane, hexadecane, or squalene [12]. For hydrocarbon oils that cannot induce IFN-I production, such as mineral oil, Ly6C^{hi} monocytes are also recruited but quickly differentiate into Ly6C^{lo} monocytes, which do not produce IFN-I but are more strongly phagocytic [12, 13]. Thus the percentage and absolute number of Ly6C^{hi} monocytes and the ratio of Ly6C^{hi} monocytes to Ly6C^{lo} monocytes is an important indicator of IFN-I production. Ly6C^{hi} monocytes have a Ly6C^{hi} CD11b^{+} Ly6G^{-} phenotype, Ly6C^{lo} monocytes are defined as Ly6C^{lo} CD11b^{+} Ly6G^{-}, and neutrophils are defined as Ly6C^{mid} CD11b^{+} Ly6G^{+} (Fig. 1a). We usually evaluate Ly6C staining as a histogram gated on CD11b^{+} Ly6G^{-} cells (Fig. 1b).
2. *Lymphocyte panel:* Detect lymphocytes by staining with the following antibodies: anti-CD3-PE, anti-CD8-APC, anti-B220-APC-CY7, anti-CD69-PE-CY7 (all from BD Bioscience), and anti-CD4-Brilliant Violet (BioLegend).
3. *pDC panel:* Detect the pDC subset within the DC population by staining with the following antibodies: anti-Ly6C-FITC, anti-B220-APC-CY7, anti-CD11c-APC (BD Bioscience), and streptavidin-PE-CY7, anti-CD11b-Brilliant Violet, and anti-PDCA-1-biotin (BioLegend).
4. *Lipogranuloma cell panel:* Approximately 3 months after pristane injection, small "lipogranulomas" form on the mesothelial surfaces of the peritoneum and the diaphragm. These structures consist of ectopic lymphoid tissue and contain autoantibody-secreting cells [14]. To analyze these lipogranuloma cells by flow cytometry or in vitro culture, the lipogranulomas are excised from the peritoneum and digested with collagenase

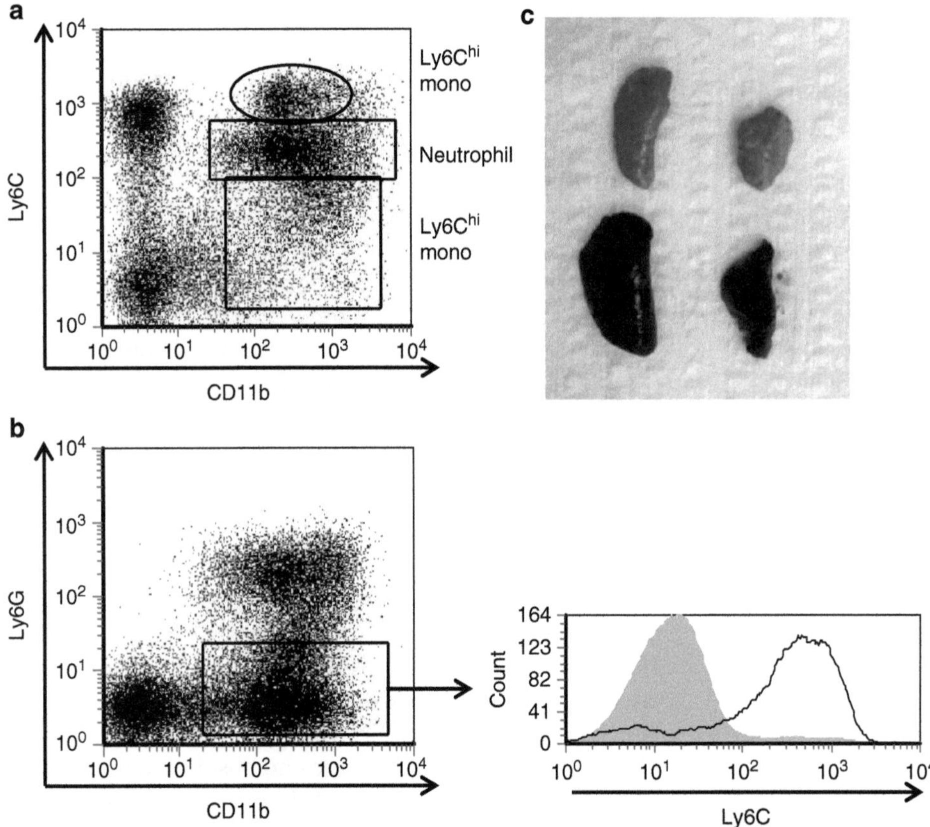

Fig. 1 (**a**) C57BL/6 (B6) mice were injected with 0.5 mL pristane, and 2 weeks later, peritoneal cells were collected and stained with CD11b, Ly6C. Three populations were identified (from *top* to *bottom*): Ly6C^{hi} monocytes, neutrophil, and Ly6C^{low} monocytes. (**b**) B6 mice were injected with 0.5 mL pristane or mineral oil and 2 weeks later, peritoneal cells were collected and stained with CD11b, Ly6G. The graph shows the expression of Ly6C gated on the CD11^{+} Ly6G^{lo} population (*shaded* histogram, mineral oil treated mice; *open line* histogram, pristane-treated mice). (**c**) Representative photograph of lung tissue from normal mice (*upper row*) and from B6 mice injected with pristane 2 weeks earlier, showing alveolar hemorrhage (*bottom row*)

(2 mg/mL) and dispase (1 mg/mL) with shaking (25 × *g*) at 37 °C for 30 min. The tissue is then gently teased apart and the cells are washed three times with PBS and 2 mmol/L ethylene diamine tetraacetic acid, before filtering through a 70 μm pore-size cell strainer (BD Falcon™ REF 352350) and resuspending in flow cytometry buffer or culture medium. Detect these cells by staining with the lymphocyte and pDC antibody panels listed above.

3.1.3 Analysis of Cytokine Production in the Peritoneal Lavage Fluid by ELISA

A variety of cytokines secreted into the peritoneum following pristane treatment [8] can be assessed by commercial ELISA using standard manufacturer protocols.

1. The highly expressed cytokine is IL-12 and is detected by ELISA (BD OptEIA™ mouse IL-12 p40 ELISA Set Cat. No. 555165).
2. The IFN-I-inducible chemokine CCL2 (MCP-1) is also produced at high levels in the peritoneum and can be measured by ELISA (BD OptEIA™ Mouse MCP-1 ELISA Set, Cat. No. 555260).
3. In pristane-induced lupus, levels of monocyte chemotactic protein-1 (MCP-1) correlate well with the percentage of Ly6C^{hi} monocytes, the major source of IFN-I [12].
4. Other cytokines such as IFNγ, IL-6, and TNFα are produced at lower levels and are measured in the peritoneal fluid by ELISA with BD OptEIA™ sets, by intracellular staining of the peritoneal cells, or by real-time RT-PCR using RNA isolated from the peritoneal exudate cells. High levels of IL-12/p40 and IL-6 are detectable by ELISA as early as 2 weeks after pristane treatment in BALB/c and B6 background mice.

3.1.4 Analysis of IFN-I Production in the Peritoneum

Although ELISA can be used to quantify IFN-I levels in peritoneal lavage fluid, there are 13 IFN-I subtypes [15], and in our hands, the ELISA has proved somewhat unreliable.

1. Quantitative (real-time) RT-PCR of the expression levels of IFN-I-inducible genes ("interferon signature"): Quantify the expression of three interferon-stimulated genes (IDGs)—*Mx1*, *Irf7*, and *Isg15*—using *β-actin* (or *18S* ribosomal RNA or *Gapdh*) as a "housekeeping gene" control.
2. Using cDNA synthesized from the peritoneal cell pellet, perform RT-PCR using the primers listed in Table 1 as previously described [12, 13]. Amplification conditions are the following: 95 °C for 10 min, followed by 45 cycles of 94 °C for 15 s, 60 °C for 25 s, and 72 °C for 25 s.
3. After the final extension (72 °C for 10 min), perform a melting-curve analysis to ensure specificity of the products.
4. Quantify the transcripts using the comparative ($2^{-\Delta\Delta Ct}$) method [16].

Table 1
RT-PCR primers used to calculate the interferon index

	Forward	Reverse
Mx1	5′-GATCCGACTTCACTTCCAGATGG	5′-CATCTCAGTGGTAGTCCAACCC
Irf7	5′-ACAGCACAGGGCGTTTTATC	5′-GAGCCCAGCATTTTCTCTTG
Isg15	5′-GAGCTAGAGCCTGCAGCAAT	5′-TAAGACCGTCCTGGAGCACT

5. A composite interferon index reflective of the total production of IFN-I is calculated as follows: For each IFN-inducible gene, an expression score is assigned representing the number of standard deviations above or below the mean expression of the control group. The composite "interferon index" is the average of the three individual expression scores (Mx1 + Irf7 + Isg15) ÷ 3.

3.1.5 Total Immunoglobulin Levels

Between 2 and 4 weeks after pristane injection, the mice develop polyclonal IgM hypergammaglobulinemia, which is followed by polyclonal IgG at 6–12 weeks and other systemic inflammatory reactions (*see* **Note 6**).

1. Determine the levels of total IgG1, IgG2a, IgG2b, IgG3, IgA, and IgM by ELISA using serum diluted 1:200,000 and/or 1:500,000 and mouse immunoglobulins as standards (mouse immunoglobulin panel, Southern Biotechnology, Birmingham, AL).
2. Coat microtiter plate wells with goat anti-mouse κ + λ light chain antibodies at a 3 μg/mL concentration incubating with diluted serum samples diluted 1:100,000 to 1:1,000,000 depending on expected serum antibody titer and wash with PBS three times.
3. To the wells add 100 μL alkaline phosphatase-conjugated goat anti-mouse antibodies specific for individual isotypes and incubate at room temperature for 2 h (Southern Biotechnology).
4. After three washes with PBS, incubate in the dark with 50 μL per well of alkaline phosphatase substrate (1 tablet of *para*-nitrophenylphosphate [PNPP] per plate diluted into 5 mL of 0.025 M bicarbonate buffer and 10 μL of 1 M $MgCl_2$) until the wells turn yellow.
5. Read the optical density at 405 nm in a visible light plate reader. Isotype standards are used for standard curve fitting and immunoglobulin concentrations are calculated using SoftMax software [17].

3.1.6 Evaluation of Late Disease Manifestations

The late manifestations of lupus 3–6 months after pristane injection include the development of IgG autoantibodies and glomerulonephritis. Autoantibodies appear in sequence: IgG anti-Su antibodies appear first (2–3 months after pristane injection), followed by anti-Sm, anti-RNP, and anti-ribosomal P (3–4 months), and then by anti-dsDNA antibodies (6 months). We have previously published detailed methods for analyzing sera for a variety of specificities by radioimmunoprecipitation assay [17] and will not review this approach further here. Certain autoantibodies can be quantified by ELISAs, including anti-DNA and anti-Sm/RNP (or U1A, a type of anti-RNP antibody). Although these are the major

Table 2
Strain difference in response to pristane injection

Pathology	C57BL/6 (B6) or C57BL/10 (B10)	BALB/c	SJL
Anti-dsDNA IgG	0 %	40 %	0 %
Anti-chromatin IgG	0 %	60 %	N/A
Anti-Sm/RNP IgG	10 %	20–40 %	10 %
Anti-Su IgG	25 %	50–70 %	10 %
Anti-ribosomal P IgG	20 %	0 %[a]	75 %
Glomerulonephritis	Mild (mesangial, class II) disease	Glomerular IgG and complement deposits, cellular proliferation, proteinuria (class IV)	Glomerular IgG and complement deposits, cellular proliferation, proteinuria (class IV)
Pulmonary hemorrhage	Severe	No	No

N/A not available
[a]BALB/cByJ 0 %; BALB/cJ 5–10 %

specificities produced by all strains tested to date, not all strains produce each antibody. Table 2 shows the specificities and their approximate prevalence in various strains of mice treated with pristane (*see* **Note 7**).

Anti-Double-Strand DNA Autoantibody ELISA

1. Dialyze calf thymus DNA (0.5 mg/mL Sigma #D4522) into 0.03 M sodium acetate 0.1 M NaCl 1 mM ZnCl pH 4.4.
2. Add S1 nuclease (Promega #M5761) to a concentration of 0.1 U/µg of DNA for 3 h at 37 °C. Dialyze the digested DNA against PBS + 0.05 % w/v NaN_3, centrifuged, and stored in aliquots at 4 °C.
3. Coat microtiter plates (Nunc Immobilizer amino F96 plates) with the following mixture: 60 µL of stock DNA (500 µg/mL) + 4.94 mL autoclaved water + 5 mL of Reacti-Bind DNA coating solution (Pierce, Cat # 17250). *It is important to mix the coating solution in a glass tube because in the presence of Reacti-Bind, the DNA will stick to anything plastic.*
4. To each well of the microtiter plate, add 100 µL of this mixture and then incubate the plate overnight at 4 °C protected from light.
5. Next wash the plate three times with TBS-Tween 20 (150 mM NaCl 20 mM Tris pH 7.5, 0.1 % v/v Tween 20).
6. Block the remaining "sticky" sites for 1–3 h (protected from light at room temperature) with 150 µL/well of 0.5 % BSA in

0.15 M NaCl, 2 mM K^+·EDTA, and 20 mM Tris pH 7.5 + 0.1 % NP40 (NET/NP-40) containing 0.05 % NaN_3.

7. Dilute the test serum samples 1:500 in 0.5 % BSA NET/NP40 0.05 % w/v NaN_3 and add 100 μL to individual wells.
8. Use a high-titer anti-DNA reference serum diluted 1:100, 1:500, 1:2,500, 1:12,500, 1:62,500, 1:312,500, and 1:1,562,500 in the same buffer to generate a standard curve.
9. Incubate the plates for 2 h at room temperature and wash before incubating for 2 h with alkaline phosphatase-conjugated goat anti-mouse IgG (appropriately diluted in 0.5 % BSA NET/NP40 0.05 % NaN_3).
10. After washing again, develop the plate using phosphatase substrate (5 mg tablets, Sigma Cat # S0942) in 5 mL diethanolamine buffer (for 1 L, 97 mL diethanolamine, 0.1 g $MgCl_2 \cdot 6H_2O$, 0.2 g NaN_3 in ~900 mL H_2O, pH 9.6 adjusted to 9.6 with HCl). Read the maximum absorbance at 405 nm in a 96-well plate reader.

Anti-Sm/RNP autoantibody ELISA:
The use of an antigen capture ELISA based on monospecific human autoimmune serum to quantify anti-Sm/RNP antibodies in mouse sera is recommended.

1. Coat MaxiSorp 96-well plates with human IgG purified from a high-titer monospecific anti-RNP serum, resuspended at 5 mg/mL in PBS, from previously frozen aliquots. To coat the wells, take the anti-RNP IgG diluted to 5 μg/mL in 20 mM Tris–HCl pH 8 and add to the wells overnight at 4 °C.
2. The next day, the wells are washed once with NET/NP40 (*see* above) and block for 1 h using 10 % calf serum in PBS 0.1 % sodium azide.
3. To prepare the antigen, add 2.5 mL of NET/NP40 directly to a frozen K562 (human erythroleukemia cell line, from ATCC) pellet of 10^8 cells (no thawing) along with 25 μL of phenylmethylsulfonyl fluoride (PMSF) in absolute ethanol (18 mg/mL) and aprotinin (Sigma A6279). Sonicate the cells for 50 s, then incubated on ice, and again sonicated for 50 s. The cell lysate is then centrifuged (10,000 × g for 30 min at 4 °C in a microcentrifuge) and the supernatant is frozen in aliquots.
4. Add the cell lysate for 1.5 h at room temperature to half of the wells of a microtiter plate (50 μL/well) and 50 μL of 0.5 % BSA NET/NP40 is added to the other half as a background control for each sample (antigen-free well).
5. Wash the plates three times with 0.5 M NaCl NET/NP40 and block with 10 % v/v bovine calf serum in PBS + 0.1 % sodium azide 150 μL/well for 5 min.

6. Add diluted serum samples for 1 h (2 h for low-titer samples) at room temperature, followed by washing and incubation for 1 h with 1:1,000 alkaline phosphatase labeled goat anti-mouse IgG (absorbed with human serum proteins) in 0.5 % BSA NET/NP40.
7. Plates are developed and read as above (*see* anti-DNA ELISA).

Anti-U1A autoantibodies and autoantibody-secreting cells:
The production of anti-U1A autoantibodies, a specific type of anti-RNP antibody, can be measured by ELISA using recombinant human U1A protein fused to a 6His sequence as antigen [14]. A plasmid containing Hu U1A-6His can be used to transform *E. coli* BL21 DE3.

1. Express the recombinant protein by growing the transformed bacteria in LB medium containing 10 μg/mL kanamycin and 2 mM IPTG.
2. Four hours later, the bacteria are lysed using 6 M guanidine HCl + 0.5 mM phenylmethylsulfonyl fluoride and 0.3 TIU/mL aprotinin.
3. Purify the recombinant protein by adherence to Ni-NTA resin columns (Sigma). Elute the His-tagged protein with 6 M urea according to the manufacturer's instructions.
4. Coat microtiter plate wells (Immobilizer Amino, Nunc) with 1 μg/mL purified recombinant U1A antigen in borate buffered saline (0.010 M borate buffer, 0.15 M NaCl, pH 8.2, tablets purchased from Sigma to be reconstituted in water) overnight at 4 °C.
5. Execute the remainder of the ELISA conducted as described above.

ELISPOT Assay for Anti-U1A Autoantibody-Forming Cells

1. Coat MultiScreen HTS plates (Millipore) overnight at 4 °C with either recombinant U1A protein or BSA (each at 5 μg/mL).
2. Wash the plate 3× with PBS. Then wash 3× with PBS 0.01 % Tween 20 (*never let ELISPOT plate dry!!!*).
3. Add 200 μL of blocking solution (RPMI 1640 with 10 % fetal calf serum or whatever media cells are cultured in).
4. Incubate at 37 °C for 2 h. Meanwhile, prepare the cell suspensions.
5. Prepare isolated lipogranuloma cells from pristane-treated BALB/cJ mice (*see* protocol above) suspension at different concentrations (i.e., 1×10^5/mL, 2×10^4/mL). Discard blocking solution and add 100 μL per well of each suspension in triplicate and incubate at 37 °C in 5 % CO_2 for at least 20 h.

6. Wash the plate 3× with PBS. Then wash 3× with PBS 0.01 % Tween 20.
7. Alkaline phosphatase-conjugated goat anti-mouse IgG or IgM Abs (1/1,000 dilution; Southern Biotechnology) are added to the wells. Incubate for 2 h at 37 °C in 5 % CO_2.
8. Wash the plate 3× with PBS 0.01 % Tween 20 and then 3× with PBS (must wash with PBS last because Tween 20 interferes with spot development).
9. Add 100 μL/well of BCIP/NBT (Pierce Chemical) and incubate in dark at room temperature for 5 min.
10. Stop spot development with distilled water and wash extensively. Blot the plate to remove excess liquid and dry the back of the wells. Let dry overnight in the dark, since spot intensity will decrease with light exposure. The number of anti-U1A-secreting lipogranuloma cells per 100,000 cells is determined by counting the spots using a dissecting microscope.

3.2 Assessment of Renal Disease

Proteinuria is evaluated on a drop of urine collected from live mice with Albustix strips (Miles Laboratories, Elkhart, IN), which provide semiquantitative measurements. Renal pathology is assessed in mice 6–8 months after pristane injection. Glomerular cellularity can be evaluated by counting the number of nuclei per glomerular cross section (20–30 glomerular cross sections per mouse) after hematoxylin and eosin (H&E) staining of paraffin-embedded kidney sections.

Glomerular Cellularity

1. Fix kidneys in 10 % formalin v/v and embed in paraffin wax.
2. Cut 3–5 μm sections lengthwise through the entire kidney and adhere the sections to Superfrost Plus microscope slides (Fisher Brand Catalog No: 12-550-15) (2–3 slides/mouse). Stain the sections with H&E.
3. Photograph 5–6 randomly selected regions of renal cortex containing well-stained glomeruli and print out the pictures. Photographs are coded and shuffled so that they can be read in a "blinded" manner.
4. Glomeruli that are cut through the center (i.e., maximum diameter) are selected for counting nuclei.
5. Using a pen to mark counted nuclei, the number of nuclei per glomerular section is determined in at least 10 mid-glomerular sections per kidney and the mean is determined.

Direct immunofluorescence of glomerular immune deposits:
For assessment of renal immune-complex deposition, 4 μm frozen sections are stained with FITC-conjugated goat anti-mouse IgG or IgM antibodies or with rabbit anti-mouse C3 antiserum and

examined by fluorescence microscopy (for a detailed protocol, see below).

Other factors to consider using a pristane inducible model of lupus (*see* **Notes 8–11**).

3.3 The B6.H-2^{bm12} cGVHD Model

Chronic GVHD models are based on the major histocompatibility complex (MHC) mismatch between the donor of transferred immune cells and the host. Two different types of GVHD inductions have been used as models of lupus, the acute GVDH parent-into-F1 (P→F1) model, which has been recently reviewed [18], and the chronic GVHD *B6.H-2^{bm12}* into B6 model, which will be reviewed here.

The B6(C)-*H2^{bm12}*/KhEgJ strain (JAX stock #001162, B6.bm12) is a strain with a B6 genetic background that carries a spontaneous 3 amino acid substitution in the class II Aβ molecule of the H-2^{b} allele. Immunological alterations have been described in this strain, such as decreased expression levels of class II H-2 molecules and decreased antigen-specific T cell responses. The bm12 mutation has also been shown to alter the development of autoimmune diseases depending of the genetic background, with a protective effect for experimental myasthenia gravis on a B6 background [19], but an accelerating effect for spontaneous lupus on an NZB background [20]. In addition, it was discovered in the early 1980s that adoptive transfers of B6.bm12 cells into congenic strains on a B6 background, or vice versa, resulted in an SLE-like syndrome, including the production of autoantibodies with specificities for nucleic acid/protein complexes (ANA, anti-dsDNA, anti-chromatin, and anti-Sm autoantibodies) that are characteristic of SLE and the development of immune-complex nephritis [21]. The model was further characterized by R. A. Eisenberg's group [22], who showed that the cGVHD reaction resulted from cognate interactions between alloreactive donor CD4^{+} T cells and host self-reactive B cells [23, 24]. The host B cells producing autoantibodies are conventional B cells [25]. Mature B cells preferentially participate in the cGVHD induction, with a predominant role of marginal zone B cells in the initiation of the response [26]. Host CD4^{+} T cells do not participate in the cGVHD induction, but their presence is absolutely required for "nurturing" B cells during early ontogeny in the form of IL-4 and/or CD40 stimulation [27–29]. The bm12-cGVHD model has now been used for over 30 years. It has many advantages, the most salient ones being:

- It is inducible in the B6 background. This grants access to a large number of strains and provides an easy and strong control to the experimental strains. It also allows for the implementation of classic immunological protocols such as bone-marrow (BM) chimeras and other types of adoptive cell transfers.

- It is easy to implement with a single i.p. injection of unfractionated splenocytes.
- Disease onset and development is quick, measured in weeks as compared to months for spontaneous SLE.
- Disease onset and development are predictable and reproducible with little interindividual variation as compared to spontaneous lupus.

3.3.1 cGVHD Induction

This model works equally well with B6.bm12 → B6 and B6 → B6.bm12, and the direction of the transfer should be selected according to the specific hypothesis tested, as illustrated in the examples in Subheading 3.3. Most published studies have been conducted with unfractionated splenocytes delivered as a RBC-depleted single-cell suspension via an i.p. injection in 200 μL of sterile PBS. The typical induction protocol is as follows:

1. Inject recipient mice i.p. with 200 μL of final donor splenocyte suspension using a 25-gauge 5/8″ needle with a 1 mL slip-tip syringe (*see* **Note 12**).

Allotypic markers can be used to distinguish donor from recipient cells, by breeding them on the experimental strain and B6 controls. Note that there is no genotyping protocol other than sequencing to detect the bm12 allele, and therefore breeding allotypic markers (or any other mutation) from a H-2^b to bm12 background would be cumbersome. To globally distinguish donor from recipient hematopoietic cells, the CD45^a allele (also known as CD45.1 or Ly5^a and encoded by the *Ptprc* gene) derived from the B6.SJL-*Ptprc*^{a} *Pep3*^{b}/BoyJ strain (JAX stock # 002014) can be used to distinguish from the B6/ B6.bm12-derived CD45^b allele. Although donor B cells have been shown not to contribute to the autoantibody production in this model, donor and recipient B cells or the antibodies they produce can be distinguished with the IgH^a allele provided by the B6.Cg-*Igh*^{a} *Thy1*^{a} *Gpi1*^{a}/J strain (JAX stock # 001317) and the IgH^b allele provided by the B6/ B6.bm12 strains. The same strain can also be used to provide the Thy1^a allotypic marker for T cells to be distinguished from the Thy1^b allele derived from the B6/ B6.bm12 strains.

3.3.2 Phenotypes Assessment

The bm12-cGVHD model induces three types of autoimmune-related phenotypes whose assessment will be described here separately.

Autoantibodies

A broad spectrum of lupus associated is produced in the bm12-cGVHD model. Typically, serum is collected starting with a collection just before cell transfer. Autoantibodies are detectable as early as 10–14 days after induction, peak around 3 weeks post-induction, and then slowly decline. The kinetics of total IgG is different, with an initial steep increase during the first 3 weeks followed by a slower increase up to 10 week post-induction [30]. Globally, these results showed that the ideal endpoint of a bm12-cGVHD experiment is 3 weeks post-induction if the main readout is autoantibody production.

Anti-dsDNA and Anti-chromatin IgG ELISA

1. Dissolve dsDNA (Sigma) in PBS to a 50 μg/mL concentration and add 50 μL to each well of an Immulon 2HB plate (Thermo Scientific).
2. Cover the plate with a plate sealer and incubate in Environ Shaker (Lab Line) for 90 min at 37 °C.
3. Discard solution from the plate and wash with PBS 3 times in a plate washer.
4. *For anti-chromatin IgG ELISA only:* Dissolve total histone (Roche) in 0.06 M bicarbonate buffer to a 10 μg/mL concentration and add 50 μL to each well. Incubate in the shaker for 90 min at 37 °C and then discard solution from the plate and wash with PBS 3 times as in Subheading 3.
5. Add 50 μL blocking buffer (3 % BSA, 3 mM EDTA, 0.1 % gelatin) to each well, incubate in the shaker for 90 min at 37 °C, and then discard the solution from the plate and wash with PBS 3 times.
6. Make 1:100 dilutions of the sera to be tested in serum diluent buffer (2 % BSA, 3 mM EDTA, 0.1 % gelatin, 0.05 % Tween 20). As a positive control and to generate a standard curve, we use pooled sera from ≥6 month old BcN/LmoJ mice (Jax Labs stock#007228). Sera from any other lupus-prone strain such as MRL/lpr or (NZB × NZW)F1 would work equally well. The standard curve is generated from four fivefold serial dilutions starting at 1:100. The volume of diluted sera should be at least 100 μL to allow duplicate well for each sample. Larger volumes can be prepared and stored at 4 °C for at least 1 week for additional assays.
7. Add 50 μL of serum dilutions and standard in duplicates to wells, leaving a blank well after your standards. Incubate in shaker for 90 min at 37 °C and then discard sera from plate and wash with PBS 3 times.
8. Make a 1:1,000 dilution of goat anti-mouse IgG AP (Millipore) in 2nd antibody diluent buffer (1 % BSA, 0.05 % Tween 20). Add 50 μL to each well, incubate in the shaker for 90 min at 37 °C, and then discard the solution from the plate and wash with PBS 3 times.
9. Prepare 5 mL of 0.025 M bicarbonate buffer, 10 μL of 1 M $MgCl_2$, and 1 *p*-nitrophenylphosphate PNPP tablet (Fisher) per plate and add 50 μL to all wells.

10. Allow the plate to develop (i.e., turn yellow) and read at wavelength of 405 nm with a plate reader. Continue reading plate periodically until any of the samples or standard reach an O.D. value ≥2.
11. Standard units for each serum sample are calculated from the average between the duplicates with a linear regression of the standard curve by setting the value of 100 U for the 1:100 dilution of the standard.

Antinuclear autoantibodies (ANA) detection by screening staining patterns on Hep-2 cells with a fluorescently labeled anti-mouse IgG monoclonal antibody [31] (*see* **Note 13**):

1. Line a 100×15 mm petri dish with a paper towel, then use ddH_2O to thoroughly soak the paper towel, and place a Hep-2 slide (Inova) into the petri dish. Each slide contains 12 wells, so the number of slides can be adjusted to the number of samples to be tested.
2. Dilute 1:40 of the test sera in PBS and then add 20 μL of each diluted sample onto the wells of the Hep-2 slide. Be careful not to touch the slide with the pipette tip but ensure that the well is entirely covered with serum sample.
3. Incubate the Hep-2 slide in the moist chamber for 30 min at room temperature and then aspirate the serum samples using a vacuum flask. Be careful not to scratch the bottom area with coated cells.
4. Use a squirt bottle to wash the slide 3–4 times with PBS one row at a time. Avoid cross contamination as much as possible and never aim the squirt bottle directly onto wells to avoid washing off the cells.
5. Remove remaining drops of PBS wash using a vacuum flask. The area between wells needs to be dry before adding the 2nd antibody.
6. Make a 1:50 dilution of anti-mouse IgG-FITC (Southern Biotech) in 0.1 % BSA in PBS and add 20 μL to each well.
7. Incubate the Hep-2 slide in the dark (the moist chamber can be covered with aluminum foil) for 30 min at room temperature.
8. Aspirate the 2nd antibody with a vacuum flask and wash 3–4 times with PBS. Remove remaining drops of PBS as before.
9. Take up Fluoromount-G (eBioscience) with an 18-gauge 1.2×25 mm needle in a 1 mL slip-tip syringe and then switch to a 25-gauge 5/8″ needle and disperse drops of about 1 mm in diameter onto the center of each well.
10. Carefully place a 24×60 mm cover slip onto the Hep-2 slide starting from one side, and make sure that the cover slip is perfectly aligned with the slide to keep it from moving and damaging the samples.

11. Invert the Hep-2 slide and press gently onto the paper towel to remove excess Fluoromount-G. Store the slides in the dark at 4 °C until analysis with a fluorescent microscope.

3.3.3 Immune Activation

In parallel to the production of autoantibody, the peak immune cell activation is achieved around 3 weeks post-induction. Splenocytes have been the most commonly used to assess immune activation, although the same results should be obtained from peripheral lymph nodes. Both donor and recipient $CD4^+$ T cells and recipient B cells undergo activation and expansion, which lead to a significant enlargement of the lymphoid organs, which can be easily measured as spleen weight or splenocytes numbers. Activation and differentiation markers can be assessed by flow cytometry on T cells (increased CD69 and CD44, decreased CD62L) and B cells (increased CD69, class II MHC, CD86, CD80, decreased CD22). The development of a germinal center response with class-switched ($GL7^+$ Fas^+ IgM^-) B cells and $CXCR5^+$ $PD\text{-}1^+$ $ICOS^+$ follicular helper T_{FH} cells has also been reported. The type of activation and differentiation markers can be tailored to the hypothesis being tested in a particular study. A typical flow cytometric analysis of immune activation protocol:

1. Prepare a single-cell suspension from spleen in RPMI 1640 medium buffered with 10 % HEPES.
2. Lyse splenocytes for 5 min in RBC lysis buffer (1 M Tris NH_4Cl) at room temperature.
3. Wash with RPMI 1640/10 % HEPES twice and count the cells.
4. Distribute $1–5 \times 10^6$ cells per stain in Eppendorf tubes and incubate with 0.5 μL purified anti-mouse CD16/32 (Fc Block, eBioscience) in FACS buffer (PBS, 5 % FBS, 10 % NaN_3) supplemented with 10 % rabbit serum for 30 min on ice.
5. Stain cells with 1 μL of primary antibody per sample on ice for 30 min in the dark before washing and resuspending in FACS buffer with 0.5 μL PercP-Cy 5.5 streptavidin (BD Bioscience) per sample. Primary antibodies from a same panel should be combined and added as a "cocktail" to the samples. The following panels have been developed to conduct analysis with a 4-color FACSCalibur cytometer. They can be adapted to combine more primary antibodies in a same panel to be used on other multi-laser cytometers. All antibodies are obtained from either BD Bioscience or eBioscience.

   GC B cell panel: anti-GL7 FITC, anti-CD23 PE, anti-CD21, anti-IgM APC.

   B cell activation panel 1: anti-CD22.2 FITC, anti-I-A/I-E PE, anti-CD86 Biotin, anti-B220 APC.

B cell activation panel 2: anti-CD69 PE, anti-CD80 Biotin, anti-CD25 APC, anti-B220 FITC.

CD4⁺ T cell activation panel: anti-CD44 FITC, anti-CD62L PE, anti-CD25 Biotin, anti-CD4 APC.

CD4⁺ T cell T_{FH} panel: anti-CD69 FITC, anti-CXCR5 PE, anti-PD1 Biotin, anti-CD4 APC.

6. Incubate on ice for 30 min in the dark, spin down, and resuspend in 100–200 μL FACS buffer. If the cells are not going to be analyzed on the same day with a flow cytometer, 1 % formalin should be added to the final FACS buffer to fix the cells, which can be then kept up to 1 week in the dark at 4 °C.

3.3.4 Clinical Disease

The bm12-cGVHD model leads to the development of immune-complex (IC) glomerulonephritis. IC deposits in the glomeruli can be detected on kidney frozen sections by immunofluorescence with anti-IgG or IgG2a and anti-C3 antibodies starting at 4–5 weeks post-induction [31] and as late as 4–6 months post-induction [24] with the following protocol (*see* **Note 14**):

Preparation of the Kidney Sections

1. Place the fresh kidney lengthwise into a disposable base mold (Fisher) and fill in the mold with Tissue-Tek (Sakura) until the kidney is covered. Submerge the base mold containing the kidney in a container filled with pentane (Fisher) previously cooled in a −80 °C freezer and store kidney at −80 °C until ready to be sectioned.
2. One hour before cutting sections, move the frozen kidney from −80 °C to −20 °C. Use a cryostat (Microm) set at −18 °C to cut two 8 μm thick sections onto a Superfrost microscope slide (Fisher). Label the slide with a pencil and use forceps or a scalpel to remove the remaining Tissue-Tek attached to the kidney sections. Submerge slide into previously cooled acetone (Fisher) and leave at 4 °C for 10 min to fix the tissue sections. Allow the slide to dry at room temperature.

Staining with Anti-C3 and Anti-IgG2a

1. Use a thin Sharpie marker to outline the sections on the back of the slide and then trace this outline on the section side with an Aqua-Hold Pap Pen (Fisher).
2. Add one drop of PBS to each section and place the slide onto a tray on ice.
3. Make IF blocking buffer (9 mL PBS, 1 mL normal rat serum [Equitech-Bio, Inc]) filtered through a 0.22 μm filter attached to a 10 mL Luer-Lock tip syringe.
4. Fling the PBS off the slide and add 50–70 μL IF blocking buffer to each section, making sure the entire section is covered, and then incubate on ice for 10 min.

5. Dilute anti-mouse C3 FITC (Cedarlane) and goat anti-mouse IgG2a FITC (Southern Biotech) at 1:100 dilution in IF blocking buffer.
6. Fling the IF blocking buffer off the slide and then add 50–70 μL of anti-C3 FITC to one section and 50–70 μL of anti-IgG2a FITC to the other section on the same slide. Leave slide in the dark for 30 min at 4 °C.
7. Fling antibody dilutions off the slide and then wash the slide with 0.1 % Tween 20 in PBS followed by PBS then ddH_2O. Use squirt bottles for washes and never aim the stream directly onto a section to avoid damage to that section.
8. Allow the slide to sit at room temperature in the dark for 10–15 min until the kidney sections are completely dry.
9. Add ~2 μL of Prolong Gold (Invitrogen) to the center of each kidney section; avoid forming bubbles.
10. Carefully place a 24 × 50 mm cover slip onto the slide; start from one side and make sure that the cover slip is perfectly aligned with the slide to keep it from moving and damaging the samples.
11. Invert the slide and press gently onto paper towel to remove excess Prolong Gold. Store slides in the dark at 4 °C until the sections can be examined with a fluorescent microscope.

3.3.5 Applications

The bm12 cGVHD-induced model of SLE is a B6-based model. Due to the large number of genetically modified strains that have been created on this genetic background, the bm12-cGVHD protocol presents an easy and rapid model to either investigate specific cellular mechanisms of autoimmunity or determine whether a specific genetic modification contribute to SLE. Consistent with direct interactions between donor $CD4^+$ T cells and host B cells being responsible for the induction of the autoimmune response in the bm12-cGVHD model, it has been mostly used to characterize either B or T cell-intrinsic phenotypes. However, this should not be a limitation, as the bm12-cGVHD model can be used to characterize extrinsic factors affecting the ability of lymphocytes to become autoreactive (*see* **Notes 15–18** for details of applications of the lupus model).

4 Notes

1. As commercial pristane is purified from shark liver oil, the cost has increased substantially as numbers of sharks have declined.
2. As in humans, female mice are more susceptible to the development of lupus. Although male mice also develop disease, we generally use only females. If both males and females are used,

it will be important to have a similar percentage of male and female mice in the experimental and control groups. Induction of lupus is less efficient in mice older than 6 months, due in part to the increased amount of fat present in the peritoneum and a somewhat decreased inflammatory response. The increased fat makes it more difficult to perform peritoneal lavage (*see* below) with complete recovery of the fluid. Loss of the lavage fluid decreases accuracy of the total peritoneal cell count.

3. The cell pellet should not contain many RBCs unless the liver has been punctured during the lavage. However, RBCs included in the pellet can be lysed with RBC lysis buffer (150 mM NH_4Cl, 10 mM $KHCO_3$, 0.1 mM EDTA) for 5 min at room temperature.
4. Initially use the concentrations of antibodies in accordance with the manufacturer's recommendations. Use more dilute or concentrated solutions of antibodies if appropriate.
5. Neutrophils, pDCs, and lymphocytes are recruited into the peritoneum following the injection of either lupus-inducing (pristane, hexadecane, squalene) or non-lupus-inducing (mineral oil) oils.
6. *Systemic inflammatory response:* Intraperitoneal injection of pristane also causes a systemic inflammatory response, which is evident in the peripheral blood. Increased numbers of circulating Ly6C^{hi} monocytes can be detected in peripheral blood by flow cytometry as described above for peritoneal cells [12]. Sca-1 (Ly6A/E) is an IFN-I-inducible gene that is a valuable marker because it can be assessed readily in small samples of peripheral blood. In B6 background mice (not in BALB/c), surface staining with anti-Sca-1-PE (BD Pharmingen™) on B cells in peripheral blood is correlated with IFN-I expression. Sca-1 expression on B cells can be determined on serial bleeds to assess the time-course of IFN-I production [13].
7. Sera are collected before pristane injection and monthly thereafter by tail-bleeding (or any other approved blood collection method). Antinuclear antibodies (ANA) can be detected by immunofluorescence using prefixed commercial slides from Inova Diagnostics (San Diego, CA), Bio-Rad (Hercules, CA), or other vendors (*see* detailed protocol in Subheading 3.2.2.1).
8. *Strain considerations:* The pristane model is a fast and convenient shortcut studying the role of a specific gene in the pathogenesis of lupus since it saves the time and trouble of making a congenic mouse in a spontaneous lupus model such as MRL/lpr. Pristane can induce lupus in essentially all non-autoimmune, immunocompetent backgrounds, including (but not limited to)

BALB/c, C57BL/6 (B6), C57BL/10 (B10), SJL, C3H, DBA/1, DBA/2, 129Sv, and others. However, different genetic backgrounds, such as BALB/C and B6, have somewhat different (quantitatively or qualitatively) disease manifestations, some of which are summarized below and in Table 2.

- Expression of Sca-1 on B6 B cells correlates strongly with the level of IFN-I production; however, Sca-1 expression does not change in BALB/c mice, which express lower levels of this antigen.
- B6 and B10 mice develop sometimes fatal pulmonary alveolar hemorrhage, which is mild or absent in BALB/c background mice. The number of mice per group will need to be increased using B6 background mice due to this problem.
- A higher percentage of BALB/c mice produce autoantibodies than B6 mice [2]. 20–40 % of BALB/c mice produce anti-Sm and 60–90 % of them produce anti-RNP antibodies, whereas only 10 and 25 % of C57BL/6 mice produce autoantibodies with these respective specificities. B6 mice do not produce anti-dsDNA or anti-chromatin IgG, which are produced by 40 and 60 % of BALB/c mice, respectively. However, C57BL/6 mice produce anti-ribosomal P antibodies, which are not produced by BALB/c. Both B6 and BALB/c mice produce anti-Su autoantibodies. The BALB/c background is ideal for examining autoantibody responses due to the higher frequency of anti-Sm/RNP and anti-DNA antibodies. If studying a particular autoantibody (such as anti-Sm/RNP), the number of B6 mice per group will need to be larger than necessary for BALB/c. However, the number of B6 mice needed can be minimized by using the production of "any autoantibody" (e.g., anti-Sm/RNP, anti-Su, or anti-ribosomal P) as a readout.
- B6 mice develop milder nephritis (mesangial, class II) than BALB/c or SJL mice (proliferative, class III or IV). The latter strains develop glomerular IgG and complement deposits, cellular proliferation, and proteinuria [32–34]. However, B6 mice still exhibit immune-complex deposition in the glomeruli, which can be detected by direct immunofluorescence.

9. *Sex differences:* We have not found any significant short-term difference between female and male mice in the production of Ly6C^{hi} monocytes, IFN-I signature, or IL-6 or IL-12p40 production. However, in the long term, female mice have more severe disease and increased levels of autoantibodies in comparison with males. Therefore, as in human SLE in which the female/male ratio is ~9:1, pristane-induced lupus is primarily a disease of females [35].

10. *Comparison with SLE patients and spontaneous models of SLE:* Pristane-treated mice develop clinical manifestations of lupus, including arthritis, immune-complex-mediated glomerulonephritis, and pulmonary capillaritis (a model for diffuse alveolar hemorrhage in SLE) as well as autoantibodies. Inflammation of the pericardium and pleura also occurs, but it is unclear whether this is autoimmune in origin. SLE is a human syndrome diagnosed using a set of 11 criteria [36]. Pristane-treated BALB/c mice meet 4 or 5 of these criteria, while B6 meet 3 or 4 of them (uncertain if serositis is autoimmune mediated). The classic (NZB × NZW)F1 spontaneous model of lupus meets 3 or 4 criteria including immune-complex nephritis, antinuclear antibody, anti-dsDNA, and in NZB mice autoimmune hemolytic anemia. However, the IFN-I signature is much weaker in (NZB × NZW)F1 mice than in pristane-induced lupus.

11. *Pristane-induced alveolar hemorrhage:* The most significant problem we have confronted with pristane-induced lupus is mortality due to pulmonary alveolar hemorrhage. This is largely specific to B6 (and B10) background mice, which represent most of the available knockout strains [11]. Since the mechanism of alveolar hemorrhage is unknown, it is difficult to completely avoid the problem. Other than planning for a loss of about 30 % of B6 mice and planning accordingly, we have used the following "tricks" to decrease mortality. The Jackson Laboratory B6 substrain seems to have a reduced susceptibility to alveolar hemorrhage and should probably be used whenever possible. However, the control substrain should be matched with that of the test strain (such as a knockout strain), making it impossible in some cases to use the JAX-derived B6 substrain. In that case, we use the following approach to minimize death from alveolar hemorrhage:
    - Pre-inject 0.1 mL of pristane and then 2 weeks later inject with 0.5 mL of pristane.
    - Filter the pristane with a 0.22 μm sterilized filter (Millipore Ireland Ltd) before injection. This method cannot totally eliminate mortality, so it is prudent to include more mice than statistically necessary to compensate for premature death.

12. *Mice used for cGVHD induction:* Donors and recipients as young as 6 weeks of age have been used [37, 38]. Older mice (6–7-month-olds have been reported in several studies) may be used if the tested phenotype is known to increase with age or to yield a larger number of donor cells. Transfers of purified $CD4^+$ T cells (either sorted by flow cytometry or enriched by negative selection with antibody-coated magnetic beads) can be used instead of whole splenocytes to specifically address the intrinsic ability of $CD4^+$ T cells with a specific mutation to induce an autoimmune response. These purified $CD4^+$ T cells

can be either injected i.p. ($1-5\times10^6$ cells) or intravenously in the caudal vein ($1-5\times10^5$ cells) if the number of cells is limiting. Although any source of T cells should be amenable to the protocol, the spleen has been used in all published studies as a convenient source of donor cells.

13. Anti-dsDNA and chromatin IgM, IgM, and IgG antibodies to ssDNA and IgM rheumatoid factor, as well as increase in total IgG, have also been detected by ELISA in some studies [30]. Anti-erythrocytes antibodies have been detected with a direct Coombs' assay [24].

14. Renal pathology by standard light microscopy and immunohistochemistry for known inflammatory mediators of lupus nephritis (infiltrating macrophages, IL-6, MCP-1, Rantes, IP-10) has been assessed as early as 11 weeks post-induction [39]. Proteinuria has been measured in a few studies, and it has been detected as early as 2 weeks post-induction with a slow increase up to 6 weeks [39] or 12 weeks post-induction [30]. It should be noted however that the proteinuria was modest (maximum in the 100–200 mg/dl range), and if this readout is selected, consideration should be given to use a true quantitative measurement of microalbuminuria by ELISA (Kamiya Biomedical Cat. # KT-343) or total protein from urine collected in metabolic cages [40]. Mortality has been reported in a few studies: A 25 % mortality starting at 6 weeks and plateauing for up to 12 weeks post-induction, which was the endpoint of the study, has been reported in bm12 → B6 mice [30]. A 50 % mortality between 9 and 16 weeks post-induction has been reported in BM chimeras in which either B6.bm12 or B6 splenocytes were transferred [24]. It should be noted however that this global endpoint assessment is less robust and has been far less used than the other autoimmune phenotypes (autoantibodies, immune activation, IC deposits) assessed at earlier time points.

15. *B cells:* To study the mechanisms by which B cell tolerance is broken, the cGVHD model has been used in mice transgenic for autoreactive B cell receptors (BCR) in which B cells are tolerized by the chronic expression of the HEL autoantigen [41–43] or by the non-autoimmune B6 genetic background for the 3H9 anti-DNA antibodies [30, 44, 45]. Alloreactive bm12 $CD4^+$ T cell stimulation breaks tolerance in these models, which allowed the characterization of signaling mechanisms of the autoreactive B cells [41, 42] as well as the role of receptor editing in maintaining tolerance [43]. T cell help was shown to activate 3H9 anti-DNA reactive B cells, suggesting that preventing T cell activation of anti-DNA-specific B cells was a tolerogenic mechanism [44]. The antigen-driven nature of the anti-DNA antibody repertoire and the role of receptor

editing in 3H9 and 3H9/56R heavy chain transgenic B cells was also characterized in details after cGVHD induction [45, 46]. Finally, the role of TLR9 in the activation of the autoreactive B cells was also investigated by inducing bm12-cGVHD in B6.TLR9$^{-/-}$ mice with or without the 3H9 transgene [30]. The bm12-cGVHD model can also be used to test how specific genes, such as *Mer* encoding for a receptor tyrosine kinase mediating phagocytosis of apoptotic cells, affect autoreactivity in B cells. B6.Mer$^{-/-}$ mice were resistant to bm12-cGVHD induction due to an intrinsic ability of Mer$^{-/-}$ B cells to produce autoantibodies [37]. This model uncovered a previously unknown function of *Mer* in regulating marginal zone B cell function through their CD1d expression [37, 47].

16. *T cells:* The bm12-cGVHD model was used to characterize a novel H1-splice isoform of Ly108 as protective for the induction of activated CD4^{+} T cells that provide help for autoreactive B cells [38]. Ly108 is the major candidate gene for the NZW-derived *Sle1b* lupus susceptibility locus. *Sle1b* CD4^{+} T cells, which are low H1 expressors, induce a significantly greater cGVDH response that B6 congenic controls when transferred into B6.bm12 recipients. The bm12-cGVHD model was also used to dissect the role of IL-21 in the activation of autoreactive B cells [48]. Donor T cells produce IL-21 and differentiate into follicular helper T cells, which depend on IL-21R expression (T_{FH}). Transfer of bm12 CD4^{+} T cells into B6.IL.21R$^{-/-}$ mice failed to activate B cells as compared to B6 recipient controls. The cGVHD model therefore contributed to show along with the P→F1 model that IL-21 promotes autoimmunity through both CD4^{+} T and B cell-intrinsic mechanisms, suggesting that IL-21 blockade may be beneficial as a treatment for SLE by targeting B cell hyperactivity and T_{FH} cells. These experiments also illustrates that transfers into B6.bm12 recipients may be best when evaluating T cell phenotypes.
17. *Nonlymphoid factors:* The bm12-cGVHD has the potential to evaluate other factors from either the innate immune system or nonimmune cells that regulate the pathogenesis of systemic autoimmunity. This has been shown for myeloid cells suppressing the ability of bm12 CD4^{+} T cells to induce B6.*Sle2c2* B cells to produce autoantibodies [49]. B6.*Sle2c2* mice are resistant to bm12-cGVHD induction, and a combination of mixed BM chimeras using B6.Rag2$^{-/-}$ (B and T cell deficient), B6.*μMT* (B cell deficient), or B6.*Tcra* (T cell deficient) mice as BM donor along with B6.*Sle2c2* or B6 showed that the cell type responsible for the suppression was nonlymphoid BM derived. The bm12-cGVHD model has also been used to evaluate how autoantibodies become pathogenic in the kidney. Fn14, the receptor for TNF-like weak inducer of apoptosis

(TWEAK), is expressed on mesangial cells and podocytes, and its level of expression is high in renal biopsies from SLE patients. bm12-cGVHD induced in B6.Fn14$^{-/-}$ mice lead to similar autoantibody production but reduced renal pathology as compared to B6, and anti-TWEAK antibody treatment was successful in reducing renal pathology [39]. The combination of the bm12-cGVHD model with BM chimeras showed that the development of nephritis required the functional expression of Fn14 on resident kidney cells and not on macrophages [50]. These studies showed that the TWEAK/Fn14 pathway is a valid therapeutic target for SLE and paved the way for other target identification/treatment studies to be conducted with the bm12-cGVHD model.

18. *Loci with unknown a priory target cells:* We have used the bm12-cGVHD model to assess the pathogenic potential of lupus susceptibility loci that we have identified in the NZM2410 spontaneous model of lupus [51]. These loci are small genomic regions of the NZM2410 genome bred onto a B6 background in a series of congenic strains that have been used to identify susceptibility genes [52]. We have characterized a spectrum of immune phenotypes associated with each of these loci, but none of them is pathogenic by itself, as it requires the combination of the three major loci, *Sle1*, *Sle2*, and *Sle3*, to achieve the full manifestation of the parental clinical disease [53]. Some of the sub-loci, such as the *Sle1*a and *Sle1c* sub-loci, result only in a modest upregulation of immune activation without a strong production of autoantibodies [54]. It was therefore important to establish that the sub-loci contribute by themselves to the autoimmune process. The *Sle1c* locus enhanced the bm12-cGVHD response [55], and this was mapped to the centromeric *Sle1c2* locus, which corresponds to enhanced CD4^{+} T cell effector functions associated with a lower expression of the *Esrrg* gene [56], but not the *Sle1c1* locus, which corresponds to altered B cell function associated with a loss of function allele of the *Cr2* gene [57]. The *Sle1a* locus also enhanced the bm12-cGVHD response, which was mapped to the *Sle1a2* region, which contains many candidate genes and target cell types [31]. The *Sle1a1* locus did not enhance the bm12-cGVHD response [31]. *Sle1a1*, which corresponds to the expression of a dominant-negative isoform of the *Pbx1* gene, intrinsically enhances CD4^{+} T cell effector functions and decreases Treg expansion [58]. It should be noted that only the bm12 → B6.*Sle1a1* experiment has been performed so far. Our results should therefore be interpreted as *Sle1a1/Pbx1* having no direct effect on enhancing the development of autoreactive B cells, but we cannot yet rule out that *Sle1a1/Pbx1*-expressing CD4^{+} T cells could provide a stronger

help to autoreactive B cells, which will be determined with *Sle1a1*→B6.bm12 transfers. The *Sle2* locus, which is associated with B cell hyperactivity, the expansion of the B1a cell subset, and the increased production of polyreactive/autoreactive IgM antibodies lead to a decreased response in the bm12-cGVHD model [49]. This surprising result was due to the presence of a suppressor locus, *Sle2c2*, that we have characterized using the bm12-cGVHD model (see above). Within the *Sle2* locus, the *Sle2c1* locus, which is the main locus responsible for the expansion of the B1a cell subset and the production of polyreactive IgM [59], has no effect on the bm12-cGVHD response (Morel et al. unpublished). One might speculate that it is due to the fact that B1a cells generate largely independent T cell responses, and therefore a T cell-dependent model of systemic autoimmunity would not be affected by the expression of *Sle2c1*. This series of experiments with the *Sle* congenic mice confirms that the bm12-cGVHD is not a general model of B and T cell hyperactivation and that it can be used to probe fine-level mechanisms of autoimmune pathogenesis.

References

1. Sang A, Yin Y, Zheng Y-Y, Morel L (2012) Animal models of molecular pathology: systemic lupus erythematosus. In: Conn PM (ed) Progress in molecular biology and translational science, vol 105. Academic Press, New York, pp 321–370
2. Reeves WH, Lee PY, Weinstein JS, Satoh M, Lu L (2009) Induction of autoimmunity by pristane and other naturally occurring hydrocarbons. Trends Immunol 30:455–464
3. Satoh M, Reeves WH (1994) Induction of lupus-associated autoantibodies in BALB/c mice by intraperitoneal injection of pristane. J Exp Med 180:2341–2346
4. Satoh M, Treadwell EL, Reeves WH (1995) Pristane induces high titers of anti-Su and anti-nRNP/Sm autoantibodies in BALB/c mice. Quantitation by antigen capture ELISAs based on monospecific human autoimmune sera. J Immunol Meth 182:51–62
5. Nacionales DC, Kelly-Scumpia KM, Lee PY, Weinstein JS, Lyons R, Sobel E et al (2007) Deficiency of the type I interferon receptor protects mice from experimental lupus. Arthritis Rheum 56:3770–3783
6. Hooks J, Moutsopoulos H, Geis S, Stahl N, Decker J, Notkins A (1979) Immune interferon in the circulation of patients with autoimmune disease. N Engl J Med 301:5–8
7. Satoh M, Kuroda Y, Yoshida H, Behney KM, Mizutani A, Akaogi J et al (2003) Induction of lupus autoantibodies by adjuvants. J Autoimmun 21:1–9
8. Kuroda Y, Nacionales DC, Akaogi J, Reeves WH, Satoh M (2004) Autoimmunity induced by adjuvant hydrocarbon oil components of vaccine. Biomed Pharmacother 58:325–337
9. Lee PY, Kumagai Y, Li Y, Takeuchi O, Yoshida H, Weinstein J et al (2008) TLR7-dependent and FcgammaR-independent production of type I interferon in experimental mouse lupus. J Exp Med 205:2995–3006
10. Xu Y, Lee PY, Li Y, Liu C, Zhuang H, Han S et al (2012) Pleiotropic IFN-dependent and -independent effects of IRF5 on the pathogenesis of experimental lupus. J Immunol 188:4113–4121
11. Barker TT, Lee PY, Kelly-Scumpia KM, Weinstein JS, Nacionales DC, Kumagai Y et al (2011) Pathogenic role of B cells in the development of diffuse alveolar hemorrhage induced by pristane. Lab Invest 91:1540–1550
12. Lee PY, Weinstein JS, Nacionales DC, Scumpia PO, Li Y, Butfiloski E et al (2008) A novel type I IFN-producing cell subset in murine lupus. J Immunol 180:5101–5108
13. Lee PY, Li Y, Kumagai Y, Xu Y, Weinstein JS, Kellner ES et al (2009) Type I interferon modulates monocyte recruitment and maturation in chronic inflammation. Am J Pathol 175: 2023–2033
14. Nacionales DC, Kelly KM, Lee PY, Zhuang H, Li Y, Weinstein JS et al (2006) Type I

interferon production by tertiary lymphoid tissue developing in response to 2,6,10,14-tetramethyl-pentadecane (pristane). Am J Pathol 168:1227–1240

15. Lee PY, Li Y, Richards HB, Chan FS, Zhuang H, Narain S et al (2007) Type I interferon as a novel risk factor for endothelial progenitor cell depletion and endothelial dysfunction in systemic lupus erythematosus. Arthritis Rheum 56:3759–3769
16. Livak KJ, Schmittgen TD (2001) Analysis of relative gene expression data using real-time quantitative PCR and the 2-ΔΔCT method. Methods 25:402–408
17. Hamilton KJ, Satoh M, Swartz J, Richards HB, Reeves WH (1998) Influence of microbial stimulation on hypergammaglobulinemia and autoantibody production in pristane-induced lupus. Clin Immunol Immunopathol 86:271–279
18. Soloviova K, Puliaiev M, Foster A, Via C (2012).The parent-into-F1 murine model in the study of lupus-like autoimmunity and CD8 cytotoxic T lymphocyte function. In: Perl A (ed) Methods in molecular biology. Methods in molecular biology, vol 900. Humana Press, Totowa, NJ, pp 253–270.
19. Christadoss P, Lindstrom JM, Melvold RW, Talal N (1985) Mutation at I-A beta chain prevents experimental autoimmune myasthenia gravis. Immunogenetics 21:33–38
20. Naiki M, Yoshida SH, Watanabe Y, Izui S, Ansari AA, Gershwin ME (1993) The contribution of I-Abm12 to phenotypic and functional alterations among T-cell subsets in NZB mice. J Autoimmun 6:131–143
21. Rolink AG, Pals ST, Gleichmann E (1983) Allosuppressor and allohelper T cells in acute and chronic graft-vs.-host disease. II. F1 recipients carrying mutations at H-2K and/or I-A. J Exp Med 157:755–771
22. Morris SC, Cohen PL, Eisenberg RA (1990) Experimental induction of systemic lupus erythematosus by recognition of foreign Ia. Clin Immunol Immunopathol 57:263–273
23. Morris SC, Cheek RL, Cohen PL, Eisenberg RA (1990) Allotype-specific immunoregulation of autoantibody production by host B cells in chronic graft-versus host disease. J Immunol 144:916–922
24. Morris SC, Cheek RL, Cohen PL, Eisenberg RA (1990) Autoantibodies in chronic graft versus host result from cognate T-B interactions. J Exp Med 171:503–517
25. Reap EA, Sobel ES, Jennette JC, Cohen PL, Eisenberg RA (1993) Conventional B cells, not B1 cells, are the source of autoantibodies in chronic graft-versus-host disease. J Immunol 151:7316–7323
26. Choudhury A, Cohen PL, Eisenberg RA (2007) Mature B cells preferentially lose tolerance in the chronic graft-versus-host disease model of systemic lupus erythematosus. J Immunol 179:5564–5570
27. Chen F, Maldonado MA, Madaio M, Eisenberg RA (1998) The role of host (endogenous) T cells in chronic graft-versus-host autoimmune disease. J Immunol 161:5880–5885
28. Choudhury A, Maldonado MA, Cohen PL, Eisenberg RA (2005) The role of host CD4 T cells in the pathogenesis of the chronic graft-versus-host model of systemic lupus erythematosus. J Immunol 174:7600–7609
29. Choudhury A, Cohen PL, Eisenberg RA (2010) B cells require "nurturing" by CD4 T cells during development in order to respond in chronic graft-versus-host model of systemic lupus erythematosus. Clin Immunol 136: 105–115
30. Ma Z, Chen F, Madaio MP, Cohen PL, Eisenberg RA (2006) Modulation of autoimmunity by TLR9 in the chronic graft-vs-host model of systemic lupus erythematosus. J Immunol 177:7444–7450
31. Cuda CM, Zeumer L, Sobel ES, Croker BP, Morel L (2010) Murine lupus susceptibility locus Sle1a requires the expression of two subloci to induce inflammatory T cells. Genes Immun 11:542–553
32. Satoh M, Kumar A, Kanwar YS, Reeves WH (1995) Anti-nuclear antibody production and immune-complex glomerulonephritis in BALB/c mice treated with pristane. Proc Natl Acad Sci U S A 92:10934–10938
33. Satoh M, Hamilton KJ, Ajmani AK, Dong X, Wang J, Kanwar YS et al (1996) Autoantibodies to ribosomal P antigens with immune complex glomerulonephritis in SJL mice treated with pristane. J Immunol 157:3200–3206
34. Chowdhary VR, Grande JP, Luthra HS, David CS (2007) Characterization of haemorrhagic pulmonary capillaritis: another manifestation of pristane-induced lupus. Rheumatology (Oxford) 46:1405–1410
35. Smith DL, Dong X, Du S, Oh M, Singh RR, Voskuhl RR (2007) A female preponderance for chemically induced lupus in SJL/J mice. Clin Immunol 122:101–107
36. Li Y, Lee PY, Kellner ES, Paulus M, Switanek J, Xu Y et al (2010) Monocyte surface expression of Fcgamma receptor RI (CD64), a biomarker reflecting type-I interferon levels in systemic lupus erythematosus. Arthritis Res Ther 12:R90
37. Shao W-H, Eisenberg RA, Cohen PL (2008) The Mer receptor tyrosine kinase is required for the loss of B cell tolerance in the chronic

graft-versus-host disease model of systemic lupus erythematosus. J Immunol 180: 7728–7735

38. Keszei M, Detre C, Rietdijk ST, Munoz P, Romero X, Berger SB et al (2011) A novel isoform of the Ly108 gene ameliorates murine lupus. J Exp Med 208:811–822
39. Zhao Z, Burkly LC, Campbell S, Schwartz N, Molano A, Choudhury A et al (2007) TWEAK/Fn14 interactions are instrumental in the pathogenesis of nephritis in the chronic graft-versus-host model of systemic lupus erythematosus. J Immunol 179:7949–7958
40. Xie C, Sharma R, Wang H, Zhou XJ, Mohan C (2004) Strain distribution pattern of susceptibility to immune-mediated nephritis. J Immunol 172:5047–5055
41. Feuerstein N, Chen F, Madaio M, Maldonado M, Eisenberg RA (1999) Induction of autoimmunity in a transgenic model of B cell receptor peripheral tolerance: changes in coreceptors and B cell receptor-induced tyrosine-phosphoproteins. J Immunol 163:5287–5297
42. Feuerstein N, Shivers D, Chen F, Eisenberg RA, Finkel TH (2003) Chronic GVH prevents anergy in bone marrow self-reactive B cells: a selective increase in post-endoplasmic reticulum processing and trafficking to the cell surface of autoreactive IgM receptors. Int Immunol 15:975–985
43. Feuerstein N, DeSimone DC, Eisenberg RA, Finkel TH (2004) Chronic graft-versus-host reaction is associated with a decrease in Ig light chain receptor editing in bone marrow self-reactive B cells. Eur J Immunol 34:1361–1370
44. Sekiguchi DR, Jainandunsing SM, Fields ML, Maldonado MA, Madaio MP, Erikson J et al (2002) Chronic graft-versus-host in Ig knockin transgenic mice abrogates B cell tolerance in anti-double-stranded DNA B cells. J Immunol 168:4142–4153
45. Sekiguchi DR, Eisenberg RA, Weigert M (2003) Secondary heavy chain rearrangement: a mechanism for generating anti-double-stranded DNA B cells. J Exp Med 197:27–39
46. Witsch EJ, Cao H, Fukuyama H, Weigert M (2006) Light chain editing generates polyreactive antibodies in chronic graft-versus-host reaction. J Exp Med 203:1761–1772
47. Shao W-H, Zhen Y, Finkelman FD, Eisenberg RA, Cohen PL (2012) Intrinsic unresponsiveness of Mertk-/- B cells to chronic graft-versus-host disease is associated with unmodulated CD1d expression. J Autoimmun 39:412–419
48. Nguyen V, Luzina I, Rus H, Tegla C, Chen C, Rus V (2012) IL-21 promotes lupus-like disease in chronic graft-versus-host disease through both CD4 T cell- and B cell-intrinsic mechanisms. J Immunol 189:1081–1093
49. Xu Z, Vallurupalli A, Fuhrman C, Ostrov D, Morel L (2011) An NZB-derived locus suppresses chronic graft versus host disease and autoantibody production through non-lymphoid bone-marrow derived cells. J Immunol 186:4130–4139
50. Molano A, Lakhani P, Aran A, Burkly LC, Michaelson JS, Putterman C (2009) TWEAK stimulation of kidney resident cells in the pathogenesis of graft versus host induced lupus nephritis. Immunol Lett 125:119–128
51. Morel L, Rudofsky UH, Longmate JA, Schiffenbauer J, Wakeland EK (1994) Polygenic control of susceptibility to murine systemic lupus erythematosus. Immunity 1:219–229
52. Morel L (2012) Mapping lupus susceptibility genes in the NZM2410 mouse model. Adv Immunol 115:113–139
53. Morel L, Croker BP, Blenman KR, Mohan C, Huang G, Gilkeson G et al (2000) Genetic reconstitution of systemic lupus erythematosus immunopathology with polycongenic murine strains. Proc Natl Acad Sci U S A 97: 6670–6675
54. Morel L, Blenman KR, Croker BP, Wakeland EK (2001) The major murine systemic lupus erythematosus susceptibility locus, Sle1, is a cluster of functionally related genes. Proc Natl Acad Sci U S A 98:1787–1792
55. Chen Y, Perry D, Boackle SA, Sobel ES, Molina H, Croker BP et al (2005) Several genes contribute to the production of autoreactive B and T cells in the murine lupus susceptibility locus Sle1c. J Immunol 175:1080–1089
56. Perry DJ, Yin Y, Telarico T, Baker HV, Dozmorov I, Perl A et al (2012) Murine lupus susceptibility locus Sle1c2 mediates CD4+ T cell activation and maps to estrogen-related receptor gamma. J Immunol 189:793–803
57. Boackle SA, Holers VM, Chen XJ, Szakonyi G, Karp DR, Wakeland EK et al (2001) Cr2, a candidate gene in the murine Sle1c lupus susceptibility locus, encodes a dysfunctional protein. Immunity 15:775–785
58. Cuda CM, Li S, Liang S, Yin Y, Potula HH, Xu Z et al (2012) Pre-B cell leukemia homeobox 1 is associated with lupus susceptibility in mice and humans. J Immunol 188:604–614
59. Xu Z, Potula HH, Vallurupalli A, Perry D, Baker H, Croker BP et al (2011) Cyclin-dependent kinase inhibitor Cdkn2c regulates B cell homeostasis and function in the NZM2410-derived murine lupus susceptibility locus Sle2c1. J Immunol 186:6673–6682

Chapter 10

Measuring Interferon Alpha and Other Cytokines in SLE

Mikhail Olferiev, Mari Lliguicota, Kyriakos A. Kirou, and Mary K. Crow

Abstract

The progression of disease in patients with systemic lupus erythematosus (SLE) is affected by production, accumulation, and actions of cytokines. Type I interferon (IFN), specifically IFN-α, is recognized as a central mediator of disease pathogenesis in SLE. We describe a functional assay to measure type I IFN activity in SLE plasma and have also measured the response of peripheral blood cells to that cytokine family. This method can be scaled to assess IFN functional activity, as well as activity and cellular response to other cytokines, in relation to cellular and serologic parameters relevant to SLE.

Key words SLE, Interferon alpha, Cytokines, Neutrophil granule signature, WISH, Gene expression, Response, qPCR, Gene expression

1 Introduction

Lupus Pathogenesis and Cytokines: Systemic lupus erythematosus (SLE) is considered a prototype systemic autoimmune disease that affects multiple organs and tissues. The pathogenesis of SLE is incompletely understood and considered to be dependent on genetic, epigenetic, and environmental factors, along with stochastic events, that result in autoimmunity and inflammation. More than half of SLE patients show increased circulating type I interferon (IFN-I) [1] and IFN-stimulated gene transcripts (ISG) in peripheral blood mononuclear cells (PBMC) [2, 3]. The activation of the IFN-I pathway in tissue from SLE patients is associated with related clinical manifestations of disease [4, 5]. The discovery of Toll-like receptors (TLRs) reactive with endogenous nucleic acids and the demonstration of endosomal TLR activation by nucleic acid-containing immune complexes [6], along with data from genome-wide association studies identifying lupus-associated genetic variants that encode components of the innate immune signaling pathways [7, 8], have revealed important mechanisms of IFN-I production and highlighted the pivotal role of IFN-I in the pathogenesis of SLE. Additional cytokines proposed to be relevant

Paul Eggleton and Frank J. Ward (eds.), *Systemic Lupus Erythematosus: Methods and Protocols*, Methods in Molecular Biology, vol. 1134, DOI 10.1007/978-1-4939-0326-9_10,

Table 1
Cytokines proposed to be involved in SLE pathogenesis

Cytokine	Proposed function in SLE
IFN-α [2]	Antiviral and proinflammatory, induces MHC expression, promotes DC and plasma cell maturation, inhibits Treg and Th17 maturation, is associated with disease activity
IP-10/CXCL10 [29]	ISG, attracts and activates human leukocytes
MIP1β/CCL4 [30]	ISG, chemoattractant for various immune cells
TNF-α [31]	Inflammatory and anti-proliferative effect. Might control IFN-α induction and modulate interferon response in SLE patients. Inhibition of sTNF-α with monoclonal antibodies could cause drug-induced SLE in some patients treated with those agents
IL-6 [12]	Promotes B cell differentiation and expansion of autoreactive B cells, blocks regulatory T helper cell differentiation
IL-10 [32]	Reduces apoptosis of B and T cells, inhibits antigen presenting cell function, supports B cell differentiation
BAFF [33]	Promotes B cell survival and differentiation to antibody producing cells
IL-21 [34]	Promotes T and B cell differentiation
IL-17; IL-23 [27]	Promotes T and B cell differentiation
IL-18 [28]	Promotes Th1 immune responses, possibly increases TNF-α production

in the pathogenesis of SLE are summarized in Table 1 and were reviewed elsewhere [9–12].

Overview of Cytokine Assays: In general, cytokines involved in SLE can be investigated by three approaches: (1) quantification of cytokine secretion, (2) quantification of cytokine accumulation, and (3) quantification of cytokine function in vivo or in vitro. The first two evaluate the concentration of free or bound cytokines in a biological sample, while the last establishes biological activity of cytokines based on their effect on cells in their microenvironment. Below we briefly overview the most popular and currently used methods and provide our protocols to evaluate the biological activity of IFN-I in SLE PBMC and plasma. We have used quantitative polymerase chain reaction (qPCR) to measure expression of IFN-inducible genes in both cases.

The qPCR assay measures the concentration of DNA or RNA molecules. For cytokine studies, qPCR measures either a specific cytokine transcript or mRNA transcripts regulated by the studied cytokine. The qPCR can also be adapted for studies of cytokine processing and mechanisms of epigenetic regulation. The specificity and sensitivity of the assay are the main advantages of the method. An important challenge is the choice of the reference ("housekeeping") gene transcript. There is no universal reference gene; thus, it is always necessary to validate several candidate genes in separate sets of experiments. The qPCR experiments should follow the Minimum Information for Publication of Quantitative Real-Time PCR (MIQE) guidelines [13]. The required standardization for a small number of samples (<20) and a large group of studied genes (>10) might be associated with an unacceptable cost. In some cases, a DNA microarray experiment could be more appropriate. The selection of informative primer pairs for the selected gene is facilitated by computer software but must be subjected to experimental validation. It is reasonable to use primers from commercial vendors when dealing with a small number of tests (usually less than 100). Nevertheless, primers sold by companies should be validated for given conditions. Validated primers for human cytokines can be found in previous publications [14, 15].

The DNA microarray assay detects multiple RNA transcripts within one experiment. The use of microarray is reasonable when (a) studying cytokine mRNA profiles in a limited number of samples, (b) studying cellular activation by cytokines (in vivo and in vitro), and (c) performing preliminary experiments with the goal to determine reference and response genes for future qPCR experiments. It should be noted that microarray experiments require a large amount of RNA per sample when compared to qPCR. For those samples with a limited amount of mRNA, kits for linear mRNA amplification are available from several companies such as the Applause™ system from NuGEN. Several platforms and approaches have been created by different companies for RNA profiling. Current microarrays cover messenger and noncoding parts of genes and allow for the measurement of alternative splicing variants. Depending on the scientific goal, one might use an inexpensive microarray and obtain results for a large number of samples or perform detailed profiling of transcripts using a more advanced array. Whichever decision is made, it is highly recommended to follow the Minimum Information About a Microarray Experiment (MIAME) guidelines [16]. Since microarray experiments require intensive probe preparation and specially designed scanners for reading microarray chips, it is common to provide RNA samples to specialized facilities which, in our opinion, is an additional benefit in comparison to qPCR. Facilities will always test the RNA integrity before performing microarray experiments and follow an established protocol. Submit all samples for one experiment at once since processing, labeling, and hybridization of RNA/DNA may slightly differ depending on the particular reagent lot.

The use of computer software is essential for microarray experiment data analysis. The "all-in-one" analysis products, such as Partek Genomic Suite™ (Parteck) or GeneSpring GX™ (Agilent), are expensive and may not be affordable for small laboratories. The major advantages of such products are a user-friendly interface and company support. Laboratories with a small budget might choose a freeware software like Expression Console™ in combination with Transcriptome Analysis™ (Affymetrix). For researchers familiar with the R statistical environment (R Development Core Team) and who desire to assure detailed control of their microarray experiment, we encourage use of a Bioconductor [17].

Grouping of genes based on the similarities of the expression profiles can identify functionally related genes. The functional analysis of gene clusters can be studied using databases. The Database for Annotation, Visualization, and Integrated Discovery, DAVID (Laboratory of Immunopathogenesis and Bioinformatics, SAIC-Frederick, Inc.), provides statistics and functional details about submitted genes [18]. The other highly recommended approach is the Ingenuity Systems (Qiagen). The enrichment of ISG can be studied using an interferome database [19].

Western blot (*WB*) is a well-established method for detecting cellular or serum proteins. The major advantage of this technique is its ability to identify proteins of defined molecular weight with high specificity and sensitivity. Separation of denatured proteins during electrophoresis demonstrates the specificity of staining as well as protein modifications such as phosphorylation and ubiquitination.

Immunoprecipitation using specific antibodies allows detection of components of precipitated protein complexes. The precipitated fractions can be studied using WB to detect the presence of interacting proteins and their molecular weight.

Enzyme-linked immunosorbent assay (ELISA) uses pairs of antibodies for adsorption and detection of target molecules. The major advantage of ELISA for cytokine detection is its high sensitivity (up to 0.1 pg/mL) and accurate quantification in a wide range of concentrations. The combination of biotin-labeled secondary antibody and streptavidin-horseradish peroxidase (HRP) provides high signal amplification and is compatible with several substrates.

The most widely used substrate for colorimetric ELISA is 3,3′,5,5′ tetramethylbenzidine (TMB) due to its fast detection and high sensitivity. When the range of detection is important, 2,2′-azino-di [3-ethyl-benzthiazoline] sulfonate (ABTS) is preferable. Cytokines present at low concentration can be measured using a luminescence detection system.

The disadvantage of ELISA is the inability to test multiple cytokines at once. The company Quansys Biosciences developed kits and a detection system for simultaneous detection of up to 16 human cytokines in one well. Compared to traditional ELISA, the multiplex ELISA significantly reduces the volume of samples.

Immunohistochemistry (IHC) is used to visualize tissue under the microscope. For example, biopsies from the kidney of an SLE patient can be stained using specific antibodies to visualize specific cytokines or their receptors. High specificity of staining depends on antibody quality and the method of tissue preparation. The sensitivity depends on the secondary antibody and the visualization method. The advantage of colorimetric detection with the use of horseradish peroxidase (HRP) conjugated to secondary antibodies and their substrate (usually 3′3-diaminobenzidine) is high sensitivity and long-term stability of obtained results. Importantly, the method permits visualization of tissue morphology when counterstained with a desired dye. The benefit of immunofluorescent staining is the ability to use several antibodies simultaneously, which allows for differentiation of cell types and organelles.

Fluorescent-activated cell sorting (*FACS*) is a procedure where a fluorochrome-labeled cell passes through a thin capillary and becomes illuminated by a laser beam. The excited fluorochromes emit light within a defined range of wavelength that is recorded by a detector. Subpopulations of peripheral blood cells represent the primary study targets for FACS. FACS allows for the simultaneous use of multiple types of fluorochromes which is necessary for studies of cytokine production or signaling within cell populations. The detected population of cells might be physically separated using FACS and studied using other methods like microarray or qPCR.

Protein Microarrays and Multiplex Bead Array Assays (*MBA*): Advances in microelectronics and microfluidics have allowed spectral analysis on a micrometer scale, raising the possibility of analyzing multiple probes at once. The principle behind the protein microarray technique is most similar to the ELISA approach, but the arrays can read thousands of parameters from a single chip. With regard to cytokine detection, protein microarrays with specific antibodies for detection are often used, although alternative approaches exist.

There are two types of protein microarrays: forward phase and reverse phase. The former allows for analysis of multiple parameters and requires the immobilization of capture agents. The second is useful when multiple samples are studied within the same chip and requires immobilization of protein extracts from multiple samples.

Bead-based microarrays represent an alternative to planar microarray. The principle behind this method is similar to that used in flow cytometry. However, instead of cells, it uses designed beads that can be distinguished either by a color code, size, or shape. By using a set of beads recognizing specific proteins, it is possible to determine the concentration of multiple cytokines in one sample.

Several platforms (Luminex, CBA BD™ Bioscience, ProcartaPlex eBiosciences etc.) allow users to analyze up to 100 parameters simultaneously. The sensitivity of bead-based immunoassays is apparently similar or even superior to traditional ELISA, since accuracy, precision, and dynamic range are often improved.

Reporter Gene Assays: Reporter gene assays study the effect of biological samples in a model system. Reporter systems, such as a stable transfected cell line, use promoters that respond to cytokine treatment by activating reporter genes. Reporter genes are usually translated to a functional protein such as firefly luciferase or green fluorescent protein. SLE studies often used reporter assays to detect the presence of IFN-I. Those assays are based on the use of HeLa or WISH cell lines transfected with a reporter vector [20, 21]. It should be noted that the WISH assay developed by us and described below is distinct from a reporter assay.

2 Materials

2.1 Preparation of Samples

- Pasteur and regular pipettes.
- Conical plastic tubes (1.5, 15 and 50 mL) with lids.
- QIA shredder columns (Qiagen).
- 16×100 mm×10.0 mL BD Vacutainer® Plus plastic plasma tube (BD Vacutainer).
- Ficoll-Paque PLUS™ (GE Healthcare Life Sciences).
- Phosphate-Buffered Saline pH 7.0 (Gibco, Life Technologies).
- MACS Bovine Serum Albumin (10 %) Stock Solution (Miltenyi Biotec).
- Red Blood Cell Lysis Buffer (eBioscience, Affymetrix).
- Hemocytometer or automatic cell counter (Life Technologies).
- Buffer RLT (Qiagen).
- 2-Mercaptoethanol 25 mL (Sigma).

2.2 Gene Expression by qPCR

2.2.1 RNA Purification

- Ethyl alcohol (ACS/USP) 200 proof (Pharmco-AAPER)
- RNeasy kit (Qiagen) including:

  RNAeasy mini columns.

  Collection tubes.

  Buffer RLT.

  RNase-free water (pH adjusted for sample elution).
- Nanodrop ND 1000 (Thermo Scientific) or any UV-light spectrophotometer.
- Any −80 °C freezer (for sample storage).

2.2.2 Complementary DNA (cDNA) Synthesis

- Good-quality 12-channel pipette 0–10 μL range.
- QuantiTech® Reverse Transcription kit (Qiagen) including:

  gDNA wipeout buffer.

  RT buffer.

  Primer mix.

  Reverse transcriptase.

Table 2
Primers used for WISH assay

Name	Sequence
HPRT1 forward	5′-TGCTCGAGATGTGATGAAGG-3′
HPRT1 reverse	5′-TCCCCTGTTGACTGGTCATT-3′
IFIT1 forward	5′-CTCCTTGGGTTCGTCTACAAATTG-3′
IFIT1 reverse	5′-AGTCAGCAGCCAGTCTCAG-3′
MX1 forward	5′-TACCAGGACTACGAGATT-3′
MX1 reverse	5′-TGCCAGGAAGGTCTATTAG-3′

Table 3
Primers used for gene expression analysis of PBMC

Name	Target sequence
HPRT1 QT00059066	NM_000194
IFIT1 QT01852466	NM_001001887, NM_001548
IFIT3 QT00100030	NM_001549

2.2.3 qPCR

- Real-time qPCR system (e.g., AB 7900 HT Fast Real-Time PCR).
- UltraPure (DNase/RNase-free distilled) water (Life Technologies).
- iTaq TM SYBR® Green Supermix with Rox (BioRad).
- 384- or 96-well qPCR compatible plates (Applied Biosystems).
- Primers (Tables 2 and 3) and *see* **Notes 1** and **2**.
- Optical Clear Adhesive Film for qPCR (Applied Biosystems).

2.3 WISH Assay

- WISH ATCC® CCL-25TM (American Type Culture Collection, Manassas, VA).
- Dulbecco's Modified Eagle Media supplemented with L-glutamine (Life Technologies).
- Fetal Bovine Serum 16,000–500 mL (Life Technologies).
- Cryovials.
- Falcon 175 cm^2 Tissue Culture Flasks.
- Trypsin-EDTA (1×): 0.25 % Trypsin, 1 mM ethylenediaminetetraacetic acid, 5.33 mM KCl, 0.44 mM KH_2PO_4, 4.17 mM $NaHCO_3$, 137.93 mM NaCl, 0.338 mM Na_2HPO_4, 5.56 mM D-glucose 100 mL (Life Technologies).
- Dimethyl sulfoxide (DMSO), BioReagent (Sigma).

- Recombinant Human Interferon-α A Pure, With Carrier (Gibco, LifeTechnologies).
- TurboCapture 384 mRNA Kit (Qiagen) includes the following items:
- TurboCapture 384 mRNA Plate.
- AlumaSealTM II Sealing Film.
- Buffer TCL (with inhibitor of RNAse).
- Buffer TCW.
- Buffer TCE.
- TaqMan Reverse Transcription Reagents (Life Technologies) includes the following items:
- MultiScribe™ Reverse Transcriptase (50 U/μL).
- RNase inhibitor (20 U/μL).
- dNTP mixture (2.5 mM each dNTP).
- Oligo d(T)16 (50 μM).
- Random hexamers (50 μM).
- 10× RT buffer.
- $MgCl_2$ solution.
- iTaq TM SYBR® Green Supermix with Rox (BioRad).
- TE buffer (10 mM Tris–HCl, 1 mM EDTA, pH 8.0).
- Custom primers (Table 2).
- 2-Mercaptoethanol 25 mL (Sigma).

3 Methods

3.1 Preparation of Samples

3.1.1 Preparation of Human Plasma from Freshly Obtained Human Blood

After obtaining IRB approval and proper informed consent, proceed to collect blood from research human subjects by venipuncture in a 10 mL BD Vacutainer sodium heparin tube. Properly fill the tube and gently invert several times to prevent the formation of fibrin clots and cytokine release due to platelet activation. Process blood within 1 h. Do not keep blood on ice.

1. Invert tube several times. Centrifuge blood for 10 min at 400 ×*g*.
2. Collect the top clear layer of blood-derived plasma in small 1.5 mL tubes. Do not pick up the thin white layer of leukocytes resting on the top of the erythrocytes.
3. Store plasma at −80 °C. Interferons are considered to be stable molecules, but other cytokines might degrade with time. Avoid freeze/thaw cycles; interferon activity in plasma may be affected.

3.1.2 PBMC Isolation and Lysis

1. Dilute plasma-depleted blood with one volume of phosphate-buffered saline (PBS, pH 7.4), mix well, and then layer carefully on 20 mL of Ficoll-Paque PLUS in a 50 mL tube (*see* **Note 3**).
2. Centrifuge blood at 400×*g* for 30 min at room temperature (RT) to separate PBMCs. Ensure that the tube is properly balanced and do not use the centrifuge brake as shaking will disturb the Ficoll layer.
3. Aspirate the top clear layer out using a vacuum, leaving a white ring of PBMC on top of the intact gradient. Collect the PBMC fraction into a separate 50 mL tube using a Pasteur pipette. Discard the rest.
4. Fill tube containing PBMCs up to 50 mL with PBS supplemented with 0.2 % BSA (PBS+0.2 % BSA). Mix tube gently. Centrifuge for 10 min at 100×*g*. All PBMCs will form a firm pellet at the bottom of the tube, and the supernatant can simply be poured out from the tube.
5. Gently disintegrate the PBMC pellet using a pipette tip in 2 mL of red blood cell (RBC) lysis buffer. Transfer cells into a new 15 mL tube and incubate for 5 min at RT. Do not exceed lysis time.
6. Fill tube up to 14 mL with PBS+0.2 % BSA. Mix gently and centrifuge at 100×*g* for 10 min.
7. Remove supernatant. Dissolve the pellet in 1 mL of PBS+0.2 % BSA. Calculate the concentration and viability of PBMCs.
8. Prepare the necessary amount of RLT buffer by adding 0.01 volume of 2-mercaptoethanol and assuming 1 mL of RLT buffer is required per 10 millions of cells.
9. Centrifuge cells at 100×*g* for 10 min. Discard supernatant and disrupt pellet in the residual volume of buffer using a vortex.
10. Carefully suspend PBMCs in RLT buffer using a pipette tip. Vortex cell suspension vigorously for 30 s and then place 0.35 mL (3.5 million cells) in the QIA shredder column.
11. Centrifuge QIA shredder columns at maximum speed in a tabletop centrifuge for about 90 s. Cap collection tubes with provided lids.
12. Store lysates in −80 °C freezer until future use.

3.2 Gene Expression by qPCR

3.2.1 RNA Purification

Several systems for cDNA purification exist. We use RNeasy Mini Kit from Qiagen because it produces high-quality mRNA and does not require use of a phenol/chloroform mix, which is hazardous for humans.

1. Thaw RNA samples. We found that it is easy to work with a group of 12–16 samples simultaneously.

2. Carefully homogenize RNA samples with 0.35 mL of 70 % ethanol.
3. Transfer sample to the top of an RNeasy Mini Column placed into a 2 mL collection tube. Centrifuge 15 s at 8,000 × *g*.
4. Wash column using 0.7 mL of RW1 buffer. Centrifuge 15 s 8,000 × *g*.
5. Wash column twice using 0.7 mL of RPE buffer. Centrifuge 15 s 8,000 × *g*.
6. Place RNeasy Mini Column into new tube and centrifuge 1 min at 8,000 × *g*.
7. Place RNeasy column into new collection tube (RNase free). Apply 40 μL of RNase-free water (provided with kit), incubate about 1 min on table, then centrifuge 1 min at 8,000 × *g*.
8. The RNA concentration is determined by measuring the optical density at 260 nm in a spectrophotometer or Nanodrop machine. The RNA concentration after purification should be more than 5 μg/mL, and the 260/280 ratio should be between 1.9 and 2.1.
9. RNA can be stored at −80 °C for a year without significant degradation.

3.2.2 cDNA Synthesis

We use the QuantiTech® Reverse Transcription kit. The kit includes an enzyme that removes any trace amount of genomic DNA from the RNA sample.

1. Thaw RNA samples and reagent provided with kit.
2. Combine 14 μL of RNA sample and 2 μL of gDNA Wipeout Buffer in 0.2 mL PCR tube or PCR plate. Note that the amount of RNA per reaction should not exceed 1 μg and all reactions should contain an equal amount of RNA.
3. Incubate exactly 2 min at 42 °C, then place on ice.
4. Combine 4 μL of RT buffer, Primer Mix 1 μL, and reverse transcriptase 1 μL with the contents of the tube.
5. Incubate 15 min at 42 °C, then place at 95 °C for 3 min to inactivate the reaction.

3.2.3 qPCR

It is important to assay each sample in triplicate (*see* **Note 4**). We recommend using plasmids containing the target gene in order to quantify the amount of target RNA correctly using the relative standard curve method (*see* **Note 5**). The standard curve should start at a concentration higher than any of the experimental samples and proceed below the concentration of the lowest sample. Always include no-template controls to avoid false-positive results.

1. Prepare master mix by combining 5 μL of iTaq TM SYBR® Green Supermix with Rox (BioRad) and 0.5 μL of titrated primer mixture.

2. Mix 4.5 μL of diluted cDNA (should be optimized) and 5.5 μL of master mix in a 384-well PCR plate. Note that the volume of master mix should cover 10 % more wells than the actual number of reactions.
3. Seal the plate with an optical-grade self-adhesive film. Spin the plate for 30 s at 400 × *g*.
4. Run the samples in your qPCR machine using the following protocol: 10 min at 95 °C, 40 cycles at 95 °C for 15 s, and 60 °C for 1 min. The last stage measures the dissociation curve in the temperature interval from 60 to 95 °C (*see* **Note 6**). The cycle parameters depend on the thermocycler and should be optimized.

3.2.4 Analysis of qPCR Results

1. The software provided with your qPCR machine is capable of quantifying the amount of cDNA in samples based on the comparative curve method.
2. Check the amplification curves from all wells for each primer set and exclude wells where no amplification curve is observed.
3. Display melting curve for each primer. Remove all samples where melting curve looks abnormal.
4. The program automatically sets the best possible threshold line (Ct values) that will horizontally intersect all amplification curves at their exponential phase.
5. Check the quality of standard curves. Normally, the angle for the standard curve should be −3.2 to −3.4 in logarithmic scale, which corresponds to 100 % efficiency. Correlation coefficient should be no less than 0.98.
6. The software should be able to automatically calculate relative quantities.

3.3 WISH Assay

The "WISH assay" measures interferon in human serum or plasma samples based on the transcriptional response of the WISH epithelial cell line [22]. In previous decades, WISH cells (*see* **Note 7**) were quite popular as an informative cell line for assay of interferon activity based on inhibition of the cytopathic effect of virus infection [23]. The current WISH assay utilizes qPCR to quantify an IFN-I response. The presence on WISH cells of IFN-I receptors and the relative absence of Toll-like receptors that might mediate induction of IFN-I in response to stimulatory TLR ligands in serum or plasma make this cell line particularly informative for measuring the functional effects of all IFN-I proteins in the test fluid, including IFN-α, IFN-β, and any other IFN-I species. The contribution of a particular subtype of interferon present in serum or plasma to the expression of ISG in WISH cells can be confirmed using neutralizing antibodies specific for those IFNs.

The interferon response of several candidate genes was screened, and the most reliable genes were chosen for inclusion in our routine assay. The WISH assay can be easily scaled to screen a large number of samples. Furthermore, the simplicity of qPCR allows for the use of the WISH assay in research and clinical studies.

3.3.1 WISH Cell Culture

WISH cells (ATCC CCL-25TM) grow in Dulbecco's Modified Eagle Media supplemented with L-glutamine and 5 % fetal bovine serum (working media). Prepare many stocks of WISH cells from the same passage in order to minimize variation between assays and store them in liquid nitrogen.

1. Establishing the WISH cell culture: Melt the arriving vial of WISH cells in a 37 °C water bath and then transfer the contents of the vial into a 50 mL conical tube. Slowly add working media up to 50 mL. Centrifuge cells at 100×*g* to remove cryopreserving agent. Resuspend the pellet in 10 mL of working media. Place 5 mL of obtained cells into 175 cm^2 tissue culture flasks filled with 10 mL of working media. Grow cells up to ~80 % confluence.
2. Passaging the WISH cells: Wash flask with 8 mL of sterile PBS quickly. Fill flask with 5 mL of warm trypsin-EDTA solution. Cells detach after 1–2 min of slow shaking. Add 12 mL of working media to stop reaction and transfer into a 50 mL conical tube. Centrifuge cells 100×*g* for 10 min. Place up to two million cells into new culture flasks filled with working media.
3. Freezing working stock of WISH cells: When the desired number of cells is obtained, make frozen stocks of WISH cells. Freeze two million cells/vial in 1 mL fetal calf serum supplemented with 10 % DMSO.
4. Prepare WISH cell assay plate: Grow WISH cells from stock in a 175 cm^2 tissue culture flask as described above for 5 days. Change media once on day 3. Seed WISH cells at a density of 0.5×10^5 per well in 200 μL of media in 96-well plates. Keep overnight in CO_2 incubator (5 % CO_2 37 °C).

3.3.2 Plasma Samples and Calibrators for WISH Assay

1. Thaw plasma slowly in RT and use promptly. Long exposure to RT may cause interferon degradation.
2. Centrifuge plasma at 10,000×*g* at 4 °C for 10 min. Discard lipid layer using pipette tip. The spontaneously formed fibrin clots, if any, will precipitate at the bottom of the tube. Collect the rest of the plasma into a new tube using small pipette tip.
3. Serial dilution of recombinant human interferon alpha (rhIFN-α) is required for assay calibration. We dilute a vial containing rhIFN-α powder with sterile working media to obtain a 10,000 IU/mL stock. Store 10 μL aliquots at −80 °C.

The top concentration of 100 IU/mL is made by addition of 10 μL of rhIFN-α solution to 1 mL of pooled healthy donor plasma. The top concentration is diluted with plasma to create concentrations of 50, 25, 12.5, and 6.25 IU/mL of rhIFN-α.

4. Plate 110 μL of samples or standards in triplicate in a new 96-well plate. Keep plate(s) at 4 °C overnight.
5. Centrifuge samples plate(s) at 400×*g* for 10 min prior to WISH cell stimulation.

3.3.3 WISH Cell Stimulation, Mature RNA Extraction, and cDNA Strand Synthesis

WISH cells firmly attach to the bottom of the well. The TurboCapture Kit (QIAGEN) is the simplest way to extract mature RNA (mRNA). The method is based on the specific binding of the polyA tail of mRNA to polyT oligonucleotides covalently attached at the base of each well.

1. Pour out media from plate with growing WISH cells on paper towels. Wash with 100 μL of sterile PBS. Place 100 μL of samples into each well from prepared 96-well plates. Use a multichannel pipette to quickly fill the whole plate.
2. Incubate plate(s) for 8 h in a CO_2 incubator to achieve maximum expression of interferon-inducible genes. Do not activate WISH cells for more than 10 h, for best results.
3. Prepare necessary amount of TCL solution by adding 100 μL of 2-mercaptoethanol to 9.9 mL of TCL buffer (sufficient for one 96-well plate). 2-mercaptoethanol is toxic and emits a foul odor. Work under a chemical hood.
4. Take plate(s) out, one by one, and proceed quickly. Pour out the plasma on tissue paper, wash twice with 100 μL of PBS (be sure to remove all residual volume of PBS by tapping the plate on a paper towel), then add 90 μL of TCL solution per well.
5. Seal the plate, place on shaker for 15 min, and then put the plate(s) at −80 °C.
6. Next day (or when you are ready), take plate(s) with lysed cells out of the freezer and thaw them for about 30 min at RT.
7. Shake plates with cell lysates on a shaker for 15 min, then transfer 20 μL of the lysates into corresponding wells in a 384 TurboCapture plate. A 384 TurboCapture plate can hold samples from four 96-well plates (*see* **Note 8**).
8. Seal plate and incubate 2 h on an orbital shaker at 100 rpm to bind mRNA to the well.
9. To elute mRNA, heat TurboCapture plate at 65 °C for 5 min (384-well thermocycler is the best choice; alternatively use a 384-well aluminum block placed in a heater). Cool down slowly to RT (*see* **Note 9**).

10. Prepare reverse transcription reagents as follow:

Component	Volume (per one well) (μL)
10× TaqMan RT buffer	1.0
25 mM $MgCl_2$	2.2
dNTP mixture	2.0
Oligo dT	0.5
RNase inhibitor	0.2
Reverse transcriptase (50 U/μL)	0.25
Total volume	6.15

Note: Total volume of reverse transcription reaction is 10 μL. A 384-well plate requires 2.6 mL of reverse transcription reagents

11. Combine 3.85 μL of eluted mRNA and mix with 6.15 μL of reverse transcription mixture in a new 384-well (or 4×96 well) plate. Place into thermocycler and incubate for 10 min at 25 °C, 30 min at 48 °C, and finally inactivate reverse transcription reaction by heating the plate for 5 min at 95 °C. Store the obtained cDNA at −20 °C until future use.

3.3.4 Detection of Interferon-Inducible Genes Using qPCR

Although there are several techniques to quantify cDNA, we measured PCR products by the amount of intercalating SYBR Green dye (*see* **Note 10**).

Several potential interferon-inducible genes were studied, including IFIT1, IFIT3, IFI44, IFI44L, MX1, and PRKR. IFIT1 and MX1 showed high response and the smallest least variance between experiments. The HPRT1 gene was selected as the reference target. The sequences for the HPRT1, IFIT1, and MX1 primers used are shown in Table 2.

Each qPCR amplification plate should include in triplicate no-template controls and high- and low-positive controls for both reference and target genes (*see* **Note 11**). The high-positive control should be ten times more concentrated than the low-positive control. Positive controls are indicators of amplification quality. Both reference and target gene primers must be located in the same plate.

1. Each amplification is performed in a total volume of 10 μL per well. For N reactions, prepare the reaction mix by combining N X 5 μL of iTaq™ SYBR® Green Supermix with ROX reagents and NX 0.5 μL of 10 μM forward and reverse primer mix. Prepare reagents for 10 % more reactions. Place 5.5 μL of polymerase reagent mixture in each well.
2. Dilute the obtained cDNA samples to either 1:10 or 1:15 with water. The exact dilution depends on the sensitivity of the thermocycler and should be estimated in preliminary experiments. Add 4.5 μL of diluted cDNA sample to the reaction mix and then seal the plate with optical film.

3. Spin plate 400×*g* at 4 °C for 3–5 min to ensure the reaction mixture is at the bottom.
4. Set up the desired program for the qPCR instrument and start amplification. The cycle provided to the instrument is 2 min at 50 °C, 10 min at 95 °C, then 40 cycles at 95 °C for 15 s and 60 °C for 1 min. The last stage measures the dissociation curve in a temperature interval from 60 to 95 °C. The cycle parameters depend on the thermocycler and should be optimized. We use the AB 7900 HT Fast Real-Time PCR System. The results of amplification should be exported in the absolute quantification format.

3.3.5 WISH Assay Data Analysis

The analysis of WISH data is simple since the percent of amplification with the use of our primers and described reagents is around 100 %±10 %. The comparative (ΔΔCt) method is the most straightforward approach to estimate relative expression. To generate Ct values (the cycle number at which signal crosses a threshold line), use the designated software provided with your qPCR system. ΔΔCt values are calculated based on the formula:

$$Fold\,change = 2^{-\Delta Ct_{treated} - \Delta Ct_{reference}}$$

where $\Delta Ct_{treated}$ is the difference between the Ct values of target and reference genes in the sample of interest and $\Delta Ct_{reference}$ is the difference between the Ct values of target and reference genes in a pooled healthy donor sample.

Based on multiple experiments, we established a polynomial dose–response model. The cubic polynomial function can be used to build the calibration curve (Fig. 1). Any computational software can be used for data analysis (Microsoft Excel, LibreOffice Calc, etc.). The R package (http://www.r-project.org) provides instruments to build a calibration curve and estimate relative expression of interferon activity. We developed an R script to perform rapid data analysis based on obtained Ct values. To use our script, no knowledge of R is required.

1. Create a data file containing the following five columns separated by a tab sign: "Position," "Sample," "Detector," "Ct," and "IFN," where "Position" is the position of the well on the qPCR plate, "Sample" is the sample name, "Detector" is the target or reference gene, "Ct" is the Ct value (see the provided example), and "IFN" is the known concentration of rhIFN-α.
2. Label the standards as desired (e.g., C000, C006, C012, C025, C050, and C100). Supply the exact concentration of rhIFN-α (IU/mL) used in the experiment in the "IFN" column in numeric format (e.g., 6.25). There should be at least six standards with increasing concentration of IFN-α to build a calibration curve. You may increase the number of standards or vary the concentration of IFN-α.

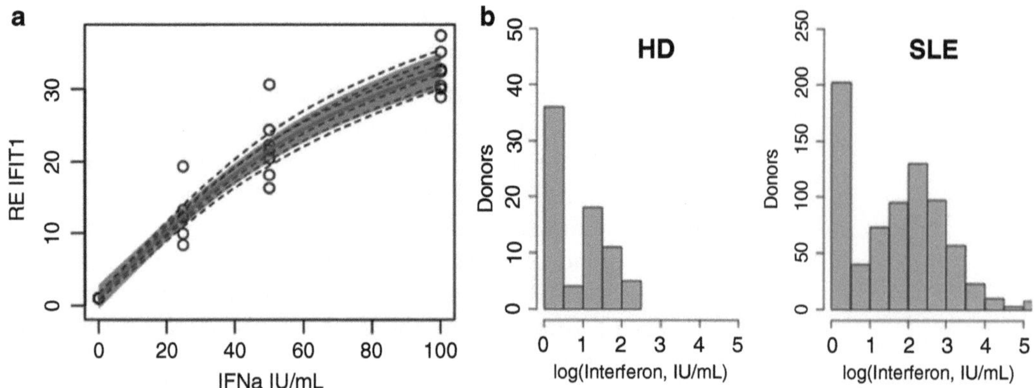

Fig. 1 (**a**) WISH assay calibration using rhIFN-α (IU/mL). The relative expression of the IFIT1 gene was measured in WISH cells stimulated with rhIFN-α. Six independent experiments were performed. *Open circles* represent actual data, *dotted lines* indicate individual spline models (package sme), *red line* and background indicate mean and confidence intervals based on all experiments. (**b**) Histograms of plasma interferon activities for healthy (*left*) and SLE (*right*) donors are shown. Some of SLE patients showed higher interferon activities compared to healthy donors

3. Samples for assessing the quality of qPCR and no-template control would be excluded from the analysis; type label "N" in IFN column.
4. Leave IFN column empty for studied plasma samples.
5. Save experimental data as a tabulated file in a new directory; name it as "<anyname>.txt." You might place data from multiple experiments in the same directory. Data may contain only one reference gene and one target gene. If you studied more than one target gene in the same qPCR experiment, use separate files for each.
6. Download and place the provided R source file (Interferon. Units.R) in the same directory.
7. Download R project for statistical computing, from http://www.r-project.org.
8. Start R, then select the directory where the source code and data are located; use Change dir (on PC) or Change Working Directory (on Mac) dialogues.
9. Open the provided source file using either File->Source R code (on PC) or File->Source File (Mac).
10. When the source starts to run, the list of files appears. Type the number corresponding to the data file (<anyname>.txt) which contains Ct values for the study.
11. The appearance of a calibration plot indicates the end of the computations. Two files will appear in the same directory after the source stops running. File "calibration.curve<anyname>. pdf" can be opened using the portable document format (pdf)

viewer and contains the calibration plot. File "interferon.values<anyname>.csv" contains the estimated concentration of interferon activities for samples in IU/mL. You can view and edit the file by using any spreadsheet programs (e.g., Microsoft Excel, LibreOffice Calc, etc.). The typical calibration curve and data distribution for HD and SLE patients are shown in Fig. 1.

4 Notes

1. Use of available primers for qPCR from commercial sources might save a significant amount of time and can be obtained from several sources (e.g., Qiagen). However, even the ready primers should be titrated in preliminary experiments. The primers purchased from Qiagen were titrated, and a 1/10 dilution was found to be optimal in the provided primer mix.
2. We order custom primers from Life Technologies and store individual primers in small aliquots in a 100 μM solution in TE buffer at −20 °C. Before each experiment, we combine the forward and reverse primers together and dilute them to a 10 μM concentration with RNase-free distilled water.
3. Tubes designed to facilitate blood layering are available in the market (e.g., SepMate™ from StemCell Technologies).
4. Always test triplicate samples to enable estimation of standard error. Low abundance genes require five or more replicates, depending on standard deviation. Standard titrations should always be included in protocols.
5. Positive controls, a bacterial plasmid carry amplified product, might be obtained once in large quantities. Inexpensive plasmids are available from several sources (e.g., www.addgene.com). Plasmids are easy to grow in large quantities, and the exact concentration can be measured.

   The top concentration for the positive control should be established in preliminary experiments. One to five serial dilutions are then performed to determine the lowest detectable concentration and range of linear amplification. Store controls in small aliquots in TE buffer at −20 °C.
6. The results of amplification should include the melting curve. A single sharp peak indicates the presence of a single product, whereas an additional small peak before the large peak suggests the presence of primer-dimers or alternative products.
7. WISH cells, originally described as a human amnion-derived cell line [24], were later identified as a HeLa contaminant, a rare type of human adenocarcinoma [25, 26]. Currently, WISH cells carry markers of HeLa cells and probably could be defined as one of the multiple clones of HeLa cells.

8. The TurboCapture mRNA Kit (Qiagen) is manufactured in two formats: 96-well and 384-well plates. Both can be used for the WISH assay.
9. For cDNA synthesis, we usually elute mRNA from a TurboCapture plate; however, it is possible to perform cDNA synthesis directly in the TurboCapture plate. In that case multiplex amplification would be performed from the same plate, saving time and reagent cost. However, the amount of cell lysate should be properly diluted to obtain meaningful results.
10. We routinely use the SYBR green detection system for qPCR quantification because of the simplicity. However, it is recommended to use a multiplex system and TaqMan probes for the WISH assay when routinely testing multiple samples. Multiplex qPCR minimizes processing time and eliminates mistakes due to variation in pipetting.
11. The specificity of amplified products for custom primers was confirmed by the melting curve and product sequencing. The amplification efficiency was close to 100 % with the described primers.

5 Conclusions

The WISH assay has advantages and disadvantages, and the information that it provides regarding IFN-I is distinct from that obtained using other techniques. The WISH assay provides a measure of the functional IFN-I activity in a serum or plasma sample (or potentially in a culture supernatant) that reflects all available subtypes of IFN-I that bind to the IFN-I receptor on the WISH cells. Other methods, such as ELISA, measure the protein concentration of the specific IFN-I types detected by the antibodies used in the assay but do not reflect functional activity of those cytokines. The IFN-I levels measured in the WISH assay show only low to moderate correlation with IFN-I-induced gene expression detected in peripheral blood cells assayed ex vivo, as many additional factors, including level of IFN-I receptor, genetic variations in signaling and regulatory gene products, and other stimulatory factors that were present in the in vivo environment, will impact that response of peripheral blood cells to a given quantity of IFN-I. Both high levels of plasma IFN-I as detected by the WISH assay and high levels of IFN-I-induced gene expression in PBMC tested ex vivo are associated with active lupus disease.

We also emphasize the value of performing sequential measures of IFN-I activity using a longitudinal study design. We find that IFN-I activity levels can fluctuate over time in some patients, providing an opportunity to assess the relationship of this important cytokine family to clinical and serologic parameters, with the goal of gaining improved understanding of lupus pathogenesis and mechanisms of lupus flare.

References

1. Becker-Merok A, Østli-Eilersten G, Lester S et al (2013) Circulating interferon-α2 levels are increased in the majority of patients with systemic lupus erythematosus and are associated with disease activity and multiple cytokine activation. Lupus 22:155–163
2. Crow MK, Wohlgemuth J (2003) Microarray analysis of gene expression in lupus. Arthritis Res Ther 5:279–287
3. Bennett L, Palucka a K, Arce E et al (2003) Interferon and granulopoiesis signatures in systemic lupus erythematosus blood. J Exp Med 197:711–723
4. Nzeusseu Toukap A, Galant C, Theate I et al (2007) Identification of distinct gene expression profiles in the synovium of patients with systemic lupus erythematosus. Arthritis Rheum 56:1579–1588
5. Crow MK (2010) Interferon-alpha: a therapeutic target in systemic lupus erythematosus. Rheum Dis Clin North Am 36:173–186
6. Lövgren T, Eloranta M-L, Båve U et al (2004) Induction of interferon-alpha production in plasmacytoid dendritic cells by immune complexes containing nucleic acid released by necrotic or late apoptotic cells and lupus IgG. Arthritis Rheum 50:1861–1872
7. Crow MK (2008) Collaboration, genetic associations, and lupus erythematosus. N Engl J Med 358:956–961
8. Wang C, Sandling JK, Hagberg N et al (2013) Genome-wide profiling of target genes for the systemic lupus erythematosus-associated transcription factors IRF5 and STAT4. Ann Rheum Dis 72:96–103
9. Connolly JJ, Hakonarson H (2012) Role of cytokines in systemic lupus erythematosus: recent progress from GWAS and sequencing. J Biomed Biotechnol 2012:1–17
10. Mikita N, Ikeda T, Ishiguro M et al (2011) Recent advances in cytokines in cutaneous and systemic lupus erythematosus. J Dermatol 38: 839–849
11. Poole BD, Niewold TB, Tsokos GC (2012) Cytokines in systemic lupus erythematosus 2011. J Biomed Biotechnol 2012:427824
12. Su D-L, Lu Z-M, Shen M-N et al (2012) Roles of pro- and anti-inflammatory cytokines in the pathogenesis of SLE. J Biomed Biotechnol 2012:347141
13. Bustin SA, Benes V, Garson JA et al (2009) The MIQE guidelines: minimum information for publication of quantitative real-time PCR experiments. Clin Chem 55(4):611–622
14. Overbergh L, Giulietti A, Valckx D et al (2003) The use of real-time reverse transcriptase PCR for the quantification of cytokine gene expression. J Biomol Tech 14:33–43
15. Boeuf P, Vigan-Womas I, Jublot D et al (2005) CyProQuant-PCR: a real time RT-PCR technique for profiling human cytokines, based on external RNA standards, readily automatable for clinical use. BMC Immunol 6:5
16. Brazma A, Hingamp P, Quackenbush J (2001) Minimum information about a microarray experiment (MIAME)-toward standards for microarray data. Nat Genet 29(4):365–371
17. Gentleman RC, Carey VJ, Bates DM et al (2004) Bioconductor: open software development for computational biology and bioinformatics. Genome Biol 5:R80
18. Huang DW, Sherman BT, Lempicki RA (2009) Systematic and integrative analysis of large gene lists using DAVID bioinformatics resources. Nat Protoc 4:44–57
19. Samarajiwa SA, Forster S, Auchettl K et al (2009) INTERFEROME: the database of interferon regulated genes. Nucleic Acids Res 37:D852–D857
20. Seo Y-J, Kim G-H, Kwak H-J et al (2009) Validation of a HeLa Mx2/Luc reporter cell line for the quantification of human type I interferons. Pharmacology 84:135–144
21. Bürgi M, Prieto C, Etcheverrigaray M et al (2012) WISH cell line: from the antiviral system to a novel reporter gene assay to test the potency of human IFN-α and IFN-β. J Immunol Methods 381:70–74
22. Hua J, Kirou K, Lee C et al (2006) Functional assay of type I interferon in systemic lupus erythematosus plasma and association with anti-RNA binding protein autoantibodies. Arthritis Rheum 54:1906–1916
23. Yousefi S, Escobar MR, Gouldin CW (1985) A practical cytopathic effect/dye-uptake interferon assay for routine use in the clinical laboratory. Am J Clin Pathol 83:735–740
24. Hayflick L (1961) The establishment of a line (WISH) of human amnion cells in continuous cultivation. Exp Cell Res 23:14–20
25. Nelson-Rees WA, Flandermeyer RR (1976) HeLa cultures defined. Science (New York, NY) 191:96–98
26. Chen TR (1988) Re-evaluation of HeLa, HeLa S3, and HEp-2 karyotypes. Cytogenet Cell Genet 48:19–24
27. Nalbandian A, Crispín JC, Tsokos GC (2009) Interleukin-17 and systemic lupus erythematosus: current concepts. Clin Exp Immunol 157:209–215
28. Novick D, Elbirt D, Miller G et al (2010) High circulating levels of free interleukin-18 in

patients with active SLE in the presence of elevated levels of interleukin-18 binding protein. J Autoimmun 34:121–126

29. Okamoto H, Katsumata Y, Nishimura K et al (2004) Interferon-inducible protein 10/CXCL10 is increased in the cerebrospinal fluid of patients with central nervous system lupus. Arthritis Rheum 50: 3731–3732
30. Vega L, Barbado J, Almansa R et al (2010) Prolonged standard treatment for systemic lupus erythematosus fails to normalize the secretion of innate immunity-related chemokines. Eur Cytokine Netw 21:71–76
31. López P, Gómez J, Prado C et al (2008) Influence of functional interleukin 10/tumor necrosis factor-alpha polymorphisms on interferon-alpha, IL-10, and regulatory T cell population in patients with systemic lupus erythematosus receiving antimalarial treatment. J Rheumatol 35:1559–1566
32. Park YB, Lee SK, Kim DS et al (1998) Elevated interleukin-10 levels correlated with disease activity in systemic lupus erythematosus. Clin Exp Rheum 16:283–288
33. George-Chandy A, Trysberg E, Eriksson K (2008) Raised intrathecal levels of APRIL and BAFF in patients with systemic lupus erythematosus: relationship to neuropsychiatric symptoms. Arthritis Res Ther 10:R97
34. Sarra M, Monteleone G (2010) Interleukin-21: a new mediator of inflammation in systemic lupus erythematosus. J Biomed Biotechnol 2010:294582

Chapter 11

Detection of SLE Antigens in Neutrophil Extracellular Traps (NETs)

Carmelo Carmona-Rivera and Mariana J. Kaplan

Abstract

Neutrophils are sentinel cells of the innate immune system with a primary role of clearing extracellular pathogens. The release of weblike structures decorated with granular proteins called neutrophil extracellular traps (NETs) has recently been implicated in the pathogenesis of inflammatory and autoimmune diseases. Indeed, NETs may represent an important source of autoantigens and immunostimulatory proteins in systemic lupus erythematosus (SLE). In this chapter, we describe protocols to isolate human peripheral neutrophils, to generate and isolate NETs, and to detect SLE antigens in NETs using immunofluorescence and immunoblot.

Key words Leukocytes, Nuclear components, Granular proteins, Reactive oxygen species

1 Introduction

Neutrophils are terminally differentiated cells that develop in the bone marrow and the most abundant white blood cells in the human circulation [1]. They have long been viewed as short-lived effector cells of the innate immune system. They play a critical role in the immune defense by killing pathogens through phagocytosis, degranulation, and the release of weblike structures called neutrophil extracellular traps (NETs) [2, 3]. NETs are composed of nuclear components (e.g., DNA and histones) associated to granular proteins from primary [myeloperoxidase (MPO), neutrophil elastase (NE), cathelicidin (LL-37)], secondary (lactoferrin), and tertiary [matrix metalloproteinases (MMPs) granules] [3, 4]. The molecular mechanisms leading to NET formation are still unraveling. It has been demonstrated that reactive oxygen species (ROS) produced by NADPH oxidase [3], histone citrullination by peptidylarginine deiminase-4 (PAD-4) [5, 6], and translocation of neutrophil elastase (NE) and myeloperoxidase (MPO) [7] appear to be important events leading to NET formation.

Paul Eggleton and Frank J. Ward (eds.), *Systemic Lupus Erythematosus: Methods and Protocols*, Methods in Molecular Biology, vol. 1134, DOI 10.1007/978-1-4939-0326-9_11, © Springer Science+Business Media New York 2014

Table 1
SLE autoantibodies directed to proteins present in NETs

NET protein	Autoantibody	Reference
α-Defensin	Yes	[11]
α-Enolase	Yes	[12]
Catalase	Yes	[13]
Cathelicidin/LL-37	Yes	[8]
C1q	Yes	[12]
Cathepsin G	Yes	[14, 15]
Elastase	Yes	[16]
Histones	Yes	[17–19]
Lactoferrin	Yes	[14, 15, 20, 21]
Myeloperoxidase	Yes	[15, 22, 23]

Recent evidence implicates externalization of nuclear material bound to neutrophil granular proteins during NET formation as an important event in the pathogenesis of autoimmune disorders including SLE [8, 9]. Indeed, proteomic and immunofluorescence analyses of NETs have demonstrated the presence of proteins known to be associated with specific autoantibody specificities in SLE [10] (Table 1).

Here, we describe some basic approaches to isolate NETs from peripheral blood (PB) neutrophils and to detect autoantigens in NETs using immunofluorescence and Western blot. These approaches should be complemented with more sophisticated techniques such as mass spectrometry and/or using recombinant proteins combined with in vitro assays.

2 Materials

2.1 Neutrophil Isolation

1. 25 mL of human blood collected in heparin-treated tube.
2. Laminal flow hood.
3. Sterile serological disposable pipettes.
4. 50 mL conical tubes.
5. 15 mL conical tubes.
6. Hemocytometer.
7. Ficoll-Paque density gradient medium.
8. Phosphate-buffered saline (PBS) 1×, pH 7.4 without calcium chloride/magnesium chloride. Store at room temperature.

9. 20 % (w/v) Dextran: Dissolve 20 g of Dextran in deionized water.
10. Filtered 0.2 % (w/v) NaCl solution: Dissolve 0.2 g of NaCl in deionized water. Store at room temperature.
11. Filtered 1.8 % (w/v) NaCl solution: Dissolve 1.8 g of NaCl in deionized water. Store at room temperature.

2.2 NET Isolation and Protein Quantification

1. Isolated neutrophils.
2. Microplate reader equipped with filter to detect absorbance 562 nm.
3. Humidified CO_2 incubator.
4. 24-well plate.
5. 96-well plate.
6. 1.5 mL microcentrifuge tubes.
7. Bicinchoninic acid (BCA) kit (Pierce).
8. Roswell Park Memorial Institute (RPMI)-1640 medium without supplements.
9. Micrococcal nuclease (10 Units/μL). Store at –20 °C.
10. Lipopolysaccharide (LPS) 1 mg/mL. Store at –20 °C.

2.3 Immunofluorescence

1. Isolated neutrophils (1×10^6 cells/mL).
2. Epifluorescence or confocal microscope equipped with filters to detect excitation/emission maxima: 350/461 nm (Hoechst), 495/519 nm (Alexa Fluor 488), 555/565 nm (Alexa Fluor 555).
3. Swiss Jewelers Forceps.
4. 12-well plate.
5. 12 mm round poly-L-lysine-coated glass coverslips.
6. 75 × 25 × 1 mm microscope slides.
7. 1.5 mL microcentrifuge tubes.
8. PBS 1×, pH 7.4. Store at room temperature.
9. 4 % (w/v) paraformaldehyde (PFA): Dissolve 4 g in 100 mL of PBS. Place the solution in a hot plate and stirrer inside the fume hood. Heat until it becomes clear. Store at 4 °C.
10. 0.2 % (v/v) Triton X-100 in PBS.
11. Blocking buffer: 0.2 % (w/v) gelatin. Dissolve 0.2 g of porcine gelatin in 100 mL of PBS. Place the solution in the microwave and heat until it completely dissolved. Store at –20 °C.
12. Fluorescent mounting medium. Store at –20 °C.
13. Hoechst 33342 (bisBenzimide H33342 trihydrochloride). Store at 4 °C.

14. Human sera from healthy and SLE donors.
15. Goat antihuman IgG Alexa Fluor 555 secondary antibody (Invitrogen). Store at −20 °C.

2.4 Western Blot (Protein Detection)

1. Protein samples.
2. Forceps.
3. Nitrocellulose or PVDF membrane.
4. Whatman 3MM filter papers.
5. 4–20 % gradient gel.
6. Running apparatus.
7. Transfer apparatus with cassettes.
8. Western blot box.
9. Orbital shaker.
10. 5× Loading buffer: 60 mM Tris–HCl (pH 6.8), 2 % sodium dodecyl sulfate (SDS), 10 % glycerol, 0.01 % bromophenol blue, and 5 % β-mercaptoethanol.
11. SDS-PAGE running buffer: 25 mM Tris–HCl, 192 mM glycine, 0.1 % SDS, pH 8.3.
12. Transfer buffer: 25 mM Tris–HCl, 192 mM glycine, 20 % methanol, pH 8.3.
13. Blocking buffer: 10 % (w/v) bovine serum albumin (BSA). Dissolve 1 g of BSA in 10 mL of PBS. Store at 4 °C.
14. Wash buffer 0.1 % (v/v) PBS-Tween.
15. Human sera from healthy and SLE donors.
16. Goat antihuman IgG HRP secondary antibody (Invitrogen). Store at −20 °C.
17. Enhanced chemiluminescence (ECL) substrate.
18. X-ray films.

3 Methods

3.1 Neutrophil Isolation

1. In a lamina flow hood, add 15 mL of Ficoll-Paque to a 50 mL conical tube.
2. Carefully add 25 mL of blood on top of the Ficoll-Paque.
3. Centrifuge at 417 × *g* for 20 min without brake and acceleration set at 3.
4. Remove the conical from the centrifuge.
5. Gently dispose of the plasma and PBMC fractions.
6. Take 5 mL of the red blood cell layer and add it to a 50 mL conical (*see* **Note 1**).

7. Add 2.5 mL of 20 % Dextran and mix gently. Leave undisturbed for 15 min (*see* **Note 2**).
8. Add 20 mL of PBS to the conical and mix by inverting the tube several times.
9. Let the solution to sediment approximately 20–30 min.
10. Take 15 mL of the cleared supernatant and transfer it to a fresh 50 mL conical.
11. Add PBS up to 50 mL.
12. Centrifuge at 515 ×*g* for 10 min at room temperature.
13. Carefully discard supernatant by decanting.
14. Resuspend the cell pellet with 20 mL of 0.2 % w/v NaCl and mix gently (*see* **Note 3**).
15. After 5 min, add 30 mL of 1.8 % NaCl.
16. Centrifuge at 515 ×*g* for 5 min at 4 °C.
17. Resuspend neutrophils with 10 mL of PBS and transfer suspension to a 15 mL conical.
18. Centrifuge cells at 515 ×*g* for 5 min.
19. Discard supernatant and resuspend cells in RPMI.
20. Count cells using a hemocytometer.

3.2 NET Isolation and Protein Quantification

1. In a laminal flow hood, seed 1×10^6 neutrophils/mL per well in a 24-well plate.
2. Add 1 μL of 1 mg/mL of LPS per well.
3. Place the plate in a humidified CO_2 incubator at 37 °C for 1 h (*see* **Note 4**).
4. After incubation, add 10 U/mL of micrococcal nuclease to each well (*see* **Note 5**).
5. Place the plate back to the humidified CO_2 incubator at 37 °C for 20 min.
6. Carefully collect the supernatant from each well in a 1.5 mL microcentrifuge tubes.
7. Centrifuge supernatants at 300 ×*g* for 5 min at 4 °C.
8. Transfer supernatant to a fresh 1.5 mL microcentrifuge tube (*see* **Note 6**).
9. Using a BCA kit, quantify NET proteins (*see* **Note 7**).
10. Take an aliquot of 10 μL and place it in a 96-well plate.
11. Mix reagents A and B in a proportion 1:50.
12. Add 200 μL of the mixture to the well containing your NET sample.
13. Incubate the plate for 30 min at 37 °C.

14. Read the plate using microplate reader equipped with filter to detect absorbance 562 nm.
15. Calculate NET concentration.

3.3 Immunofluorescence

1. Place one poly-L-lysine-coated glass coverslip into each well of the 12-well plate.
2. Add 1 μL of LPS (1 mg/mL) to 1 mL of isolated neutrophils (1×10^6 cells/mL) (*see* **Note 8**).
3. Pipette 50 μL of the suspension onto the center of the poly-l-lysine-coated coverslips.
4. Incubate for 1 h in a humidified incubator (37 °C, 5 % CO_2).
5. Transfer the cell plate to a fume hood and fix cells by adding 500 μL of 4 % PFA (*see* **Note 9**).
6. Gently aspirate the PFA and add 500 μL of PBS.
7. Permeabilize cells by adding 500 μL of 0.2 % Triton X-100 to each well and incubate for 10 min at room temperature.
8. Aspirate the solution and wash coverslips with PBS for 5 min.
9. Block nonspecific sites with 500 μL of 0.2 % gelatin for 30 min at room temperature (*see* **Note 10**).
10. Prepare two 10 % dilutions containing serum from healthy or SLE donors in 0.2 % gelatin.
11. Place a 45 μL drop of the diluted serum in the humid chamber.
12. Using Swiss Jewelers Forceps, transfer coverslip from the plate to the humid chamber. Place the coverslip upside down.
13. Place the humid chamber inside the incubator (37 °C) for 1 h.
14. Place coverslips back to the 12-well plate containing PBS.
15. Wash coverslips with 500 μL of PBS for 5 min three times.
16. Prepare goat antihuman IgG Alexa Fluor 555 (1:400 dilution) in 0.2 % gelatin.
17. Place a 45 μL drop of the diluted secondary antibodies in the humid chamber.
18. Using Swiss Jewelers Forceps, transfer coverslip from the plate to the humid chamber. Place the coverslip upside down.
19. Place the humid chamber inside the incubator (37 °C) for 30 min.
20. Place coverslips back to the 12-well plate containing PBS.
21. Wash coverslips with 500 μL of PBS for 5 min three times.
22. To counterstain the DNA, prepare DNA staining solution, Hoechst (1:1,000 dilution in PBS).
23. Aspirate PBS and add 1 mL of DNA staining dilution to each coverslips.

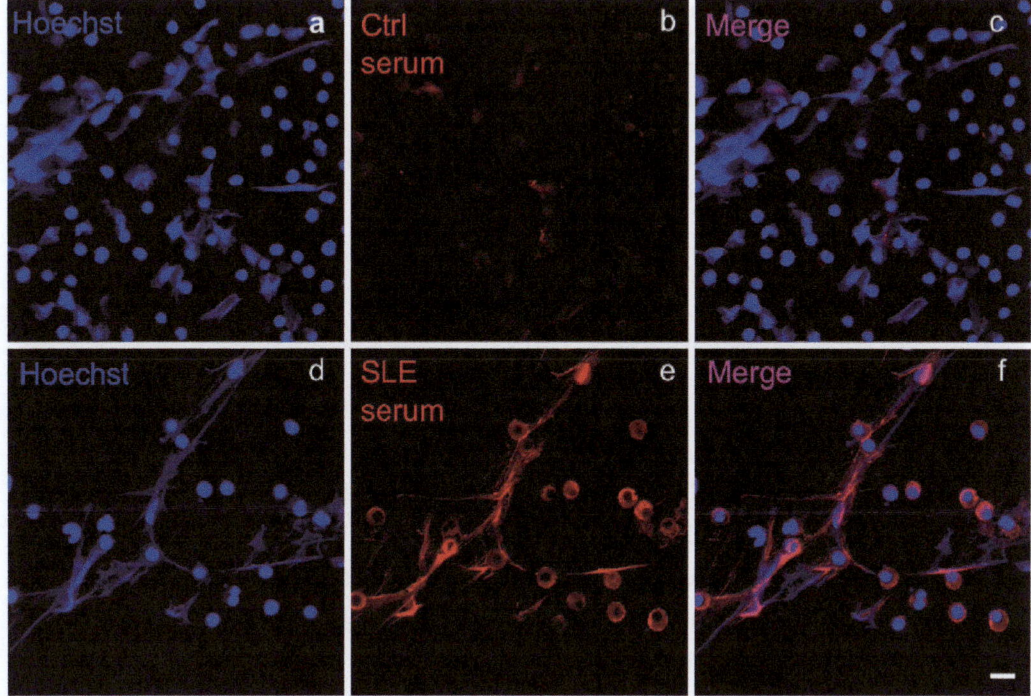

Fig. 1 Visualization of human peripheral blood (PB)-derived NETs by immunofluorescence microscopy. PB neutrophils were stimulated with LPS 1 μg for 1 h at 37 °C. Cells were fixed and immunostained with healthy donor (*Ctrl*; **b**) or SLE sera (*red*; **e**) and for DNA (Hoechst, *blue*; **a**, **d**). Scale bar 10 μm

24. Incubate for 10 min at room temperature.
25. Aspirate DNA staining solution and wash coverslips for 5 min with PBS three times at room temperature.
26. Mount coverslips using a 6 μL drop of anti-fade ProLong gold mounting medium per microscope slide. Allow the medium to dry overnight protected from light at room temperature.
27. Visualize staining on a confocal or epifluorescence microscope (Fig. 1).

3.4 Western Blot (Protein Detection)

1. Mix the NET proteins with 5 μL of loading buffer.
2. Heat samples at 100 °C for 5 min.
3. Meanwhile, fit the gradient gel plate within the running apparatus. Pour SDS-PAGE running buffer.
4. Clean the wells and load the samples inside the wells.
5. Run gel at 100 V until the bromophenol blue frontline reaches about 5 mm near the bottom.
6. Turn off the power supply and remove the plate.
7. Cut the nitrocellulose or PVDF membrane equal to the size of the gel.

8. Cut 6 Whatman 3MM filter paper equal to the size of the gel.
9. Separate the two plates of the gradient gel with a spatula.
10. Open a transfer cassette and make the "sandwich" in the following order, starting from the black side of the cassette. Wet filter paper and membrane in transfer buffer before assembling the "sandwich":
    (a) Foam.
    (b) 3 Whatman filter papers.
    (c) Gel upside down.
    (d) Membrane.
    (e) 3 Whatman filter papers.
    (f) Foam.
11. Close the cassette and place it inside the transfer apparatus.
12. Fill out with transfer buffer.
13. Connect the transfer apparatus to a power supply.
14. Run transfer at 360 mA for 60 min.
15. Disassemble the "sandwich."
16. Take the membrane with forceps and place it in western blot box containing PBS (*see* **Note 11**).
17. Wash the membrane for 5 min at room temperature.
18. Block the membrane with 10 % BSA for 30 min at room temperature (*see* **Note 12**).
19. Prepare two 1:250 dilutions containing serum from healthy or SLE donors in 5 % BSA.
20. Cut the membrane with scissors in two halves.
21. Incubate half of the membrane with control serum and the other half with SLE serum overnight at 4 °C on an orbital shaker.
22. Discard serum dilutions and wash the membranes with PBS-Tween for 5 min at room temperature three times in an orbital shaker.
23. Prepare a dilution of 1: 20,000 of the secondary antibody in 5 % BSA.
24. Incubate membrane with secondary antibody for 2 h at room temperature on an orbital shaker.
25. Discard secondary antibody and wash the membrane with PBS-Tween for 5 min at room temperature three times in an orbital shaker.
26. Prepare a 1:1 dilution of ECL substrates.
27. Incubate the membrane with ECL substrate for 1 min at room temperature with gentle agitation.

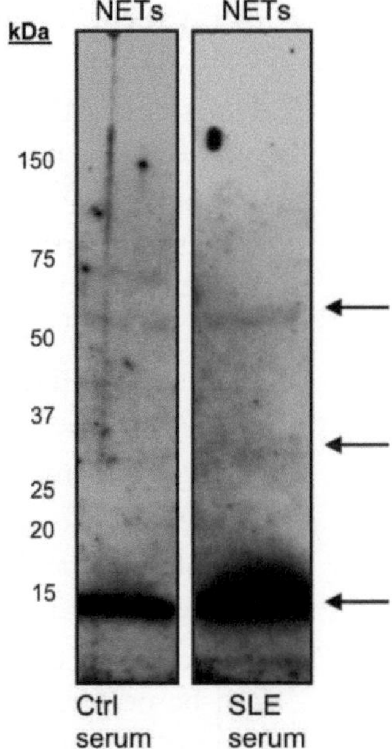

Fig. 2 Detection of SLE autoantigens in NETs by Western blot. NETs were resolved in a 4–20 % gradient gel. Proteins were transferred onto a nitrocellulose membrane. Nitrocellulose was cut in half and incubated with 1:250 dilution of healthy donor or SLE sera. Horseradish peroxidase-conjugated secondary antibodies were used to detect control (*Ctrl*) and SLE IgGs. *Arrows* indicate the antigens recognized in the NETs by SLE autoantibodies

28. Place the membrane between two sheets of transparency using forceps.
29. Place it in an X-ray cassette.
30. In a dark room, place an X-ray film on top of the membrane to capture the chemiluminescent signal (Fig. 2).
31. Place the X-ray film in a developing machine.

4 Notes

1. To avoid contamination with the interphase between the Ficoll and red blood cell layer, insert the pipette to the bottom of the tube and aspirate the sample.
2. Do not leave samples without processing for more than 15 min since the neutrophil recovering yield will decrease.
3. While typically red blood cells will be lysed within a minute, sometimes longer incubation period is required to get rid of all red blood cells.
4. Incubation periods range from 1 to 4 h depending on the condition utilized, the source of neutrophils (e.g., healthy donor,

SLE patient, mouse), and the type of stimulation (e.g., LPS, PMA, IL-8).

5. DNase I or MNase can be used in this protocol. However, it is important to note that DNAse I will completely degrade the DNA, while MNase will generate nucleosomal fragments.
6. When transferring the supernatant, do not disturb the bottom where intact cells and debris are present. If not used immediately, store the NETs at −20 °C and quantify them later.
7. Follow BCA kit instructions, which include preparation of standards.
8. Under experimental conditions, a non-treated control should be added.
9. Samples can be fixed overnight at 4 °C or for 20 min at room temperature.
10. To detect specific proteins within the NETs, double staining can be performed. Nonspecific staining (false-positive signal) can occur. Therefore, controls should be included accordingly and results should be confirmed using a different biochemical approach such as Western blot.
11. To ensure protein transfer, stain the membrane with Ponceau S solution, a red dye that can be washed out with buffer and will not interfere with protein detection.
12. Nonfat dry milk can be used instead of BSA.

References

1. Borregaard N (2010) Neutrophils, from marrow to microbes. Immunity 33:657–670
2. Amulic B, Cazalet C, Hayes GL, Metzler KD, Zychlinsky A (2012) Neutrophil function: from mechanisms to disease. Annu Rev Immunol 30:459–489
3. Brinkmann V, Reichard U, Goosmann C, Fauler B, Uhlemann Y, Weiss DS, Weinrauch Y, Zychlinsky A (2004) Neutrophil extracellular traps kill bacteria. Science 303:1532–1535
4. Villanueva E, Yalavarthi S, Berthier CC, Hodgin JB, Khandpur R, Lin AM, Rubin CJ, Zhao W, Olsen SH, Klinker M, Shealy D, Denny MF, Plumas J, Chaperot L, Kretzler M, Bruce AT, Kaplan MJ (2011) Netting neutrophils induce endothelial damage, infiltrate tissues, and expose immunostimulatory molecules in systemic lupus erythematosus. J Immunol 187:538–552
5. Wang Y, Li M, Stadler S, Correll S, Li P, Wang D, Hayama R, Leonelli L, Han H, Grigoryev SA, Allis CD, Coonrod SA (2009) Histone hypercitrullination mediates chromatin decondensation and neutrophil extracellular trap formation. J Cell Biol 184:205–213
6. Knight JS, Zhao W, Luo W, Subramanian V, O'Dell AA, Yalavarthi S, Hodgin JB, Eitzman DT, Thompson PR, Kaplan MJ (2013) Peptidylarginine deiminase inhibition is immunomodulatory and vasculoprotective in murine lupus. J Clin Invest 123(7):2981–2983
7. Papayannopoulos V, Metzler KD, Hakkim A, Zychlinsky A (2010) Neutrophil elastase and myeloperoxidase regulate the formation of neutrophil extracellular traps. J Cell Biol 191:677–691
8. Lande R, Ganguly D, Facchinetti V, Frasca L, Conrad C, Gregorio J, Meller S, Chamilos G, Sebasigari R, Riccieri V, Bassett R, Amuro H, Fukuhara S, Ito T, Liu YJ, Gilliet M (2011) Neutrophils activate plasmacytoid dendritic cells by releasing self-DNA-peptide complexes in systemic lupus erythematosus. Sci Transl Med 3:73ra19
9. Kahlenberg JM, Carmona-Rivera C, Smith CK, Kaplan MJ (2012) Neutrophil extracellular

trap-associated protein activation of the NLRP3 inflammasome is enhanced in lupus macrophages. J Immunol 190(3):1217–1226

10. Knight JS, Carmona-Rivera C, Kaplan MJ (2012) Proteins derived from neutrophil extracellular traps may serve as self-antigens and mediate organ damage in autoimmune diseases. Front Immunol 3:380
11. Tamiya H, Tani K, Miyata J, Sato K, Urata T, Lkhagvaa B, Otsuka S, Shigekiyo S, Sone S (2006) Defensins- and cathepsin G-ANCA in systemic lupus erythematosus. Rheumatol Int 27:147–152
12. Mosca M, Chimenti D, Pratesi F, Baldini C, Anzilotti C, Bombardieri S, Migliorini P (2006) Prevalence and clinico-serological correlations of anti-alpha-enolase, anti-C1q, and anti-dsDNA antibodies in patients with systemic lupus erythematosus. J Rheumatol 33:695–697
13. Mansour RB, Lassoued S, Gargouri B, El Gaid A, Attia H, Fakhfakh F (2008) Increased levels of autoantibodies against catalase and superoxide dismutase associated with oxidative stress in patients with rheumatoid arthritis and systemic lupus erythematosus. Scand J Rheumatol 37:103–108
14. Zhao MH, Liu N, Zhang YK, Wang HY (1998) Antineutrophil cytoplasmic autoantibodies (ANCA) and their target antigens in Chinese patients with lupus nephritis. Nephrol Dial Transplant 13:2821–2824
15. Manolova I, Dancheva M, Halacheva K (2001) Antineutrophil cytoplasmic antibodies in patients with systemic lupus erythematosus: prevalence, antigen specificity, and clinical associations. Rheumatol Int 20:197–204
16. Nassberger L, Jonsson H, Sjoholm AG, Sturfelt G, Heubner A (1989) Circulating anti-elastase in systemic lupus erythematosus. Lancet 1:509
17. Monestier M, Decker P, Briand JP, Gabriel JL, Muller S (2000) Molecular and structural properties of three autoimmune IgG monoclonal antibodies to histone H2B. J Biol Chem 275:13558–13563
18. Robinson WH, DiGennaro C, Hueber W, Haab BB, Kamachi M, Dean EJ, Fournel S, Fong D, Genovese MC, de Vegvar HE, Skriner K, Hirschberg DL, Morris RI, Muller S, Pruijn GJ, van Venrooij WJ, Smolen JS, Brown PO, Steinman L, Utz PJ (2002) Autoantigen microarrays for multiplex characterization of autoantibody responses. Nat Med 8:295–301
19. van Bavel CC, Dieker JW, Kroeze Y, Tamboer WP, Voll R, Muller S, Berden JH, van der Vlag J (2011) Apoptosis-induced histone H3 methylation is targeted by autoantibodies in systemic lupus erythematosus. Ann Rheum Dis 70:201–207
20. Lee SS, Lawton JW, Chan CE, Li CS, Kwan TH, Chau KF (1992) Antilactoferrin antibody in systemic lupus erythematosus. Br J Rheumatol 31:669–673
21. Caccavo D, Rigon A, Picardi A, Galluzzo S, Vadacca M, Ferri GM, Amoroso A, Afeltra A (2005) Anti-lactoferrin antibodies in systemic lupus erythematosus: isotypes and clinical correlates. Clin Rheumatol 24:381–387
22. Nassberger L, Sjoholm AG, Jonsson H, Sturfelt G, Akesson A (1990) Autoantibodies against neutrophil cytoplasm components in systemic lupus erythematosus and in hydralazine-induced lupus. Clin Exp Immunol 81: 380–383
23. Cambridge G, Wallace H, Bernstein RM, Leaker B (1994) Autoantibodies to myeloperoxidase in idiopathic and drug-induced systemic lupus erythematosus and vasculitis. Br J Rheumatol 33:109–114

Chapter 12

Detection and Characterization of Autoantibodies Against Modified Self-Proteins in SLE Sera After Exposure to Reactive Oxygen and Nitrogen Species

Brent J. Ryan and Paul Eggleton

Abstract

There are over 120 types of autoantibodies found in the blood of SLE patients against cellular and extracellular components in both their native and posttranslationally modified forms. In recent years, these autoantibodies have provoked interest as initiators of pathology and as biomarkers of disease activity. Often, the host antigens employed in lab-based and commercially developed immunoassays use non-human antigen or non-modified host antigen as a probe for autoantibodies. Here, we describe methods to posttranslationally modify host antigens, which better represent the antigen recognized by autoantibodies in vivo. This has implications in developing immunoassay with greater sensitivity and specificity.

Key words Autoantigens, Complement proteins, ELISA, Immunoblotting, Mass spectroscopy, Posttranslational modification

1 Introduction

The measurement of autoantibodies against one or more common host antigens is often used to clinically diagnose autoimmune diseases [1–3]. Normally, autoantibodies to host proteins are IgM isotype and in low abundance in healthy individuals. The low levels of autoantibodies produced by B cells in healthy individuals is due to infrequent interaction with cells that aid autoantibody production; such as antigen-presenting cells (APCs) and T cells, that are eradicated by clonal deletion early in development or silenced by clonal anergy. These processes mean that as T cells survey host peptide fragments present on MHC-II molecules, they remain unresponsive to them, unless they appear "foreign" or altered. SLE patients are known to generate a greater amount of oxidative stress in their tissues, in which excess reactive species, including reactive oxygen species (ROS), reactive nitrogen species (NOS), and reactive chlorine species (RCS), are able to interact with amino acids,

Paul Eggleton and Frank J. Ward (eds.), *Systemic Lupus Erythematosus: Methods and Protocols*, Methods in Molecular Biology, vol. 1134, DOI 10.1007/978-1-4939-0326-9_12, © Springer Science+Business Media New York 2014

lipids, and nucleic acids [4, 5]. A consequence of this posttranslational modification (PTM) of individual amino acids in proteins leads to self-peptide sequences appearing as "nonself" to the immune system and initiation of an adaptive immune response [6, 7]. Indeed, several studies have demonstrated posttranslationally modified antigens to be superior to their native counterparts in autoimmune disease [8–10].

The monitoring of a number of autoantibodies has proved useful in the diagnosis (anti-double-stranded DNA; ds-DNA) of SLE and onset of nephritis (anti-C1q) in SLE patients [11–14]. However, the measurement of autoantibody titers is not relied on for routine monitoring of the clinical course of SLE. One of the reasons for this may be the lack of clinical sensitivity and specificity in test results correlating to disease activity. A number of factors may contribute to the lack of prognostic value of these assays in clinical practice. For example, when one examines the antigens used in enzyme-linked immunosorbent assays (ELISAs) to quantify specific autoantibody levels, they comprise of unmodified antigen from various animal sources or human recombinant protein made in bacteria. The use of PTM antigens may be a more representative antigen source with which to probe for autoantibodies against a specific antigen. Indeed, in some cases, PTM antigens may be the initiating antigen in the immune response, and therefore, autoantibodies to these PTM forms of an antigen may represent a more clinically relevant biomarker [15].

In the inflammatory environment generated during SLE pathology, a greater amount of ROS, RNS, and RCS may be generated, resulting in the formation of a number of PTM to amino acids [16]. For example, exposed cysteine present in SH groups upon exposure to ROS can be oxidized to form disulfides with other SH groups or be oxidized cysteine sulfenic, sulfinic, and sulfonic acid derivatives. The amino acid methionine is also highly susceptible to oxidation resulting in the generation of methionine sulfoxide or methionine sulfone. Chlorination of the side chains of lysine and histidine can occur resulting in the formation of chloramines. Nitrating species (such as peroxynitrite) may mediate the formation of the stable end products of nitration such as 3-nitrotyrosine (3-NT). Peptides bearing 3-NT have been shown to be immunogenic, evoke anti-3NT antibody responses, and induce a prolonged immune response [17, 18]. The result of protein exposure to a variety of reactive species may lead to significant changes in protein structure, the consequence of which may be the generation or exposure of peptides that are more antigenic than unmodified proteins, resulting in an autoimmune response. This may lead to unwanted production and accumulation of autoantibodies to "self-proteins." However, we can exploit this aberration in immune tolerance to detect specific autoantibodies to PTM host proteins, with the view to correlate their production with disease activity.

2 Materials

All reagents used were analytical grade and solutions should be prepared using ultrapure water (prepared by purifying deionized water to attain a sensitivity of 18 MΩ cm at 25 °C). Treatment of solid-phase proteins requires the use of reactive species prepared in Chelex-200 treated water (to prevent spontaneous Fenton reaction generation of $^{\cdot}OH$ from H_2O_2, $ONOO^-$ or HOCl).

2.1 Reactive Species Reagents

Posttranslation modification of proteins may be achieved by exposure to a number of reactive species. We routinely expose proteins to peroxynitrite ($ONOO^-$), hydrogen peroxide (H_2O_2), hypochlorus acid (HOCl), and hydroxyl radical ($^{\cdot}OH$).

1. Peroxynitrite $ONOO^-$ synthesis.

   Peroxynitrite can be purchased commercially in small quantities, but can be made in the laboratory (*see* **Note 1**).

   (a) In a fume hood, 50 mL of 600 mM HCl, and 700 mM H_2O_2 is added to 50 mL 600 mM $NaNO_2$, on a magnetic stirring plate and then immediately added to 50 mL 1.2 M NaOH. A yellow $ONOO^-$ solution will form. To neutralize excess H_2O_2, add MnO_2 powder (~10 g) and mix for 30 min. Next, remove the MnO_2 by filtering the peroxynitrite solution through general use filter paper. The resulting supernatant is concentrated by overnight freezing at −20 °C, then the yellow-colored $ONOO^-$ solution is decanted during thawing.

   (b) The concentration of the $ONOO^-$ solution is determined spectrophotometrically at an absorbance setting of 302 nm, using the Beer-Lambert equation ($\varepsilon = 1{,}670\ M^{-1}\ cm^{-1}$) to estimate the concentration. A cuvette containing 0.4 M NaOH should act as a blank. The $ONOO^-$ aliquots can be stably stored at −80 °C for up to 6 months.

2. Both H_2O_2 and HOCl can be purchased relatively cheaply from general lab suppliers.
3. The use of 1 M H_2O_2 with and without 0.1 mM $CuCl_2$ enables the generation of $^{\cdot}OH$ to be generated through the Fenton reaction with the Cu^{2+} acting catalytically.

2.2 Modification of Solid-Phase Proteins by Reactive Species

2.2.1 Binding of Proteins of Interest to 96-Well Plates

1. Prepare sufficient sodium carbonate buffer to dilute a protein to bind to a 96-well MaxiSorp plate (Nunc). For 100 mL of buffer, add 0.1575 g Na_2CO_3 and 0.294 g $NaHCO_3$ to 100 mL of double-distilled water. The pH of the sodium carbonate buffer should be pH 9.6, adjust with 1 M HCl, if necessary. Prepare 2 μg of protein of interest in sodium carbonate buffer, pH 9.6 to a final volume of 100 μL (*see* **Note 2**).

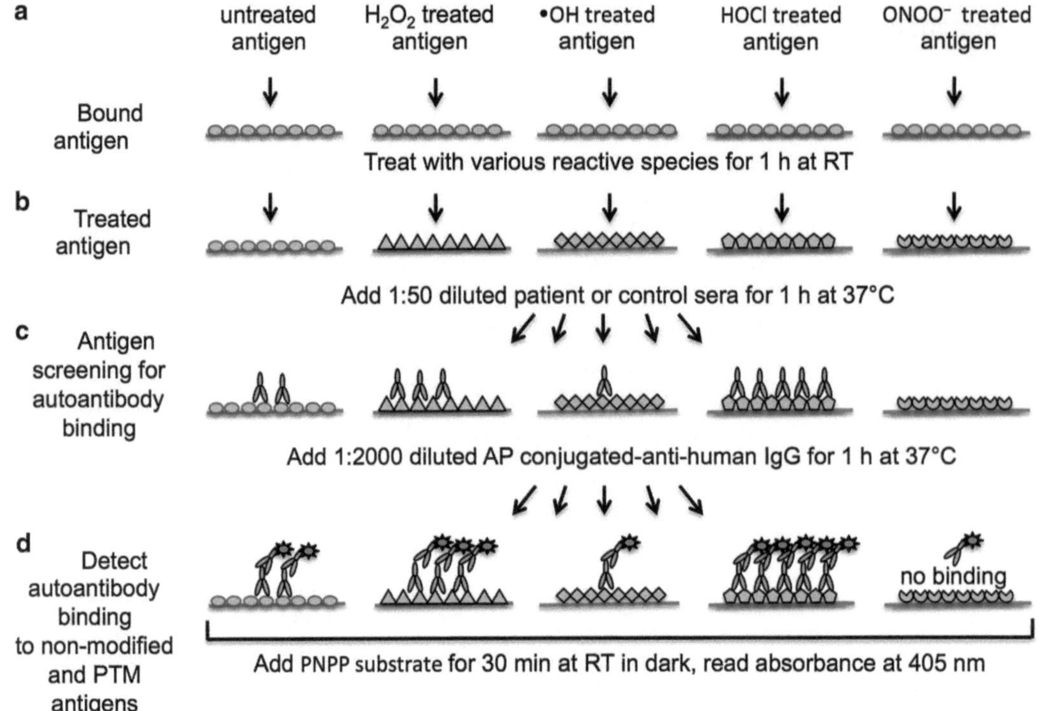

Fig. 1 Schematic outline of suggested modifications of solid-phase bound host protein by reactive species and testing for autoantibodies against PTM forms of antigen. (**a**) Proteins of interest are first bound to a 96-well plate. (**b**) The target protein is then modified. (**c**) Patient or control sera are exposed to the unmodified and modified forms of antigen and autoantibodies that recognize various form of the protein bind. (**d**) The amount of autoantibody recognizing various PTM forms of the protein is quantified spectrophotometrically

2. Allow the protein to bind to the plates overnight at 4 °C, then wash each well twice with 150 μL phosphate-buffered saline pH 7.5 containing 0.075 % v/v Tween-20 (PBST).

2.2.2 Reactive Species Treatment of Bound Proteins of Interest

3. The solid-phase proteins can now be modified by addition of various reactive species (Fig. 1). To generate a large proportion of PTM protein, a nonphysiological concentration of reactive species will be more effective than a physiological concentration (*see* **Note 3**). Initially, try exposing bound protein to 50 mM H_2O_2 (± 0.1 mM $CuCl_2$), 0.1 mM HOCl, or 0.5 mM $ONOO^-$ prepared in 200 mM phosphate buffer (*see* **Note 4**), for 1 h at room temperature.
4. Wash the plates containing unmodified and modified proteins three times with PBST, and then block each well with 5 % (w/v) dried milk powder in PBS for 2 h at 37 °C. Next, wash the plates twice more with PBST. The plates are now ready to test with autoimmune and control serum samples.

3 Methods

3.1 Enzyme-Linked Immunosorbent Assay (ELISA) for Antibodies Against PTM Proteins in SLE Serum

1. Following binding and PTM of proteins of interest to a 96-well plate, add control and patient serum (Fig. 2). Initially, make a 1:50 dilution of patient serum in PBST containing 5 % (w/v) dried milk powder. For example, dilute 20 μL of serum in 980 μL of PBST containing 3 % (w/v) dried milk powder, and add 100 μL of the diluted serum to each well for 1 h at 37 °C. As a negative control add 100 μL of 40 μg/mL human IgG prepared in PBST containing 5 % (w/v) milk powder to separate wells containing test proteins.

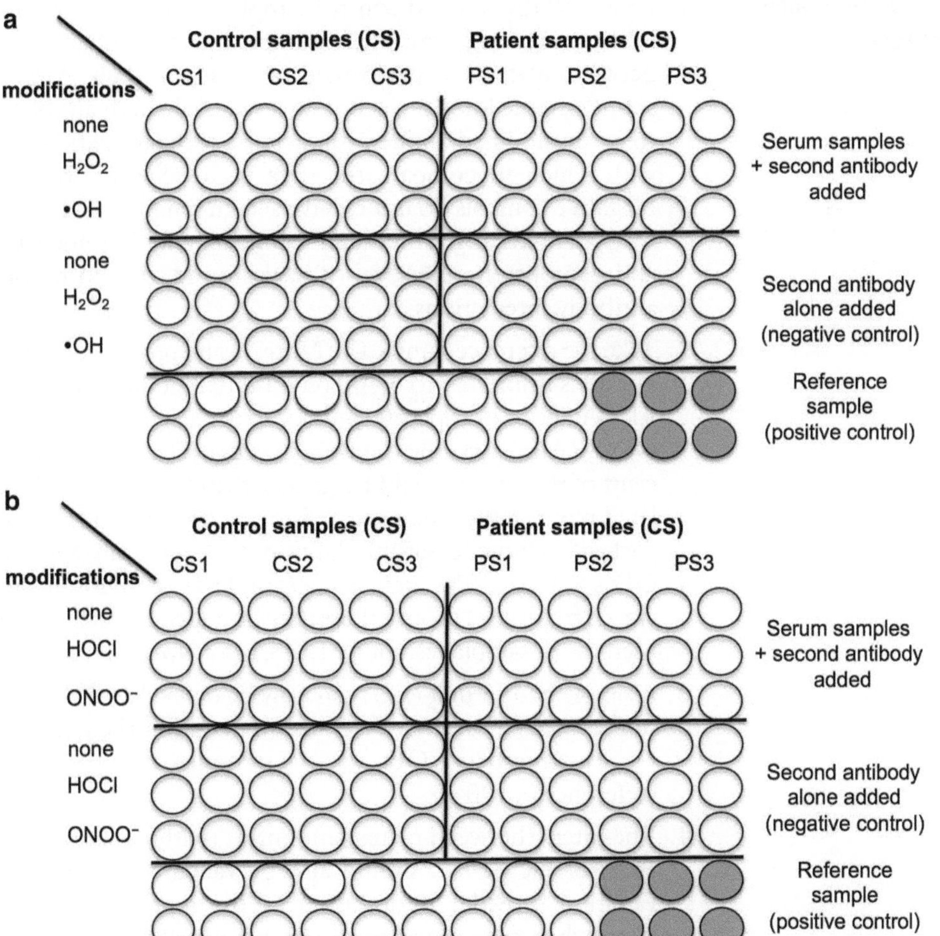

Fig. 2 Suggested layout of samples and controls for screening patient sera for autoantibodies against PTM self-antigens. (**a**) Unmodified protein and two PTM-proteins can be prepared on each plate. (**b**) Additional PTM forms of a protein can be placed on a second 96-well plate along with controls and reference samples for comparison with the first plate. *Shaded* wells represent a known positive reference sample run on each plate in sextruplicate used to standardize the ELISA

2. Wash the wells twice with PBST and add 100 μL alkaline phosphatase-conjugated goat antihuman IgG antibody (*see* **Note 5**), diluted 1:2,000 in PBST containing 5 % (w/v) milk powder for 1 h at 37 °C.
3. Wash each well twice with PBST, then add 100 μL *p-nitrophenyl* phosphate (PNPP) substrate (dilute in accordance with manufacturer's instructions) and incubate in the dark for 30 min. The reaction is terminated by addition of 11 μL 500 mM NaOH (50 mM NaOH final concentration).
4. Read the yellow-colored product at an absorbance maximum of 405 nm in a 96-well plate reader (*see* **Note 6**).

3.2 Standardization of the ELISA

1. Unless all the test and control samples are run on a single plate in replicate on a single day, it is important to standardize results between plates and performed on different days. A reference serum sample known to contain a relatively high antibody titer to an unmodified antigen can act as a standardization control, with which to compare the data with PTM of the antigen. Negative controls do not receive serum samples, but do receive wash and blocking buffers and secondary antibody and substrate and demonstrate the level of background, due to nonspecific antibody interactions.
2. Take the reference sample (*see* **Note 7**) and prepare twofold serial dilutions from 1:25 to 6,400 (eight different dilutions). Perform ELISA above in triplicate and construct a standard curve of the OD_{405} (*Y*-axis) vs. the dilution (*X*-axis). The correlation coefficient of the curve should be greater than 0.95 and can be calculated plotting the data using Prism 5 software or other statistical package. Chose a serum dilution that gives an approximate $OD_{405} = 1$ AU. This reference sample at the chosen dilution (in sextruplicate) should thereafter be added to each plate being used for all sample testing by ELISA (*see* **Note 8**).
3. A simple ELISA unit (EU) can now be defined as the percentage of the OD_{405nm} of the reference sample using the equation: $EU = \text{mean } OD_{405nm} (\text{sample}) / \text{mean } OD_{405nm} (\text{reference}) \times 100$
4. The inter- (between plates) and intra- (within plate) assay variation of the ELISA should also be validated. The inter-assay variation provides information of the reproducibility of the assay when performed on different plates, at different times, using different batches of buffers and the influence of different operators. The intra-assay variation provides information on pipetting error, mixing, timing, and influence of well positions. To assess the inter-assay variation, run a positive and negative control standard and zero analyte (buffers only) at least 20 times on 5 separate plates in five consecutive days. For intra-assay variation, run the above in a single plate. Read the plates and

calculate the mean OD ± standard deviation (SD) of the positive, negative, and blank control samples. The SD is an estimate of reproducibility of the replicate data points and is a useful tool for estimating the variability of replicate results normally calculated as the coefficient of variation (CV). The CV is calculated as %CV = SD/mean × 100 (*see* **Note 9**).

3.3 Statistics

To test the comparison of autoantibody titers to PTM antigen compared to untreated antigen, use an ANOVA for nonparametric data (Friedman test) with Dunn posttest (if multiple groups are being compared).

3.4 Interpretation

The objective of this method is to make comparative evaluations of antibody levels against various forms of host antigens that may or may not have undergone PTM during the course of the disease. By measuring a PTM form of antigen, it may increase the specificity or sensitivity of the ELISA with respect to (a) predicting onset of disease activity, e.g., nephritis, and (b) monitoring efficacy of treatment, e.g., reduction in acute-phase response or efficiency of B cell depletion.

1. Sensitivity and specificity. Determination of a positive or negative antibody titer by ELISA requires the establishment of an arbitrary "cutoff" titer. Often it is only possible retrospectively to calculate the clinical sensitivity and specificity of an assay. The actual proportions of positives that are correctly identified as positive define the clinical sensitivity of the assay, while the actual number of negatives that are identified as truly negative provide the basis of the clinical specificity.
2. Application of receiver operating characteristics (ROC) curves. ROC curves are a way of plotting specificity against sensitivity to determine optimal cutoff values for an assay [19]. Various graphical software programs (e.g., GraphPad Prism V5) can be used to construct such curves. In addition, the area under ROC curves may be used to assess if PTM of an antigen increases its diagnostic utility through increased clinical sensitivity or specificity, when compared to the unmodified antigen. Therefore, ROC curves provide a useful statistical tool to retain or discard assays that improve the accuracy of the method (in terms of increased specificity or sensitivity) to monitor disease activity.

4 Notes

1. A number of manufacturers sell peroxynitrite and these may be easily found on the Internet.
2. A 96-well can only absorb a limited amount of protein. Proteins prepared in sodium carbonate buffer at 2 μg/100 μL will likely

be in excess of the maximum amount of protein that can bind to a well, allowing saturated binding of protein to each well.

3. The concentrations of reactive species cited in our hands are sufficient to cause PTM of proteins that are detectable by mass spectrometry, without removing the bound protein from the wells of the plate, although these concentrations need to be validated for each protein of interest.
4. It is important to prepare the reactive species in 200 mM phosphate buffer (pH 7.4) in Chelex-200-treated water. Pass Milli-Q double-distilled water through a prepacked column containing Chelex-200 resin into a container that has been washed with 5 mM EDTA (pH 7.0). To prepare the sodium phosphate buffer, prepare two solutions: A and B. Solution A is comprised of 5.52 $NaH_2PO_4{\cdot}H_2O$/100 mL of Chelex-200-treated H_2O (400 mM). Solution B is prepared by adding 10.73 g $Na_2HPO_4{\cdot}7H_2O$/100 mL Chelex-200-treated H_2O (400 mM). To obtain the desired pH of 7.4, mix 3.8 mL of solution A to 10.1 mL of solution B, then dilute to 200 mL with Chelex-200-treated water. Check the pH of the buffer, and adjust volumes of solutions A and B.
5. Do not use Chelex-treated water-based buffers to dilute secondary antibodies conjugated to alkaline phosphatase (AP). AP is a zinc metaloenzyme that requires the presence of zinc to activate the active site of the enzyme when it interacts with substrate.
6. Ensure the contents of each well are completely mixed, but ensure there are no air bubbles in the wells, as this will affect the spectrophotometric readout. Do not vary the time of the substrate incubation, as this will increase variation in the data.
7. The reference sample could be a large batch of a single serum sample or a pooled sample of several patients who have relatively high antibody titers against the antigen of interest.
8. If the OD results of the reference sample are not consistent between plates (within the inter-assay variation), repeat the assay until consistent results are obtained.
9. As a rough estimate if the intra- or inter-assay individual control results lie outside a mean value ± 2 SD, then you can be confident 95 % of the time the result is unreliable. If an individual result lies outside a mean value ± 3 SD, then you can be confident 99 % of the time the result is unreliable.

Acknowledgements

This work was supported by an Arthritis Research UK grant (No. 17966), the Torbay Medical Research Fund and Northcott Devon Medical Foundation and a travel fellowship from the Alberta Innovates Health Solutions.

References

1. Peters MJ, Van Halm VP, Nurmohamed MT, Damoiseaux J, Tervaert JW, Twisk JW et al (2008) Relations between autoantibodies against oxidized low-density lipoprotein, inflammation, subclinical atherosclerosis, and cardiovascular disease in rheumatoid arthritis. J Rheumatol 35:1495–1499
2. Shi J, Knevel R, Suwannalai P, Van Der Linden MP, Janssen GM, Van Veelen PA et al (2011) Autoantibodies recognizing carbamylated proteins are present in sera of patients with rheumatoid arthritis and predict joint damage. Proc Natl Acad Sci U S A 108:17372–17377
3. Zendman AJ, Van Venrooij WJ, Pruijn GJ (2006) Use and significance of anti-CCP autoantibodies in rheumatoid arthritis. Rheumatology (Oxford) 45:20–25
4. Morgan PE, Sturgess AD, Davies MJ (2009) Evidence for chronically elevated serum protein oxidation in systemic lupus erythematosus patients. Free Radic Res 43:117–127
5. Morgan PE, Sturgess AD, Hennessy A, Davies MJ (2007) Serum protein oxidation and apolipoprotein CIII levels in people with systemic lupus erythematosus with and without nephritis. Free Radic Res 41:1301–1312
6. Eggleton P (2003) Stress protein-polypeptide complexes acting as autoimmune triggers. Clin Exp Immunol 134:6–8
7. Eggleton P, Haigh R, Winyard PG (2008) Consequence of neo-antigenicity of the 'altered self'. Rheumatology (Oxford) 47:567–571
8. Bashir S, Harris G, Denman MA, Blake DR, Winyard PG (1993) Oxidative DNA damage and cellular sensitivity to oxidative stress in human autoimmune diseases. Ann Rheum Dis 52:659–666
9. Griffiths HR, Lunec J (1996) The C1q binding activity of IgG is modified in vitro by reactive oxygen species: implications for rheumatoid arthritis. FEBS Lett 388:161–164
10. Strollo R, Ponchel F, Malmstrom V, Rizzo P, Bombardieri M, Wenham CY et al (2013) Autoantibodies to posttranslationally modified type II collagen as potential biomarkers for rheumatoid arthritis. Arthritis Rheum 65: 1702–1712
11. Ru JL, Wei H, Lu ZQ, Zhao CY, Li XF (2009) Role of DNA-associated autoantibodies to cell membrane in the diagnosis of juvenile systemic lupus erythematosus. Zhonghua Er Ke Za Zhi 47:820–823
12. Fragoso-Loyo H, Cabiedes J, Orozco-Narvaez A, Davila-Maldonado L, Atisha-Fregoso Y, Diamond B et al (2008) Serum and cerebrospinal fluid autoantibodies in patients with neuropsychiatric lupus erythematosus. Implications for diagnosis and pathogenesis. PLoS One 3:e3347
13. Hanly JG, Urowitz MB, Siannis F, Farewell V, Gordon C, Bae SC et al (2008) Autoantibodies and neuropsychiatric events at the time of systemic lupus erythematosus diagnosis: results from an international inception cohort study. Arthritis Rheum 58:843–853
14. Heinlen LD, Mcclain MT, Merrill J, Akbarali YW, Edgerton CC, Harley JB et al (2007) Clinical criteria for systemic lupus erythematosus precede diagnosis, and associated autoantibodies are present before clinical symptoms. Arthritis Rheum 56:2344–2351
15. Doyle HA, Mamula MJ (2001) Post-translational protein modifications in antigen recognition and autoimmunity. Trends Immunol 22:443–449
16. Morgan PE, Sturgess AD, Davies MJ (2005) Increased levels of serum protein oxidation and correlation with disease activity in systemic lupus erythematosus. Arthritis Rheum 52: 2069–2079
17. Ohmori H, Oka M, Nishikawa Y, Shigemitsu H, Takeuchi M, Magari M et al (2005) Immunogenicity of autologous IgG bearing the inflammation-associated marker 3-nitrotyrosine. Immunol Lett 96:47–54
18. Birnboim HC, Lemay AM, Lam DK, Goldstein R, Webb JR (2003) Cutting edge: MHC class II-restricted peptides containing the inflammation-associated marker 3-nitrotyrosine evade central tolerance and elicit a robust cell-mediated immune response. J Immunol 171:528–532
19. Nettleman MD (1988) Receiver operator characteristic (ROC) curves. Infect Control Hosp Epidemiol 9:374–377

Chapter 13

Generation of Self-Peptides to Treat Systemic Lupus Erythematosus

Jean-Paul Briand, Nicolas Schall, and Sylviane Muller

Abstract

Synthetic peptides are attracting increasing attention as therapeutics. Despite their potential, however, only a few selected peptides have been able to enter in clinical trials for chronic autoimmune diseases and systemic lupus erythematosus (SLE) in particular. Here, we describe and discuss a series of assays, which may help in characterizing valuable candidate peptides that were applied in our laboratory to develop the lupus P140 peptide program. The different steps of selection include the choice of the initial autoantigen, the design, synthesis and purification of peptides, their preliminary screen by measuring cytokines produced ex vivo by T cells and their binding to major histocompatibility complex class II (MHCII) molecules, their capacity to lower peripheral cell hyperproliferation in lupus-prone MRL/lpr mice, and, as a final step, their ability to slow down the development of lupus disease in model animals.

Key words Therapeutic peptides, Systemic lupus erythematosus, Murine models of lupus, Cytokines assays, MHC peptide binding assay, P140 peptide

1 Introduction

In the arsenal of therapeutics developed to treat patients with inflammatory autoimmune diseases, to dispose of unique synthetic peptides with specific targeted and safe properties is much sought-after. Peptides present valuable advantages over other drug candidates [e.g., therapeutic fusion proteins or monoclonal antibodies (mAb)] including higher activity per unit mass, increased selectivity and specificity, greater stability at storage, weaker immunogenicity, and better organ penetration. Also in the balance is their cost of production and purification and the possibility to produce large amounts of drug substance under good manufacturing practice conditions. Furthermore, peptides bearing natural (i.e., post-translational) or nonnatural modifications, as well as peptide mimics of protein or nonprotein antigens (DNA, RNA, carbohydrates), can be designed and may potentially replace native antigens. Their use, however, also has several inherent limitations.

Paul Eggleton and Frank J. Ward (eds.), *Systemic Lupus Erythematosus: Methods and Protocols*, Methods in Molecular Biology, vol. 1134, DOI 10.1007/978-1-4939-0326-9_13, © Springer Science+Business Media New York 2014

They generally suffer from a relatively low stability in vivo, weak oral bioavailability, and low cross-membrane delivery. Their solubility in physiological milieu can also represent a major drawback [1]. Hence, a panoply of expert tips and tricks have been introduced over time and minimize some of these difficulties [2–4]. Thus, among the strategies developed to treat patients with chronic inflammatory diseases, synthetic peptide-based immune intervention provides a serious option for addressing new therapeutic challenges [5–7]. The central question at this point remains how to identify such unique peptides and to possess a number of "go-no go" screens to transform a bioactive peptide into a therapeutic peptide. In this chapter, we describe a number of such tests that were used to design, synthesize, and biologically and preclinically evaluate the 21-mer peptide P140/Lupuzor™ that has successfully completed phase IIb clinical trials in patients with SLE [8].

2 Materials

In a general manner, prepare all solutions using analytical grade reagents and ultrapure water prepared by purifying deionized water to attain a high resistivity, preferably 16–18 MΩ/cm at room temperature (RT). Follow all waste disposal regulations, both for chemicals and biological (cell culture) materials. Also carefully follow specific, local regulations regarding animals and experimental/ethical conditions.

2.1 Materials and Reagents for the Generation of Peptides

1. Special equipment: The fully automatic multichannel peptide synthesizer used in our own studies is a homemade machine [9]. Other systems like the Symphony apparatus from Peptide Technology (Tucson, AZ) or the MiniBlock from Mettler Toledo (Quebec City, Canada) are commercially available. Analytical and preparative high-performance liquid chromatography (formerly referred to as high-pressure liquid chromatography, HPLC) systems are from Beckman (Gagny, France).
2. Solvents: Dichloromethane, dimethylformamide, piperidine, as well as acetonitrile are from Carlo Erba (France). Trifluoroacetic acid is from Acros Organics (Belgium). Amino acid derivatives, resins, and peptide reagents are from Polypeptide (Strasbourg, France). Analytical and preparative HPLC C_{18} columns are from Macherey-Nagel (Hoerdt, France).
3. Analyses: Homogeneity of peptides is checked by analytical HPLC (Beckman). Their identity is assessed by mass spectrometry (LC/MS) on a Finnigan LCQ Advantage Max system (Villebon-sur-Yvette, France) and/or by matrix-assisted laser desorption and ionization time-of-flight MS using a Protein TOF apparatus (Bruker Spectrospin, Wissembourg, France).

2.2 Reagents Required for T Cell Epitope Mapping

1. Special equipment: Sterile laminar flow cabinet, humidified incubator at 37 °C with 5 % CO_2, microscope, 96-well harvester (e.g., Packard, Meriden, CT), beta-counter (Matrix 9600 direct beta-counter, Packard), centrifuge, sterile pipettes and tubes, and culture plates (96-well flat bottom microplates; BD Biosciences, Franklin Lakes, NJ).
2. Cell culture reagents: Culture medium [L-alanyl-L-glutamine-enriched RPMI 1640 medium containing 10 % (v/v) fetal calf serum (FCS), 10 μg/mL gentamicin, 10 mM HEPES, and 5×10^{-5} M β-mercaptoethanol], pH 7.4 phosphate-buffered saline (PBS).
3. Methyl-[^{3}H] thymidine (aqueous solution containing 2 % ethanol), specific activity ~5–7 Ci/mmol (PerkinElmer, Waltham, MA).
4. Concanavalin-A (Con-A; Sigma, St Louis, MO).
5. Peptides of high purity (>90 % by HPLC) and checked by MS.

2.3 Reagents Required for IL-2 (and IL-4) Bioassays

1. Special equipment: Sterile laminar flow cabinet, humidified incubator at 37 °C with 5 % CO_2, microscope, 96-well harvester (e.g., Packard), beta-counter (e.g., Matrix 9600 direct beta-counter, Packard), centrifuge, sterile pipettes and tubes, and culture flasks and plates (96-well flat bottom microplates, BD Biosciences).
2. Cell culture reagents: Culture medium, FCS, PBS.
3. CTL-L cells obtained from the American Tissue Culture Collection (ref. TIB-214).
4. Recombinant IL-2 (or IL-4) to establish the standard curves (PharMingen, San Diego, CA).
5. Methyl-[^{3}H] thymidine (*see* Subheading 2.2).
6. Peptides of high purity (>90 % by HPLC) and checked by MS.

2.4 Reagents Required for Cytokine Measurements by ELISA

1. Special equipment: Incubator (37 °C), pipettes, microtubes, and polyvinyl microtiter plates (BD Biosciences).
2. Buffers and reagents: PBS, Tween 20, bovine serum albumin (BSA; ref. 10735094001, Roche, Tucson, AZ), 3,3′,5,5′-tetramethylbenzidine (TMB), H_2O_2, and HCl.
3. Recombinant cytokines to establish the standard curves (PharMingen).
4. Abs for coating and cytokines detection (PharMingen).
5. ELISA microplate reader (Multiskan EX, Labsystems, Kennett Square, PA).

2.5 Reagents Required for Cytokine Membrane Array Measurements

1. Special equipment: Sterile laminar flow cabinet, humidified incubator at 37 °C with 5 % CO_2, microscope, centrifuge, sterile pipettes and tubes, Malassez counting chamber (VWR, Arlington Heights, IL), and plates (24-well, flat bottom cell culture plates, BD Biosciences).
2. Cell culture reagents: Culture medium, FCS, PBS, and Ficoll (Lympholyte-M, $d = 1.0875$; Cedarlane, Burlington, Ontario, Canada).
3. Mice: MRL/lpr lupus mice and CBA/J mice (or another MHC-matched strain).
4. Peptides of high purity (>90 % by HPLC) and checked by MS.
5. Kit RayBio® cytokine antibody array (RayBiotech, Norcross, GA).

2.6 Reagents Required for Cytokine Measurements by Bead-Based Flow Cytometric Assay

1. Special equipment: Sterile laminar flow cabinet, humidified incubator at 37 °C with 5 % CO_2, microscope, centrifuge, sterile pipettes and tubes, Malassez counting chamber, and plates (24-well flat bottom cell culture plate, BD Biosciences).
2. Cell culture reagents: Culture medium, FCS, PBS, mitomycin-C (Sigma), and ACK (ammonium-chloride-potassium, for red blood cells lysis).
3. Mice: MRL/lpr lupus mice and CBA/J mice (or another MHC-matched strain).
4. Peptides of high purity (>90 % by HPLC) and checked by MS.
5. Cytometric cytokines array (BD Cytometric Bead Array Mouse Th1/Th2/Th17 cytokine kit, PharMingen).
6. FACSCalibur flow cytometer (BD Biosciences).

2.7 Reagents Required for Measuring the Binding of Peptide Analogues to MHC Class II Molecules

1. Special equipment for cell culture: Sterile laminar flow cabinet, humidified incubator at 37 °C with 5 % CO_2, microscope, centrifuge, sterile pipettes and tubes, culture flasks, and plates (96-well flat bottom microplates, BD Biosciences).
2. Special equipment for ELISA (*see* Subheading 2.4).
3. Cell culture reagents: Culture medium, FCS, and PBS.
4. Mouse L fibroblasts transfected by either class II molecules, I-A^d, I-E^d, I-A^k, or I-E^k and respective T cell hybridomas and respective test peptides (*see* Table 1).
5. High purity test peptides (>90 % by HPLC and checked by MS).

2.8 Reagents Required for the Hyperproliferation Assay

1. Special equipment: Sterile laminar flow cabinet, humidified incubator at 37 °C with 5 % CO_2, microscope, centrifuge, sterile pipettes and tubes, and Malassez counting chamber.
2. Cell culture reagents: Culture medium, FCS, PBS, and Turk blue.

Table 1
Binding of peptide analogues to murine MHC class II molecules

MHC class II-transfected cells	Hybridoma	Test peptide
I-A^d (**RT 2.3.3H**)	26.2	^{12}LEDARRLKAIYEKKK^{26} of bacteriophage λ repressor (cI)
I-E^d (**10.3H2**)	26.1	^{12}LEDARRLKAIYEKKK^{26} cI
I-A^k	E7E9	β2 adrenergic receptor peptide (human) ^{16}GSHAPDHDVTQQRDEVWV^{33}C
I-E^k	8I	^{12}LEDARRLKAIYEKKK^{26} cI

Refs. 6, 42–45

3. EasyLyse (Ref. S2364, DAKO, Glostrup, Denmark) for lysing red blood cells.
4. Mice: MRL/lpr lupus mice and CBA/J mice (or another MHC-matched strain).
5. Peptides of high purity (>90 % by HPLC) and checked by MS.

3 Methods

3.1 Method for Generating Self-Peptides (see Note 1)

Assay Principle: The introduction in 1963 of the concept of solid-phase peptide synthesis (SPPS) by Merrifield considerably modified the existing state of the art [10]. This methodology revolutionized the synthesis of peptides and allowed the rapid production of synthetic antigens, biologically active peptides, artificial proteins, active enzymes, and peptide libraries. However, in spite of the rapidity and efficiency of classical SPPS, the amount of work required for synthesizing the hundreds and thousands of different peptides and peptide analogues needed for epitope mapping and for screening immunological and biological activities of proteins has become quickly prohibitive. For many preliminary studies, only a small amount (few mgs) of each peptide is required. As the result, considerable efforts have been made to develop supports and techniques for multiple peptide synthesis (reviewed in [2]).

1. If possible, use a peptide synthesis facility equipped with a fully automated simultaneous multichannel synthesizer, which allows chemists to prepare up to 40–80 test peptides of 15–20 residues in amounts of 10–20 mg in reduced lapse of time (1 month).
2. Peptides are assembled using classical 9-fluorenylmethyloxycarbonyl (Fmoc) chemistry. This method of synthesis uses the Fmoc group for protecting the α-NH_2 function [11] and the *tert*-butyl group for protecting the side chain functionalities of the amino acid residues.

3. At the completion of synthesis, cleave the peptides from the resin and de-protect them using trifluoroacetic acid/dithiothreitol/triisopropylsilane/water cleavage cocktail for 2.5 h. After filtration from the resin, add cold ether to the cocktail solution to precipitate the peptide.
4. After low speed centrifugation, dissolve the pellets in a water/acetonitrile/acetic acid (75/20/10; v/v/v) mixture and lyophilize.
5. Purify the peptides by preparative reversed-phase chromatography and keep them lyophilized at −20 °C.
6. For use, prepare a stock solution of each peptide (in general 1 mM). First, let the vials containing peptides at RT for 30 min before opening to avoid moisture. Weigh the amount of peptide necessary for the experiment. If the peptide is hydrophilic, add ultrapure water, gently mix the tube (or better sonicate) until the powder is completely dissolved. When the peptide is hydrophobic, add first pure dimethyl sulfoxide (DMSO), sonicate and then add ultrapure water to obtain a final concentration of 10 % (v/v) DMSO. Let the peptide solution 10 min at RT to make sure the peptide is completely dissolved. This stock solution can then be diluted in culture medium.

3.2 Method for T Cell Epitope Mapping (See Notes 2–4)

Assay Principle: The general strategy in T cell epitope mapping is to design a peptide library consisting of overlapping peptide sequences that cover the entire protein of interest. Through the use of such overlapping peptide sets, epitopes can be identified in a systematic and thorough manner. $CD4^+$ T cells recognize MHC class II-bound peptide fragments of 15–25 amino acid length. Therefore, we generally realize helper T cell autoepitope mapping by using peptide sequences based on a peptide length around 20 residues and amino acid overlaps of 5–10 (for a detailed procedure, *see* [12]).

1. Isolate peripheral blood mononuclear cell (PBMCs; fraction containing any blood cell having a round nucleus) or peripheral blood lymphocytes (PBLs; fraction containing mature lymphocytes) and wash them three times in enriched RPMI 1640 medium.
2. Resuspend cells at 3×10^6 cells/mL in the above medium (in the case of peptides from the U1-70K protein, and for the screening step, the proliferative response to overlapping peptides was measured in duplicate using 3×10^5 cells/well and a single peptide 120 μM-concentration).
3. After 72 h, pulse the cultures during 18 h with [^{3}H] thymidine (1 μCi/well) and measure DNA-incorporated radioactivity. Cytokine secretion can be measured in the supernatants using the assays described below (*see* Subheadings 3.3–3.6).

4. Control: Introduce several wells containing Con-A (100 μL/well; 5 μg/mL; as positive control) during the time (90 h) of the culture or no peptide (as negative control). Additional control can be anti-CD4 mAb GK1.5 (PharMingen, 10 μg/mL) added to the culture.
5. Data analysis: Express the results both in terms of cpm and as stimulation index corresponding to cpm in the cultures with peptide/cpm in the cultures without peptide. A mean stimulation index >3 can be considered to be positive in the case of autoreactive T cells. The average [^{3}H]-thymidine incorporation in the absence of peptide is low (~100 cpm in our own experiments). The standard deviation (SD) of duplicate cultures should always remain below 20 % of the mean.
6. Repeat the assay several times in independent experiments as important variations can occur, mostly depending on individual mice. Note also that the age of mice is a crucial point. A series of preliminary experiments at different ages should be processed to evaluate the best window for testing. Ideally, for each antigen to be analyzed, strains of mice of different MHC haplotypes and different ages should be tested.

3.3 IL-2 (and IL-4) Bioassay (see Note 5)

Assay Principle: Murine IL-2 secretion can be evaluated using CTL-L cells that are dependent on IL-2 for growing (cytotoxic T cell clone derived from a C57BL/6 mouse; [13]).

1. Prepare CTL-L IL-2-dependent cells by amplifying 1×10^5 cells/mL in the presence of mouse recombinant IL-2 (10 U/mL of culture) in culture flasks and incubate at 37 °C.
2. After 2 days, collect CTL-L cells and wash them at least three times in medium without IL-2. Thaw supernatants and prepare a standard scale beginning at 90 U/mL and diluted 1/2, with recombinant IL-2 as control.
3. Dispense 1×10^4 CTL-L cells per well (in 50 μL of culture medium) and incubate at 37 °C for 24 h. Add 50 μL of [^{3}H]-thymidine to each well (1 μCi/well) and return the plates to the incubator for approximately 6 h.
4. Harvest the contents of each well onto filter mats using an automated cell harvester and determine the radioactivity with a beta-counter.
5. Secretion of IL-4 can be assayed using the same principle by adding culture supernatant to 1×10^4 IL-4-dependent CT4.S cells/well [14].
6. Control: As a control, replace the peptide of interest by a scrambled peptide (that has the same composition in amino acid residues but in a scrambled order).
7. Data analysis: Incorporate a standard curve by making serial dilutions of an IL-2 solution of known concentration

(e.g., commercial IL-2 from PharMingen). Plot standard curves as the standard cytokine protein concentration (U/mL of IL-2) versus the corresponding mean cpm of replicates, ideally triplicates. The concentration of IL-2 in the supernatants is interpolated from this standard curve (use a computer software program that facilitates data analysis). Also perform a dilution series of the unknown culture supernatants to be assured that the cpm values will fall within the linear portion of the standard curve.

3.4 Cytokine ELISAs

Assay Principle: Cytokine secretion can also be evaluated by double-sandwich ELISA using commercial Abs and self-coated polyvinyl or polystyrene plates, or commercial ELISA kits containing all required reagents and devices. Standard curves are performed with known concentrations of commercially available recombinant cytokines. In our own conditions, the minimal levels of detectable mouse cytokines are 3 U/mL IFN-γ, 0.5 U/mL IL-4, 0.3 U/mL IL-6, and 5 U/mL IL-10. Conditions used for IL-4, described below as an example, are as follows:

1. Pre-sensitize polyvinyl microtiter plates (Falcon) overnight at 4 °C with 50 μL of a rat anti-mouse IL-4 Ab (PharMingen) at 2 μg/mL in 0.05 M carbonate buffer, pH 9.6.
2. After three washings of the microtiter plates with PBS containing 0.05 % Tween (PBS-T), add BSA (1 % w/v) in PBS-T (PBS-T-BSA) for 2 h at RT.
3. After repeated washings, add 50 μL supernatant or 50 μL recombinant IL-4 (0–300 U/mL; PharMingen) used as control for 4 h at RT.
4. After three washings with PBS-T, add 100 μL of a rat anti-mouse IL-4 Ab conjugated to biotin (PharMingen) diluted 1/1,000 in PBS-T-BSA for 45 min at RT.
5. After repeated washings, positive reactions are detected by adding avidin conjugated to peroxidase (Sigma) at a 1/50,000 dilution for 30 min at RT.
6. To visualize the final reaction, add TMB as chromogen and H_2O_2 as substrate. TMB yields soluble blue end product that can be analyzed kinetically (note that because it is soluble this chromogenic substance of peroxidase is not appropriate for membrane applications or immunohistochemistry).
7. After 15 min (for end-point reaction), stop the reaction by adding 1.0 M HCl yielding in deep yellow color.
8. Measure the resulting absorbance at 450 nm on a plate reader.
9. Control: When serum cytokine levels are measured, include serum (or a pool of sera) of untreated mice as control. When culture supernatants are tested, include supernatants of untreated cells as control.

10. Data analysis: Incorporate a standard curve by making serial dilutions of an IL-4 solution of known concentration (commercial IL-4 from PharMingen). Plot standard curves as the standard cytokine protein concentration (pg or U/mL of IL-4) versus the corresponding mean OD value of replicates. The concentration of IL-4-containing samples is interpolated from this standard curve (use a computer software program that facilitates data analysis). Also perform serial dilutions of the unknown samples to be assured that the OD values will fall within the linear portion of the standard curve.

By convention, determine the sensitivity of the assay in choosing the lowest cytokine concentration that gives a signal which is at least 2–3 SD above the mean background signal value.

3.5 Method for Cytokine Membrane Array Measurements

Assay Principle: A wide assortment of tests have been devised for multiplex cytokine analysis. Such assays permit the measurement of several cytokines and chemokines simultaneously in the same small-volume biological samples (e.g., serum/plasma or cell lysates). They are either multiplex sandwich ELISAs combined with microspot technology (this section) or bead-based assays (*see* Subheading 3.6). Regarding array-based multiplex sandwich ELISA systems, several types of assays are commercially available. They combine the high specificity/sensitivity criteria of ELISAs and the high throughput potential of the arrays. Like traditional sandwich-based ELISAs, they are based on a pair of cytokine-/chemokine-specific Abs for detection. A capture Ab is first bound to the surface (e.g., a membrane or a glass solid support). After incubation with the sample, the target cytokine/chemokine present in the serum/plasma or cell lysates is trapped on the solid surface. A second biotin-labeled detection Ab is then added, which can recognize a distinct region of the target cytokine/chemokine. The binding of the latter can then be visualized through the addition of the streptavidin-labeled fluorescent dye using a laser scanner. By arraying multiple cytokine-/chemokine-specific capture Abs onto the solid support, multiplex detection of cytokines/chemokines in a single experiment is made possible (*see* **Note 6**).

Since some of these multiplex assays are relatively expensive, different approaches can be followed; the one we employ for screening potentially active peptides is based on semiquantitative methods.

1. Isolate PBMCs or PBLs from MRL/lpr lupus-prone mice (3×10^6 cells/mL) and incubate cells with individual peptides for 48 h. It is not pertinent to mix different peptides since some of them may have antagonist activities or act as partial agonists of the T cell receptor, modulating the cytokine profile and therefore interfering with the cytokines induced by other peptides of the mix.

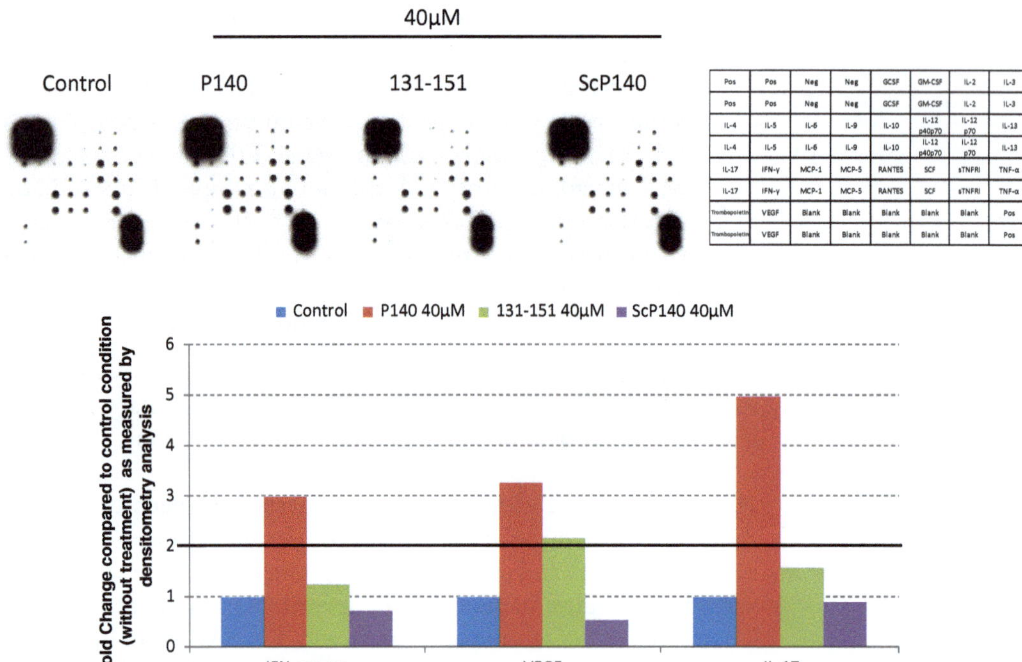

Pos	Pos	Neg	Neg	GCSF	GM-CSF	IL-2	IL-3
Pos	Pos	Neg	Neg	GCSF	GM-CSF	IL-2	IL-3
IL-4	IL-5	IL-6	IL-9	IL-10	IL-12 p40p70	IL-12 p70	IL-13
IL-4	IL-5	IL-6	IL-9	IL-10	IL-12 p40p70	IL-12 p70	IL-13
IL-17	IFN-γ	MCP-1	MCP-5	RANTES	SCF	sTNFRI	TNF-α
IL-17	IFN-γ	MCP-1	MCP-5	RANTES	SCF	sTNFRI	TNF-α
Trombopoietin	VEGF	Blank	Blank	Blank	Blank	Blank	Pos
Trombopoietin	VEGF	Blank	Blank	Blank	Blank	Blank	Pos

Fig. 1 Ex vivo cytokine measurements using an array-based multiplex ELISA system on membranes. PBMCs collected from a MRL/lpr mouse (3×10^6 cells/mL) were incubated for 48 h with 40 μM of either phosphorylated peptide P140 or the non-phosphorylated form of the peptide (i.e., peptide 131-151) or the scrambled peptide P140 (ScP140) right (top) panel. The supernatants were incubated with membranes (here displaying 22 different cytokines) following the instructions of the supplier (kit RayBio® cytokine antibody array). Controls are supernatants from cells incubated without peptide. The position of cytokines and controls is indicated on the *right* panel

2. Spin the cells down (320×*g*, 5 min) and collect the supernatants.
3. Incubate the supernatants with membranes and perform the test strictly according to the manufacturer's protocol (recommended sample dilutions, standard curve concentration, duplicates).
4. Controls: Supernatants from cells incubated without peptide (Fig. 1; kit RayBio® cytokine antibody array).
5. Control: Fresh medium containing FCS used for culturing cells.
6. Data analysis: Analyze spot intensity by densitometry (Image J, NIH) and express the results by subtracting density of blank and control from each cytokine density value.

3.6 Method for Cytokine Measurement by Bead-Based Flow Cytometric Assay

Assay Principle: In this test format, capture Abs specific for distinct cytokines are covalently linked to beads of different sizes that are differentiated on FL-3 cytometer channel. After incubation with sample, phycoerythrin (PE)-linked Ab conjugates (emitting in the FL-2 channel) that are specific for individual cytokine ensure

FL-2 signal. Fluorescence intensity for each of cytokines is obtained by plotting FL-2 versus FL-3 signals. This cytometric method allows obtaining very high sensibility and reproducibility of data; it is quantitative and automatable [15–17]. The procedure described below allows quantitative detection of seven cytokines simultaneously, namely, IL-2, IL-4, IL-6, IFN-γ, TNF, IL-17A, and IL-10.

1. The assay detailed below (BD Cytometric Bead Array Mouse Thl/Th2/Th17 cytokine kit from PharMingen) is run according to the instructions provided by the manufacturer.
2. Open one vial of lyophilized mouse Thl/Th2/Th17 standard and reconstitute with 2.0 mL of assay diluent. Transfer 300 μL to the 1:2 dilution tube and mix thoroughly. Dilute 1:1 until the 1:256 dilution.
3. Add a 10 μL aliquot of each capture bead to each assay tube into a single tube labeled "mixed capture beads."
4. Use undiluted samples (MRL/lpr lupus-prone serum or culture supernatant).
5. Mix (Vortex) the mixed capture beads and add 50 μL to each of assay tubes. Add 50 μL of the mouse Thl/Th2/Th17 cytokine standard dilutions to the control tube (the cytokine standard dilution 1:1 corresponds to 5,000 pg/mL and therefore the 1:256 dilution to ~20 pg/mL). Add 50 μL of each MRL/lpr serum or culture supernatant to the appropriately labeled sample assay tubes.
6. Add 50 μL of the mouse Thl/Th2/Th17 PE detection reagent to each assay tubes. Incubate for 2 h at RT (protected from light).
7. Add 1 mL of wash buffer to each assay tube and centrifuge at 200 × *g* for 5 min. Carefully discard the supernatant from each assay tube and add 300 μL of wash buffer per tube to resuspend the bead pellet.
8. Perform analysis on cytometer.
9. Control: For standard, use assay diluent only as negative control (0 pg/mL). For MRL/lpr mice, use the serum of lupus mice that were not treated with the therapeutic peptide, for example, and/or from normal mice. For culture supernatant, use the supernatant of cells that were not treated with the peptide, for example.
10. Data analysis: Plot standard curves as the standard cytokine concentration (pg/mL) versus the corresponding geometric mean. The concentration of unknown sample (supernatant or serum) is interpolated from each cytokine standard curve.

3.7 Binding of Self-Peptides to Murine MHC Class II Molecules

Assay Principle: The capacity of peptides to bind MHCII molecule is measured by their ability to inhibit IL-2 secreted by a specific T cell hybridoma that recognizes a test peptide presented in the context of the said MHCII molecule (mouse L fibroblasts transfected by either class II molecules, I-A^d, I-E^d, I-A^k, or I-E^k, used as antigen-presenting cells, APCs; Table 1). The conditions described below have been used with success to identify MHC restriction usage of peptides from different self-peptides [12, 18–20].

1. Add increasing concentrations (0–90 μM) of peptide to wells of 96-well flat bottom microplates (BD Biosciences) and allow them to incubate at 37 °C with individual T cell hybridoma and respective class II molecules transfected cells (5×10^4 cells/well for each cell type) in the presence of test peptide.
2. Collect the culture supernatants 24 h later (centrifuge at $320 \times g$ for 5 min), and use a double-sandwich ELISA or a bioassay to measure IL-2 secretion using known concentrations of recombinant IL-2 (PharMingen) as the test calibration (see above).
3. Control: As control, replace the peptide of interest by a scrambled peptide; use a peptide that is not normally recognized in the context of the APCs that is tested or by the hybridoma that is used to reveal the reaction.
4. Data analysis: Analyze dose-response curves using a three-parameter sigmoid curve (Sigmaplot, SPSS, Chicago, IL).

3.8 Hyperproliferation Measurement

Assay Principle: MRL/lpr lupus-prone mice, which are the most commonly studied mice model of the disease, bear an autosomic recessive mutation in the gene encoding Fas [21]. The MRL$^{+/+}$ background is responsible for the development of autoimmune kidney disease, and the lymphoproliferation (lpr)/*Fas* mutation converts a mild nephritis into a much severe disease, with a 50 % mortality rate at 24 weeks of age [22, 23]. In vivo properties of test peptides can be easily evaluated by measuring the decrease of abnormal peripheral hypercellularity in mice post peptide in vivo exposure [6].

1. Inject 11–13-week-old MRL/lpr mice intravenously with peptides of interest (100 μg peptide/mouse; 10 mice/condition) and administrate saline only in the so-called nontreated group.
2. Five days after peptide injection, collect 200 μL of blood from each mouse. Lyse red blood cells using DAKO EasyLyse (Code-Nr. S2364) according to the manufacturer's protocol (use the procedure "B" on lysing procedure protocol).
3. Suspend cells in 200 μL PBS containing 2 % (v/v) FCS and dilute them in Turk blue (ultrapure water, 0.5 % acetic acid, 0.01 % methyl violet) (50 μL cells + 50 μL Turk blue) to visualize cells.

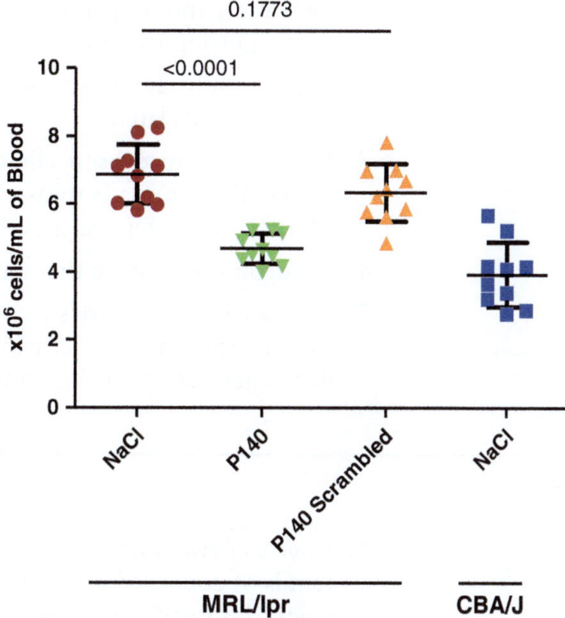

Fig. 2 In vivo effect of P140 peptide on peripheral hypercellularity. 11–13-week-old female MRL/lpr received intravenously a single administration of peptides in saline, either peptide P140 or scrambled peptide P140 (ScP140) used as a control peptide or saline only. The number of leukocytes/mL was evaluated by counting cells 5 days later. Each symbol represents one individual mouse (ten mice/group). *Horizontal bars* represent the respective average cell count values. Statistical significance was assessed using the Student's *t*-test. The number of peripheral leukocytes/mL in a healthy mouse (CBA/J mouse) is shown for comparison

4. Count cells using a Malassez counting chamber.
5. Control: CBA/J mice (or another MHC-matched strain) should be tested as healthy control group.
6. Data analysis: express results as the number of cells per mL/blood. The blood from mice that received saline only is used as control. Statistical significance in the measurement of cellularity is assessed using the Student's *t*-test. An example of result is shown in Fig. 2.

3.9 Application of Therapy in Model Animals (See Notes 7 and 8)

Assay Principle: In the case of peptide P140, the protocol adopted was as follows [24, 25]. Young pre-lupus female MRL/lpr mice receive four times the peptide P140 in saline via the intravenous route. A control group is given saline only. Measurements of outcome include the evaluation of survival, proteinuria, dermatitis, vasculitis, and serum Ab levels, in particular anti-dsDNA Abs that are biomarkers of the lupus disease.

1. Administer the peptide intravenously to 4-week-old female MRL/lpr mice (100 μg/mouse; groups of a minimum of ten

mice per peptide; peptide in saline). Inject saline only to the control group (ten mice).

2. Repeat these administrations twice at 2-week intervals and again 4 weeks later.
3. Follow the mice both clinically and biologically for several weeks. Proteinuria is measured on a fresh urine sample using Albutix (Bayer Diagnostics, Basingstoke, UK).
4. Control: Lupus mice that receive saline only.
5. Data analysis: Analyze survival of control and peptide-treated mice by the Kaplan-Meier method. Determine significance of differences using the log-rank test.

4 Notes

1. *Choice of Autoantigen*: The antigen selected as cognate protein is of course of prime importance. In peptide-based strategies designed to immunomodulate autoreactive T cells, sequences encompassing T cell epitopes already localized in key antigens can be used (e.g., [26–29]). If not known, or if proprietary sequences are preferred, a first identification of T cell epitopes recognized by $CD4^+$ T cells has to be envisaged. "Key antigens" can be proteins known to be recognized by autoAbs since it has been found that B and T cell epitopes often overlap in autoantigens [27]. It was our own starting point when we engaged ourselves in the P140 program in using the spliceosomal U1-70K small nuclear ribonucleoprotein. The latter is one of the major spliceosomal autoantigens, for which autoAbs can be found in 30 % of patients with SLE and 100 % of patients with mixed connective tissue disease.
2. *T Cell Epitope Mapping Strategy*: This strategy has been applied, for example, to the murine spliceosomal U1-70K [20] and heterogeneous nuclear ribonucleoprotein A2 [30].
3. *Synthetic Peptides Bearing Posttranslational Modifications*: Most of the primary amino acid residues are susceptible to undergo some types of posttranslational modification (acetylation, phosphorylation, methylation, deamination, ubiquitination, etc.). Solid-phase peptide chemistry offers the possibility of introducing during synthesis-modified residues and cofactors that are normally or abnormally present in numerous biological molecules or added at specific stages of the cell cycle. This strategy is particularly attractive since several antigens targeted by autoAbs contain such modified residues and cofactors and since there is evidence that modified self-antigens play an important role in disease pathogenesis [27, 31–34].

Two-dimensional gel analysis of U1-70K protein has revealed the existence of at least 13 isoelectric variants which are all phosphorylated in the cell at four (or more) serine residues. However, the origin of most of the isoelectric variants is another type of posttranslational modifications such as acetylation of lysine residues [35, 36]. In the context of our study, when the "lead" peptide 131–151 encompassing a $CD4^+$ T cell epitope had been delineated, it was tempting to rationally introduce such individual modifications, which may have varying effects on MHC class II binding and/or T cell recognition. Two peptides bearing a phospho group on Ser^{137} or Ser^{140} and two peptides bearing an acetyl group on Lys^{137} or Lys^{142} were synthesized and evaluated [24].

4. *Quality of Peptides, Peptide Purification*: Despite all the refinements brought to peptide chemistry, side reactions still occur during synthesis and cleavage of peptides. On the other hand, crude or improperly purified peptides generally rapidly degrade, even if they are kept freeze-dried. It is thus necessary that each peptide follows a careful purification process. When used as antigens in culture supernatant for sensitizing target cells or with APCs for T cell recognition, synthetic peptides need to display a purity of at least 85 %. When used for therapeutic approaches into animal models, peptides should be at an even higher purity (>95 %). Peptides of the U1-70K protein were systematically purified by preparative reversed-phase chromatography on a C18-silica matrix (C8 or C4 when peptide was highly hydrophobic). Integrity of each peptide was confirmed by mass spectrometry.
5. *IL-2 Secretion*: IL2 secretion test has to be very sensitive because it is well known that in lupus mice IL-2 production is weak in response to stimulation. IL-2-dependent CTL-L cells have to be used for assay on the day they are to be fed and a careful calibration is required. In particular, do not use the cells if the amplification in the presence of IL-2 was less than 10. Peptide dose-dependent response should be checked to conclude that the peptide effectively contains a specific epitope for Th cells.
6. *Cytokine Assay Choice*: Qualitative or semiquantitative approaches have to be considered as a screening method. Additional methods should be used to confirm and quantitate the amount of cytokines that are secreted. Densitometry studies of spots can be made but they remain indicative, not quantitatively relevant. In our hands, the levels of cytokines circulating in the sera of MRL/lpr were too weak to allow reliable detection. Although expensive for such a peptide screening phase, high sensitivity multiplex cytokine and chemokine assays that are quantitative can also be used in a first

intention tests. They allow testing much more cytokines and chemokines in parallel, and a quantitative measurement of their level can be studied. Such assays are available from Bio-Rad, Biosource/Invitrogen, and Lino/Millipore, for example. Multisite comparisons of different high sensitivity multiplex cytokine assays have been made that highlight the interest and some limitations of such methods and suggest recommendations [15, 16].

7. *An Appropriate Animal Model*: A large part of success in the quest of potential drug substances discovery depends on the availability of relevant animal models. The latter are used not only to test the therapeutic efficacy of new molecules but also to evaluate their toxicity and possible long-lasting effects in the pathophysiological context of the disease and in the absence of any other treatment. It is also crucial to determine quickly and at an early time of screening whether the molecules under study have the potential to be safe and well tolerated in addition to be effective. Choosing an appropriate animal model is therefore central in the development of therapeutics, particularly in the context of autoimmunity, since the immune system and many other cellular dysfunctions coexist and spiral out of control. While there are a variety of induced mouse models that develop rheumatoid arthritis-like diseases, for example, readily available mouse strains that naturally display lupus features or that are experimentally induced to develop the disease are much more seldom [37]. Some of them, such as MRL/lpr mice and (NZBxNZW)F1 (NZB/W) mice, are commercially available, others are not, an additional complication when large groups of animals of the same age are required to test different parameters in statistically compatible conditions. A minimum of ten animals of the same age and sex (ideally females to mimic the human lupus disease) should be included per arm to evaluate one test condition, and experiments have to be repeated several times to prevent any cage, season, and estrous cycle influence. Series of 100 or more mice of the same age and sex are often required to evaluate a few conditions and include control arms.

   Although mouse models of lupus have been pivotal to our current understanding of lupus pathogenesis, none of them is totally satisfactory. We have to admit that due to the highly complex nature of SLE, it is virtually impossible to generate a model mouse that recapitulates all the typical features, and only those of this multifactorial syndrome. Thus, MRL/lpr mice (H-2^k haplotype) develop an SLE-like phenotype that differs from the human disease by features such as a massive T cell proliferation due to the recessive autosomal mutation *lpr*, which alters transcription of the Fas receptor, circulating IgM and IgG rheumatoid factors, and gene alterations that have not been detected so far in lupus patients. Both males and females are affected and both develop spontaneous arthritis similar to those observed in rheumatoid arthritis. NZB/W mice (H-$2^{d/z}$ haplotype) lack autoAbs reacting to spliceosomal ribonucleoproteins that are frequent in lupus patients and MRL/lpr mice. This absence of Ab reactivity, while largely reported in the literature, should be reconsidered, however, following our own observations that NZB/W mice, as MRL/lpr mice, do produce Ab reacting with several distinct small nuclear and heterogeneous nuclear ribonucleoproteins [38]. Male BXSB mouse, a recombinant inbred strain issued from a cross between C57BL/6 and SB/Le strains, develops a severe form of lupus-like disease, which is largely dependent on the Y chromosome associated with accelerated autoimmunity (*Yaa*) gene (female develops a very mild disease only). The proliferating cells in BXSB mice are rather of B type, while they are mainly of T type in MRL/lpr mice.

A few lupus-induced models have been developed. They include chronic graft versus host disease model [19, 39] and normal mice in which substances such as pristane, mercury chloride, or DNA peptide mimics are administrated [37, 40]. They offer the unique opportunity to allow testing several biological parameters before and after induction and might be used to evaluate potential therapeutic molecules. In practice, they are seldom used if any for this purpose, in part because it is difficult to generate sufficient groups of animals for large-scale studies.

Ideally, an appropriate mouse model should display a clinical and biological phenotype as close as possible from the one observed in the human disease. The disease should progress relatively rapidly (to facilitate visualizing the delay of symptom appearance) and should affect the very large majority of individuals. The selected strain should also present a relatively normal rate of fertility to generate enough recipients. Finally, biomarkers easy to measure with sensitive routine assays should be available to follow the course of the disease and its improvement. In the P140 peptide program, we opted for female MRL/lpr mice because they meet a large number of these criteria. Half of MRL/lpr mice remains at 21 weeks compared to 34 weeks in the case of female NZB/W mice [41]. The beneficial effect of the peptide P140 was routinely followed by measuring white cell counts in the peripheral blood (reduction of hyperproliferation), autoAb production (anti-dsDNA Abs),

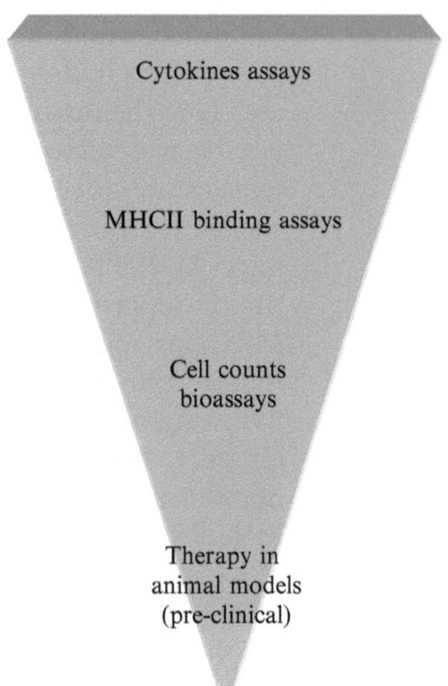

Fig. 3 "Go-no go" screens used in the P140 peptide program for lupus

proteinuria, and survival after peptide administration into prediseased, young MRL/lpr mice (Fig. 3).

8. Discovery of self-peptides to treat SLE requires possessing expertise in terms of peptide chemistry, immunochemistry, and cell biology to elaborate on potentially decisive pathways. It requires also a part of luck and observation capability as some peptide tools can emerge serendipitously from experiments that were not initially designed to this end. Wishing strictly predetermine a chart for discovering new pharmacological tools is not a warrant for success. Yet, when a potential peptide is discovered, key determining steps have to be strictly fulfilled to ensure it is "the" candidate. The road is long, the obstacles are numerous, sometimes trivial. Bringing a new molecule to the market, particularly in chronic diseases such as SLE, remains a real challenge.

Acknowledgments

Research in the authors' laboratory is financially supported by the French Centre National de la Recherche Scientifique, the Laboratory of Excellence Medalis (ANR-10-LABX-0034), Initiative of Excellence (IdEx), Strasbourg University, Région Alsace, and ImmuPharma France.

References

1. Zompra AA, Galanis AS, Werbitzky O, Albericio F (2009) Manufacturing peptides as active pharmaceutical ingredients. Future Med Chem 1:361–377
2. Briand JP, Muller S (2005) Synthetic peptides for the analysis of B-cell epitopes in autoantigens. In: Pollard KM (ed) Autoantibodies and autoimmunity: molecular mechanisms in health and disease. Weinheim, Wiley-VCH, pp 189–224
3. Gentilucci L, De Marco R, Cerisoli L (2010) Chemical modifications designed to improve peptide stability: incorporation of non-natural amino acids, pseudo-peptide bonds, and cyclization. Curr Pharm Des 16:3185–3203
4. Partidos CD, Beignon AS, Semetey V, Briand JP, Muller S (2001) The bare skin and the nose as non-invasive routes for administering peptide vaccines. Vaccine 19:2708–2715
5. Briand JP, Muller S (2010) Emerging peptide therapeutics for inflammatory autoimmune diseases. Curr Pharm Des 16:1136–1142
6. Schall N, Page N, Macri C, Chaloin O, Briand JP, Muller S (2012) Peptide-based approaches to treat lupus and other autoimmune diseases. J Autoimmun 39:143–153
7. Steinman L, Merrill JT, Mcinnes IB, Peakman M (2012) Optimization of current and future therapy for autoimmune diseases. Nat Med 18:59–65
8. Zimmer R, Scherbarth HR, Rillo OL, Gomez-Reino JJ, Muller S (2013) Lupuzor/P140 peptide in patients with systemic lupus erythematosus: a randomised, double-blind, placebo-controlled phase IIb clinical trial. Ann Rheum Dis 72:1830–1835
9. Neimark J, Briand JP (1993) Development of a fully automated multichannel peptide synthesizer with integrated TFA cleavage capability. Pept Res 6:219–228
10. Merrifield RB (1963) Solid phase peptide synthesis. I. The synthesis of a tetrapeptide. J Am Chem Soc 85:2149–2154
11. Carpino LA, Han GY (1970) The 9-fluorenylmethoxycarbonyl function, a new base-sensitive amino-protecting group. J Am Chem Soc 92:5748–5749
12. Monneaux F, Muller S (2000) Laboratory protocols for the identification of Th cell epitopes on self-antigens in mice with systemic autoimmune diseases. J Immunol Methods 244:195–204
13. Baker PE, Gillis S, Smith KA (1979) Monoclonal cytolytic T-cell lines. J Exp Med 149:273–278
14. Hu-Li J, Ohara J, Watson C, Tsang W, Paul WE (1989) Derivation of a T cell line that is highly responsive to IL-4 and IL-2 (CT.4R) and of an IL-2 hyporesponsive mutant of that line (CT.4S). J Immunol 142:800–807
15. Breen EC, Reynolds SM, Cox C, Jacobson LP, Magpantay L, Mulder CB et al (2011) Multisite comparison of high-sensitivity multiplex cytokine assays. Clin Vaccine Immunol 18:1229–1242
16. Lash GE, Scaife PJ, Innes BA, Otun HA, Robson SC, Searle RF et al (2006) Comparison of three multiplex cytokine analysis systems: Luminex, SearchLight and FAST Quant. J Immunol Methods 309:205–208
17. Morgan E, Varro R, Sepulveda H, Ember JA, Apgar J, Wilson J et al (2004) Cytometric bead array: a multiplexed assay platform with applications in various areas of biology. Clin Immunol 110:252–266
18. Dali H, Busnel O, Hoebeke J, Bi L, Decker P, Briand JP et al (2007) Heteroclitic properties of mixed alpha- and aza-beta3-peptides mimicking a supradominant CD4 T cell epitope presented by nucleosome. Mol Immunol 44:3024–3036
19. Mézière C, Stockl F, Batsford S, Vogt A, Muller S (1994) Antibodies to DNA, chromatin core particles and histones in mice with graft-versus-host disease and their involvement in glomerular injury. Clin Exp Immunol 98:287–294
20. Monneaux F, Briand JP, Muller S (2000) B and T cell immune response to small nuclear ribonucleoprotein particles in lupus mice: autoreactive CD4(+) T cells recognize a T cell epitope located within the RNP80 motif of the 70K protein. Eur J Immunol 30:2191–2200
21. Nagata S, Suda T (1995) Fas and Fas ligand: lpr and gld mutations. Immunol Today 16:39–43
22. Cohen PL, Eisenberg RA (1991) Lpr and gld: single gene models of systemic autoimmunity and lymphoproliferative disease. Annu Rev Immunol 9:243–269
23. Theofilopoulos AN, Dixon FJ (1985) Murine models of systemic lupus erythematosus. Adv Immunol 37:269–390
24. Monneaux F, Lozano JM, Patarroyo ME, Briand JP, Muller S (2003) T cell recognition and therapeutic effect of a phosphorylated synthetic peptide of the 70K snRNP protein administered in MR/lpr mice. Eur J Immunol 33:287–296
25. Page N, Gros F, Schall N, Décossas M, Bagnard D, Briand JP et al (2011) HSC70 blockade by the therapeutic peptide P140

affects autophagic processes and endogenous MHCII presentation in murine lupus. Ann Rheum Dis 70:837–843

26. Fournel S, Neichel S, Dali H, Farci S, Maillère B, Briand JP et al (2003) CD4+ T cells from (New Zealand Black x New Zealand White) F1 lupus mice and normal mice immunized against apoptotic nucleosomes recognize similar Th cell epitopes in the C terminus of histone H3. J Immunol 171:636–644
27. Hoffmann MH, Trembleau S, Muller S, Steiner G (2010) Nucleic acid-associated autoantigens: pathogenic involvement and therapeutic potential. J Autoimmun 34:J178–J206
28. Kaliyaperumal A, Michaels MA, Datta SK (1999) Antigen-specific therapy of murine lupus nephritis using nucleosomal peptides: tolerance spreading impairs pathogenic function of autoimmune T and B cells. J Immunol 162:5775–5783
29. Suen JL, Chuang YH, Tsai BY, Yau PM, Chiang BL (2004) Treatment of murine lupus using nucleosomal T cell epitopes identified by bone marrow-derived dendritic cells. Arthritis Rheum 50:3250–3259
30. Dumortier H, Monneaux F, Jahn-Schmid B, Briand JP, Skriner K, Cohen PL et al (2000) B and T cell responses to the spliceosomal heterogeneous nuclear ribonucleoproteins A2 and B1 in normal and lupus mice. J Immunol 165:2297–2305
31. Dieker JW, Fransen JH, Van Bavel CC, Briand JP, Jacobs CW, Muller S et al (2007) Apoptosis-induced acetylation of histones is pathogenic in systemic lupus erythematosus. Arthritis Rheum 56:1921–1933
32. Plaué S, Muller S, Van Regenmortel MH (1989) A branched, synthetic octapeptide of ubiquitinated histone H2A as target of autoantibodies. J Exp Med 169:1607–1617
33. Van Bavel CC, Dieker JW, Kroeze Y, Tamboer WP, Voll R, Muller S et al (2011) Apoptosis-induced histone H3 methylation is targeted by autoantibodies in systemic lupus erythematosus. Ann Rheum Dis 70:201–207
34. Dieker J, Muller S (2010) Epigenetic histone code and autoimmunity. Clin Rev Allergy Immunol 39:78–84
35. Woppmann A, Patschinsky T, Bringmann P, Godt F, Lührmann R (1990) Characterisation of human and murine snRNP proteins by two-dimensional gel electrophoresis and phosphopeptide analysis of U1-specific 70K protein variants. Nucleic Acids Res 18:4427–4438
36. Woppmann A, Will CL, Kornstadt U, Zuo P, Manley JL, Lührmann R (1993) Identification of an snRNP-associated kinase activity that phosphorylates arginine/serine rich domains typical of splicing factors. Nucleic Acids Res 21:2815–2822
37. Perry D, Sang A, Yin Y, Zheng YY, Morel L (2011) Murine models of systemic lupus erythematosus. J Biomed Biotechnol 2011: 271694
38. Monneaux F, Dumortier H, Steiner G, Briand JP, Muller S (2001) Murine models of systemic lupus erythematosus: B and T cell responses to spliceosomal ribonucleoproteins in MRL/Fas(lpr) and (NZB x NZW)F(1) lupus mice. Int Immunol 13:1155–1163
39. Schroeder MA, Dipersio JF (2011) Mouse models of graft-versus-host disease: advances and limitations. Dis Model Mech 4:318–333
40. Rottman JB, Willis CR (2010) Mouse models of systemic lupus erythematosus reveal a complex pathogenesis. Vet Pathol 47:664–676
41. Dixon FJ (1981) Murine systemic lupus erythematosus. Immunol Today 2:8–9
42. Guillet JG, Lai MZ, Briner TJ, Buus S, Sette A, Grey HM et al (1987) Immunological self, nonself discrimination. Science 235:865–870
43. Lai MZ, Ross DT, Guillet JG, Briner TJ, Gefter ML, Smith JA (1987) T lymphocyte response to bacteriophage lambda repressor cI protein. Recognition of the same peptide presented by Ia molecules of different haplotypes. J Immunol 139:3973–3980
44. Mézière C, Viguier M, Dumortier H, Lo-Man R, Leclerc C, Guillet JG et al (1997) In vivo T helper cell response to retro-inverso peptidomimetics. J Immunol 159:3230–3237
45. Ngo-Giang-Huong N, Kayibanda M, Deprez B, Levy JP, Guillet JG, Tilkin AF (1995) Mutations in residue 61 of H-Ras p21 protein influence MHC class II presentation. Int Immunol 7:269–275

Chapter 14

Measurement of Malondialdehyde, Glutathione, and Glutathione Peroxidase in SLE Patients

Tamer A. Gheita and Sanaa A. Kenawy

Abstract

Oxidative stress contributes to chronic inflammation of tissues and plays a central role in immunomodulation, which may lead to autoimmune diseases such as systemic lupus erythematosus (SLE) and antiphospholipid syndrome. Markers of oxidative damage include malondialdehyde (MDA), antioxidant scavengers as glutathione (GSH), and glutathione peroxidase (GSH Px), which all correlate well with SLE disease activity. Amelioration of some clinical manifestations of SLE may be expected by targeting lipid peroxidation with dietary or pharmacological antioxidants.

Here, we describe the detection of the key players of oxidant/antioxidant imbalance in SLE.

Key words Systemic lupus erythematosus (SLE), Oxidative stress, Malondialdehyde (MDA), Glutathione (GSH), Glutathione peroxidase (GSH Px)

1 Introduction

Systemic lupus erythematosus (SLE) is a multisystemic chronic inflammatory autoimmune disease characterized by the dysfunction of T-cells, B-cells, and dendritic cells with the production of antinuclear autoantibodies and the loss of self-tolerance, revealing defective immune regulatory mechanisms [1] and increased oxidative damage (*see* **Notes 1** and **2**) [2, 3]. There have been major advancements in the pathological mechanisms of SLE. Reactive oxygen species (ROS) have been considered as risk and enhancer factors for autoimmune diseases [4], and free radical-mediated reactions are implicated in SLE. Oxidative stress has a potential to elicit an autoimmune response and to contribute to the disease pathogenesis thus being useful when determining its prognosis [5]. Alopecia and lupus nephritis are remarkably associated with oxidative stress and impaired antioxidant systems in SLE patients [4].

Oxidative stress with an increase in malondialdehyde (MDA) and a decrease in antioxidant thiols plays a strong role in the progression of SLE disease [6]. Inhibition of oxidative stress may

Paul Eggleton and Frank J. Ward (eds.), *Systemic Lupus Erythematosus: Methods and Protocols*, Methods in Molecular Biology, vol. 1134, DOI 10.1007/978-1-4939-0326-9_14, © Springer Science+Business Media New York 2014

represent newly discovered molecular and cellular targets for the treatment of SLE [1]. Imbalance of oxidative status, represented by increased plasma MDA and impaired glutathione (GSH) and glutathione peroxidase (GSH Px), is one possible cause of SLE disease activity [7] which is also associated with fatigue [8].

The administration of biological drugs seems to have a role in increasing the mechanism of the barrier, which the body possesses against oxidative stress [9]. Antioxidants may protect against development of SLE by combating oxidative stress [10]. An understanding of the complex interactions between ROS and inflammatory pathways might be useful for the development of novel therapeutic strategies [11]. Exclusion criteria for patients and controls comprise other chronic disorders (diabetes, hypertension, malignancy, hepatitis, and bronchial asthma) and glucose-6-phosphate dehydrogenase (G6PD) deficiency.

2 Materials (*See* Note 3)

Prepare all solutions in deionized water and use analytical grade reagents. Prepare and store all reagents as instructed in methods.

2.1 Lipid Peroxide Reagents

1. Pre-boiling serum additives: Weigh 1.0 g of orthophosphoric acid in a glass beaker and add 100 ml water and mix to obtain a 1 % w/v solution. In a separate glass beaker, add 0.6 g of thiobarbituric acid and make up to 100 ml with water, to provide a 0.6 % w/v solution. Store both reagents at 4 °C. The pH of the solution does not need adjusting. The samples should be protected from light to avoid photooxidation.
2. Post-boiling serum additives: A solution of *n*-butanol is purchased commercially and used neat.

2.2 Blood Glutathione Reagents

1. Precipitating solution: Add 1.67 g glacial metaphosphoric acid, 0.20 g disodium or dipotassium ethylenediaminetetraacetic acid (EDTA), and 30.0 g of sodium chloride in a glass beaker. Add 100 ml of bidistilled water. There is no need to adjust pH.
2. Phosphate solution: Prepare a 0.3 M Na_2HPO_4 solution in water by weighing out 42.58 g Na_2HPO_4 in a glass beaker and add 100 ml water. Adjust pH to 7.4 with 1 M HCl.
3. Standard GSH: Weigh out 3.75 mg of reduced GSH and add to 100 ml 1 % w/v *m*-phosphoric acid.
4. DTNB reagent: Weigh out 40 mg 5,5′-dithiobis-(2-nitrobenzoic acid) and add to100 ml of 1 % w/v sodium citrate. There is no need to adjust pH.

2.3 Glutathione Peroxidase Kit Reagents

1. Reagent:
   Glutathione (4 nmol/L)
   Glutathione reductase (≥0.5 U/L)
   NADPH (0.28 nmol/L)
2. Phosphate buffer (0.05 mol/L, pH 7.2).
3. EDTA (4.3 nmol/L).
4. Cumene hydroperoxide (0.18 nmol/L).
5. Diluting agent.
6. Drabkin's reagent (a solution that consists of sodium bicarbonate, potassium cyanide, and potassium ferricyanide).

3 Methods (*See* Notes 4–6)

3.1 Determination of Serum Lipid Peroxides (After Uchiyama and Mihara [12])

3.1.1 Principle

The method depends on the determination of the level of thiobarbituric acid reactive substance (TBARS) that is measured as malondialdehyde (MDA). The reaction of TBARS with thiobarbituric acid in acidic medium at high temperature results in a pink pigment product, which is colorimetrically determined. In order to increase the specificity and sensitivity of the method, the resultant color product is extracted in *n*-butanol and measured at two wavelengths, namely, 535 and 520 nm, to exclude interfering substances.

3.1.2 Procedure

1. 3 ml 1 % orthophosphoric acid and 1 ml of 0.6 % thiobarbituric acid are added to 0.5 ml serum, placed in a 10 ml glass tube. Mix thoroughly and heat for 45 min in a boiling water bath.
2. Allow cooling, then add 4 ml *n*-butanol, and mixed vigorously.
3. Separate the *n*-butanol layer by centrifugation at 3,000 rpm for 15 min. Retain this layer for spectrometric analysis.
4. Measure the absorbance of the pink-colored product within the butanol at 535 and 520 nm against blank containing 0.5 ml distilled water, instead of the sample, using a Shimadzu double beam spectrophotometer (UV-150-02) or alternative.
5. The difference in optical densities between the two readings ($\Delta A535 - 520$) is taken as the level of TBARS in the sample.
6. Prepare serial dilutions of MDA in concentrations ranging from 0.808 to 12.92 nmol/ml by dissolving 1,1-3,3-tetramethoxypropane in water. When dissolved in water, 1,1-3,3-tetramethoxypropane is hydrolyzed to produce standard MDA solutions.

3.1.3 Calculation

The concentration of thiobarbituric acid reactive substance (TBARS) in the sample solution is expressed as nmol/ml using a standard solution containing a known concentration of MDA.

The following equation is used:

MDA (nmol/ml) = $(\Delta A535-520)T/(\Delta A535-520)S \times$ standard concentration

$(\Delta A535-520)T$ = difference in absorbance at 535 and 520 nm of the test sample

$(\Delta A535-520)S$ = difference in absorbance at 535 and 520 nm of the standard sample

Determination of Blood Glutathione (GSH) (After Beutler et al. [13])

3.1.4 Principle

Almost all the reduced glutathione (GSH) in blood is found within the erythrocytes and the nonprotein SH group reacts with 5,5′-dithiobis-(2-nitrobenzoic acid) (DTNB) to yield a stable yellow color which is related to the amount of glutathione.

3.1.5 Procedure

1. Whole blood (0.2 ml) was added to 1.8 ml bidistilled water and then 3 ml of the precipitating solution was mixed with the hemolysate.
2. The mixture was allowed to stand about 5 min and then centrifuged.
3. 2 ml of the supernatant was added to 8 ml of phosphate solution and then 1 ml of DTNB was added.
4. A blank was prepared with 8 ml of phosphate solution, 2 ml of the dilute precipitating solution (3 parts to 2 parts bidistilled water), and 1 ml of the DTNB reagent.
5. The optical density of the sample was measured at 412 nm against blank.
6. A standard GSH was made by mixing 2 ml standard with 8 ml disodium phosphate and 1 ml DTNB and then measured at 412 with 5 min against a blank using 2 ml bidistilled water instead of the standard.

3.1.6 Calculation

The following equation was used:

$$mg\%GSH = \frac{Absorbance\ of\ test}{Absorbance\ of\ standard} \times 75 \times 5 / 2 \times 100 / 0.2 \times 1 / 1{,}000$$

Determination of Blood Glutathione Peroxidase (GSH Px) (Paglia and Valentine [14])

3.1.7 Principle

Glutathione peroxidase (GSH Px) catalyses the oxidation of glutathione (GSH) by cumene hydroperoxide. In the presence of glutathione reductase (GR) and NADPH, the oxidized glutathione (GSSG) is immediately converted to the reduced form with concomitant oxidation of NADPH to $NADP^+$. The decrease in absorbance at 340 nm is measured.

$$2GSH + ROOH \xrightarrow{GSH\ PX} ROH + GSSG + H_2O$$

$$GSSG + NADPH + H^- ROOH \xrightarrow{GR} NADP^+ + 2GSH$$

It is recommended that Drabkin's reagent be used for dilution in case of human heparinized whole blood. This is due to the presence of peroxidases in human blood, which may give falsely elevated results; the addition of cyanide serves to inhibit this positive interference. Dilution of the blood with a diluting agent is necessary prior to addition of Drabkin's reagent, to convert the glutathione peroxidase to the reduced form; cyanide will quickly lead to inactivation.

3.1.8 Preparation of Solutions

1. Reconstituted one vial of glutathione is supplemented with appropriate volume of ethylenediaminetetraacetic acid (EDTA), pH 7.0.
2. Add 10 μl of cumene hydroperoxide to 10 ml of water and mixed thoroughly by shaking vigorously to prepare a 1:1,000 stock dilution.
3. The content of one vial of the diluting agent is reconstituted with 200 ml of bidistilled water to produce the diluting agents.
4. Reconstitute one vial of Drabkin's reagent with 500 ml water.

3.1.9 Procedure

1. Add 0.05 ml of heparinized whole blood to 1 ml diluting agent and incubate for 5 min at RT and then add 1 ml of double strength Drabkin's reagent.
2. Into a cuvette, add 0.05 ml of the above diluted sample to 2.5 ml reagent and 0.1 ml cumene hydroperoxide and then mix thoroughly.
3. The initial absorbance of the sample and a reagent blank (0.05 ml water) is read after 1 min and simultaneously read again after 1 and 2 min.
4. The reagent blank value is subtracted from that of the sample.

3.1.10 Calculation

Glutathione peroxidase activity can be calculated from the following formula:

$$\mathrm{U} / \mathrm{L}\ \textit{of hemolysate} = 8{,}412 \times \Delta A340nm / \min$$

4 Notes

1. The primary factor causing oxidative stress observed in SLE is excessive free radical production rather than impaired antioxidant activity [4].
2. On comparing MDA, GSH, and GSH Px in SLE patients and controls, there was a significant alteration in all parameters [3].
3. Imbalance between oxidative stress and helper T-cell (Th1)-derived cytokines is one possible cause for the pathogenesis of SLE. The activities of antioxidant enzymes, including GSH

Px, and antioxidant molecules such as GSH are significantly reduced in erythrocytes [15, 16] and lymphocytes [17], and the levels of lipid peroxidation, measured as MDA, are significantly higher in SLE patients [5, 15].

4. The markers of increased oxidative stress and impaired antioxidant capacity significantly correlated with disease activity in SLE. The SLE disease activity index (SLEDAI) score significantly correlates with the MDA [5, 15] and negatively with GSH, suggesting a possible causal relationship and involvement in its pathogenesis. Severity of the disease might be enhanced by the imbalance between oxidative stress and helper T-cell (Th1)-derived cytokines in SLE [15]. The SLEDAI correlates with serum markers of oxidant stress in SLE [18] and correlated negatively with levels of GSH and GSH Px [16] which may aid in the evaluation of treatment effectiveness [7]. It is suggested that in active SLE, oxidative status is increased without a corresponding elevation of the antioxidants, which verifies the value of using potent antioxidant therapy in preventing oxidative damage in SLE [19].
5. The mean MDA level is significantly higher and the GSH Px activity reduced in SLE patients with nephritis. Increased oxidative stress is a hallmark of SLE with a more obvious effect, especially in patients with lupus nephritis [20].
6. Further study on the role of antioxidants in novel therapeutic strategies should be considered in SLE patients.

Acknowledgment

The authors would like to thank Dr. Rehab W El Sisi and Dr. Heba A Gheita for their effort in revising the content of this chapter.

References

1. Perl A (2009) Emerging new pathways of pathogenesis and targets for treatment in systemic lupus erythematosus and Sjögren's syndrome. Curr Opin Rheumatol 21:443–447
2. Sheikh Z, Ahmad R, Sheikh N, Ali R (2007) Enhanced recognition of reactive oxygen species damaged human serum albumin by circulating systemic lupus erythematosus autoantibodies. Autoimmunity 40:512–520
3. Hassan SZ, Gheita TA, Kenawy SA, Fahim AT, El-Sorougy IM, Abdou MS (2011) Oxidative stress in systemic lupus erythematosus and rheumatoid arthritis patients: relationship to disease manifestations and activity. Int J Rheum Dis 14(4):325–331
4. Mansour RB, Lassoued S, Gargouri B, El Gaid A, Attia H, Fakhfakh F (2008) Increased levels of autoantibodies against catalase and superoxide dismutase associated with oxidative stress in patients with rheumatoid arthritis and systemic lupus erythematosus. Scand J Rheumatol 37:103–108
5. Wang G, Pierangeli SS, Papalardo E, Ansari GA, Khan MF (2010) Markers of oxidative and nitrosative stress in systemic lupus erythematosus: correlation with disease activity. Arthritis Rheum 62:2064–2072
6. Ben Mansour R, Lassoued S, Elgaied A, Haddouk S, Marzouk S, Bahloul Z et al (2010) Enhanced reactivity to malondialdehyde-modified proteins by systemic lupus erythematosus autoantibodies. Scand J Rheumatol 39:247–253
7. Tewthanom K, Janwityanuchit S, Totemchockchyakarn K, Panomvana D (2008)

Correlation of lipid peroxidation and glutathione levels with severity of systemic lupus erythematosus: a pilot study from single center. J Pharm Pharm Sci 11:30–34

8. Chung CP, Titova D, Oeser A, Randels M, Avalos I, Milne GL et al (2009) Oxidative stress in fibromyalgia and its relationship to symptoms. Clin Rheumatol 28:435–438
9. Coaccioli S, Panaccione A, Biondi R, Sabatini C, Landucci P, Del Giorno R et al (2009) Evaluation of oxidative stress in rheumatoid and psoriatic arthritis and psoriasis. Clin Ter 160:467–472
10. Costenbader KH, Kang JH, Karlson EW (2010) Antioxidant intake and risks of rheumatoid arthritis and systemic lupus erythematosus in women. Am J Epidemiol 172:205–216
11. Filippin LI, Vercelino R, Marroni NP, Xavier RM (2008) Redox signalling and the inflammatory response in rheumatoid arthritis. Clin Exp Immunol 152:415–422
12. Uchiyama M, Mihara M (1978) Determination of malonaldehyde precursor in tissue by thiobarbituric acid test. Anal Biochem 86: 271–278
13. Beutler E, Duron O, Kelley BM (1963) Improved method for the determination of blood glutathione. J Lab Clin Med 61:882–888
14. Paglia DE, Valentine WN (1967) Studies on the quantitative and qualitative characterization of erythrocyte glutathione peroxidase. J Lab Clin Med 70:158
15. Shah D, Kiran R, Wanchu A, Bhatnagar A (2010) Oxidative stress in systemic lupus erythematosus: relationship to Th1 cytokine and disease activity. Immunol Lett 129:7–12
16. Zhang Q, Ye DQ, Chen GP, Zheng Y (2010) Oxidative protein damage and antioxidant status in systemic lupus erythematosus. Clin Exp Dermatol 35:287–294
17. Gergely P Jr, Grossman C, Niland B, Puskas F, Neupane H, Allam F et al (2002) Mitochondrial hyperpolarization and ATP depletion in patients with systemic lupus erythematosus. Arthritis Rheum 46:175–190
18. Morgan PE, Sturgess AD, Davies MJ (2009) Evidence for chronically elevated serum protein oxidation in systemic lupus erythematosus patients. Free Radic Res 43:117–127
19. Huang WN, Tso TK, Huang HY (2007) Enhanced oxidative status but not corresponding elevated antioxidative status by anticardiolipin antibody and disease activity in patients with systemic lupus erythematosus. Rheumatol Int 27:453–458
20. Morgan PE, Sturgess AD, Hennessy A, Davies MJ (2007) Serum protein oxidation and apolipoprotein CIII levels in people with systemic lupus erythematosus with and without nephritis. Free Radic Res 41:1301–1312

Chapter 15

Evaluating a Particular Circulating MicroRNA Species from an SLE Patient Using Stem-Loop qRT-PCR

Weiguo Sui, Fuhua Liu, Jiejing Chen, Minglin Ou, and Yong Dai

Abstract

Systemic lupus erythematosus (SLE) is a complex autoimmune disease, and correct judgment of SLE activity is very important in guiding precise clinical treatment. Circulating microRNAs (miRNAs) could serve as potential biomarkers of disease activity or status in SLE, and here we describe a modified qRT-PCR method for detecting them. Stem loop has become one of the most powerful methods for determining miRNA expression because it is highly sensitive and accurate and requires only small amount of sample. In this chapter, we focus on a stem-loop reverse transcription-bound SYBR green qRT-PCR protocol for evaluating a particular circulating miRNA species in SLE patients.

Key words qRT-PCR, Systemic lupus erythematosus, SLE, Circulating miRNA

1 Introduction

Systemic lupus erythematosus (SLE) is a complex autoimmune disease, often occurring in females during their reproductive years. While the pathogenesis of lupus is unclear, among the many aspects of its pathophysiology is the production of autoantibodies specific for a host of nuclear antigens and immune complex deposition [1–3]. The complexity of SLE means that correct judgment of disease activity is very important in guiding clinical treatment. Renal biopsy is a direct and effective method to judge disease activity but is often limited by both the patient's condition and the willingness to comply with this procedure. So there is a requirement for biological markers specific to SLE, which are more sensitive and can objectively reflect the presence and degree of disease activity.

MiRNAs are noncoding RNAs typically comprising approximately 21–24 nucleotides that regulate a broad range of physiological and pathological processes [4, 5] (*see* **Note 1**). In lupus, many miRNAs have drawn the attention of researchers and several have a regulatory role in SLE (*see* Table 1). For example, some studies have shown that miRNAs have the potential to regulate

Paul Eggleton and Frank J. Ward (eds.), *Systemic Lupus Erythematosus: Methods and Protocols*, Methods in Molecular Biology, vol. 1134, DOI 10.1007/978-1-4939-0326-9_15, © Springer Science+Business Media New York 2014

Table 1
Some of the miRNAs associated with SLE

miRNA	Role in SLE	References
miR-126	Regulates DNA methylation in CD4+ T cells and contributes to T cell autoreactivity in SLE by directly targeting Dnmt1; circulating miRNA is significantly enriched in SLE patients and may be a biomarker of SLE	[12, 23]
miR-146a	Down regulated in SLE and is negatively correlated with clinical disease activity and with interferon (IFN) levels	[3]
miR-182	Directly dependent on STAT5 activation and promotes the clonal expansion of murine activated CD4+ T cells	[24]
miR-125b	Down regulated in SLE T cells, regulating the expression of ETS1 and STAT3	[25]
miR-21	Overexpressed in CD4+ T cells of SLE patients, regulates the expression of PDCD4, and promotes cell hypomethylation by repressing DNA methyltransferase 1 (DNMT1) expression	[26, 27]
miR-148a	Overexpressed in CD4+ T cells of SLE patients, promotes cell hypomethylation by repressing DNA methyltransferase 1 (DNMT1) expression	[27]
miR-145	Expressed specifically in SLE T cells, regulates the expression of STAT1	[28]
miR-224	Expressed specifically in SLE T cells, regulates the expression of API5	[28]
miR-30a	Expressed specifically in SLE T cells, promotes proliferation of B cells and the production of IgG	[29]
miR-31	Significantly decreased in lupus T cells and promotes the expression of IL-2	[30]
miR-155	Involved in regulating Treg cell phenotype	[31]

both signaling pathways and autoimmune genes [6–9]. Further, accumulating evidence also demonstrates that miRNAs are remarkably stable in the blood and can even withstand repeated freeze/thaw cycles [10–12]. It seems that specific circulating miRNAs could serve as potential biomarkers for various diseases and the detection of circulating miRNAs could have important novel implications for understanding disease processes [4, 11, 13].

Northern blotting techniques and quantitative real-time reverse transcription polymerase chain reaction (qRT-PCR) are used as the major methods for miRNA detection [14, 15], but currently, qRT-PCR has become one of the most powerful methods for determining miRNA expression. This is largely because only a small amount of sample is required to accurately pinpoint activity levels associated with a variety of biological and metabolic processes. A key obstacle in analyzing miRNAs by qRT-PCR is their

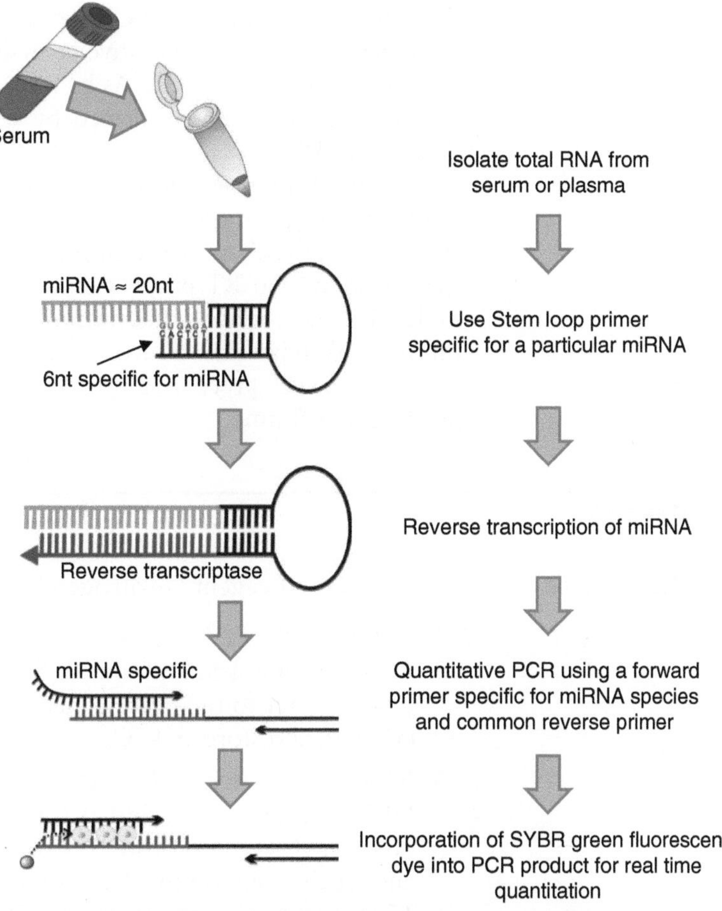

Fig. 1 Schematic diagram of the stem-loop qRT-PCR procedure. The use of stem-loop primers allows detection of mature miRNAs using just six nucleotide long primers. The resulting product can then be amplified by conventional reverse transcriptase to replicate the miRNA under investigation

typically short length, which precludes the use of standard primer pairs, which are themselves typically longer than the miRNA target. The use of stem-loop primers provides a solution to this problem. Stem-loop primers can selectively detect mature miRNA using just six several nucleotides to provide specificity for any particular miRNA species (*see* Fig. 1 for overview). The stem-loop structure provides enough stability to allow reverse transcriptase to replicate the miRNA, while providing extra length to the cDNA product so that it can be analyzed by conventional qRT-PCR [16].

There are several qRT-PCR protocols for miRNA detection, reflecting different experimental objectives, but two main steps are similar: The first step is reverse transcription, which reverse transcribes RNA into cDNA, and the second step is qRT-PCR. In the second step, fluorophores are added into the PCR reaction system. The instrument can base on accumulating fluorescent signal to monitor the entire PCR process in real time and to generate a standard curve for quantitative analysis of the test samples. Real-time quantification of miRNAs by stem-loop RT-PCR is a reliable method that has been confirmed by several researchers independently [16–18].

In this chapter, we focus on a stem-loop reverse transcription-bound SYBR green qRT-PCR protocol for evaluating a particular circulating miRNA species in SLE patients. In the first step, target-specific stem-loop RT primers bind to the 3′ portion of miRNA molecules and reverse transcription is performed using Moloney murine leukemia virus (M-MLV) reverse transcriptase. In the second step, SYBR green is used to detect and quantify the PCR product in real time.

2 Materials

2.1 RNA Isolation

1. TRIZOL® Reagent (Invitrogen life technologies).
2. Chloroform.
3. 75 % Ethanol: Add 78.9 ml 95 % ethanol and 21.1 ml DEPC-treated water to the beaker, mix and then transfer to a 100 ml cylinder, and store at 4 °C.
4. RNase-free water: 0.1 % DEPC-treated water. To prepare DEPC-treated water, add 0.1 ml DEPC to 100 ml of the ddH_2O, shake vigorously to bring the DEPC into solution, and let the solution incubate for 12 h at 37 °C. Autoclave for 15 min to remove any trace of DEPC.
5. SiO_2 adsorption liquid.
6. *Caenorhabditis elegans* lin-4(Cel-lin-4) (Shanghai jima).

2.2 Reverse Transcription

1. dNTP (Promega, 10 mM).
2. RNase inhibitor (Promega, 40 U/μl).
3. 0.5 M EDTA (pH 8.0) solution. Weigh 18.61 g EDTA and transfer to 100 ml cylinder. Add approximately 90 ml DEPC-treated water. Adjust the pH to 8.0 and add DEPC-treated water to 100 ml. Autoclave and store at RT.
4. Tris–HCl (pH 8.0) solution. Weigh 121.1 g Tris and transfer to 1 L beaker, add about 800 ml ddH_2O to dissolve it, mix and adjust pH with HCl, make up to 1 L with ultrapure water. Autoclave and store at 4 °C.
5. TE (Tris–EDTA) buffer (10 mM Tris–HCl pH 8.0, 1 mM EDTA): aliquots of 0.5 ml 1 mol/L Tris–HCl (pH 8.0) and 1 ml 0.5 mol/L EDTA (pH 8.0), respectively, are transferred to a 500 ml cylinder and made up to 500 ml with ddH_2O, autoclaved, and stored at 4 °C.

6. Target-specific stem-loop reverse transcription primer of the circulating miRNA species of interest dissolved and diluted to 10 μM with TE buffer.
7. *C. elegans* lin-4(Cel-lin-4) stem-loop reverse transcription primer diluted to 10 μM with TE buffer.
8. M-MLV reverse transcriptase and 5× buffer (Promega).
9. RNase-free water.

2.3 Quantitative Real-Time PCR

1. The target-specific forward primer of the cDNA reverse transcript from the specific serum miRNA of interest is dissolved and diluted to 10 μM with TE buffer.
2. Reverse primer: miRNA_R:5′ CTCAACTGGTGTCGTGGA is dissolved and diluted to 10 μM with TE buffer.
3. Cel-lin-4 forward primer (ACACTCCAGCTGGGTCCCTG AGACCTCAAGTG) is dissolved and diluted to 10 μM with TE buffer.
4. 2× SYBR Green PCR Master Mix.
5. RNase-free water.

3 Methods

RNAs are isolated from serum samples using TRIZOL® according to the manufacturer's protocol. Target-specific stem-loop RT primers that bind to the 3′ portion of miRNA molecules are used, reverse transcription is performed using M-MLV, and SYBR green is used to detect and quantify the PCR product in real time (*see* **Notes 2–4**).

3.1 Serum Collection

1. Whole blood (2.5 ml) is collected via direct venous puncture into collection tubes, allowed to clot, and processed for isolation of serum within 4 h.
2. Samples are centrifuged at 3,000 ×*g* for 5 min at RT to obtain the serum, transferred to a fresh RNase-free tube, and stored at −80 °C.

3.2 RNA Isolation

1. Serum is thawed on ice before 1.2 ml TRIZOL® is added to 300 μl serum aliquots together with 2 μl cel-lin-4 miRNA (*see* **Note 5**).
2. Tubes are shaken vigorously for 30 s, 200 μl chloroform added, and shaken vigorously again for a further 20 s, incubated at RT for 3 min to permit complete dissociation of nucleoprotein complexes, and then centrifuged at 14,000 ×*g* for 10 min, RT.
3. The aqueous phase, excluding the interphase, is transferred to a fresh tube and 10 μl SiO_2 adsorption liquid added, mixed,

and the solution centrifuged at 14,000 × *g* for 10 min (*see* **Notes 6** and **7**).

4. The supernatant is discarded and replaced with 400 μl 75 % alcohol, before centrifuging at 14,000 × *g* for 5 min.
5. At the end of the procedure, the RNA pellet is air-dried for 5–10 min (*see* **Note 8**) and dissolved in 25 μl RNase-free water by passing the solution a few times through a pipette tip to solubilize and incubating for 10 min at 55–60 °C. RNA can be stored at −80 °C.

3.3 Reverse Transcription

The stem-loop method to target specific stem-loop RT primers that bind the 3′ portion of miRNA molecules and M-MLV is used for reverse transcription (*see* **Note 9**).

1. Reagents are combined according to Table 2 in a clean RNase-free tube and the total volume marked "*V*1" (*see* **Note 10**), while 10 μl total RNA and an appropriate amount of DEPC-treated water (*see* **Note 11**) are added to a new tube, with the total volume marked as "*V*2."
2. Tube 2 is mixed and incubated at 85 °C for 5 min to open the RNA secondary structure and then placed on ice immediately to prevent RNA refolding and recovery of its secondary structure.
3. The solution from tube 1 is then added to tube 2, mixed, and incubated at 42 °C for 60 min to allow reverse transcription to occur. Finally, the mix is incubated at 85 °C for 10 min to inactivate the reverse transcription enzyme.

Table 2
Reagents list for tube "*V*1" (*see* Notes 10 and 11)

Reagents	Vol (μl)
10 mM dNTP (1 mM final conc)	2
RNase inhibitor	0.5
miR-X1 RT primer of interest	0.5
miR-Xn RT primer of interest	0.5
Cel-lin-4 RT primer	0.5
M-MLV 5× PCR buffer[a]	5.0
M-MLV reverse transcriptase (200 U)	1.0
Total volume	9 + 0.5 n

[a]250 mM Tris–HCl (pH 8.3), 375 mM KCl, 15 mM $MgCl_2$, 50 mM DTT

3.4 Quantitative Real-Time PCR

SYBR green is a cyanine-type fluorescent dye used in qRT-PCR protocol because of its high affinity for nucleic acids and, in particular, double-stranded DNA. Increases in fluorescence after binding double-stranded DNA provide an accurate means of quantifying the PCR product in real time.

1. The cDNA obtained from the reverse transcription process is diluted by adding 0.25 μl cDNA to 4.75 μl RNA-free water in a clean tube, mixed, and put on ice.
2. Next, the forward and reverse primers (0.5 μl each) chosen for the investigation are added together with 10 μl 2× SYBR Green PCR Master Mix (*see* **Notes 12** and **13**) and the volume of the reaction system made up to 20 μl with RNA-free water.
3. The samples are transferred to a 96 well plate and analyzed using a qRT-PCR system.
4. Typical reaction conditions are 95 °C for 5 min, followed by 40 cycles of 95 °C for 15 s, 65 °C for 15 s, and 72 °C "plate reading" for 32 s (*see* **Note 14**).
5. For data analysis, obtain the primary curve, C_T value, and melting curve (60–95 °C) while the reaction completes. Values are normalized to the cel-lin-4 internal reference and calculated according to the comparative $2^{-\Delta\Delta CT}$ method (*see* **Note 15**).

4 Notes

1. Information on most aspects of miRNA can be found on the miRBase miRNA database (http://www.mirbase.org/index.shtml).
2. Experiments should be conducted in a dedicated area to avoid RNase contamination. RNA isolations should be conducted in laminar airflow cabinets that have been wiped with alcohol before the experiment.
3. If proprietary RNase-free products are not available, plastic products and tips should be soaked with 0.1 % DEPC water overnight before use, while glass and iron utensils roasted at 160 °C for 4 h, rinsed thoroughly with RNA-free water, and autoclaved to remove any RNA enzyme.
4. Change gloves frequently during the experiment.
5. The cel-lin-4 acts as internal reference control. We choose cel-lin-4 as it has been reported widely as a reference control [16, 19]. It is also stably expressed in serum. However, other controls can be used such as U6 [20].
6. Following centrifugation, the mixture separates into a lower red, phenol–chloroform phase, an interphase, and a colorless upper aqueous phase. RNA remains exclusively in the aqueous phase.

7. Don't take the interphase.
8. Do not dry the RNA by centrifugation under vacuum. It is important not to let the RNA pellet dry completely as this will greatly decrease its solubility.
9. We find that it is the best to separate the reverse transcription area and the RT-PCR area.
10. MiR-X1 to MiR-Xn are the miRNAs that researchers want to investigate, the RT primers are required to add to the reaction system.
11. The total volume of the reverse transcription system ($V1 + V2$) is 25 μl, $V_{DEPC\text{-treated water}} = 25\text{-}V_1\text{-}V_{RNA}$. We often add 10μl RNA.
12. We find it best to conduct this procedure on ice.
13. The forward primer is specific to the circulating miRNA of interest and the reverse primer we used was miRNA_R:5′ CTCAACTGGTGTCGTGGA common reverse primer.
14. Each sample is analyzed three times.
15. $2^{-\Delta\Delta CT}$ method is a convenient way to analyze the relative changes in gene expression from real-time quantitative PCR experiments, $2^{-\Delta\Delta CT} = [(C_T$ gene of interest $- C_T$ internal control) sample A $-$ (C_T gene of interest $- C_T$ internal control) sample B] [21, 22].

References

1. Petri M (2010) Systemic lupus erythematosus. In: Stone J et al (eds) A clinician's pearls and myths in rheumatology. Springer, London, pp 131–159
2. Pan Y, Sawalha AH (2009) Epigenetic regulation and the pathogenesis of systemic lupus erythematosus. Transl Res 153:4–10
3. Te JL et al (2010) Identification of unique microRNA signature associated with lupus nephritis. PLoS One 5:e10344
4. Wang H et al (2012) Circulating levels of inflammation-associated miR-155 and endothelial-enriched miR-126 in patients with end-stage renal disease. Braz J Med Biol Res 45(12):1308–1314
5. Esquela-Kerscher A, Slack FJ (2006) Oncomirs [mdash] microRNAs with a role in cancer. Nat Rev Cancer 6:259–269
6. Bartel DP (2004) MicroRNAs: genomics biogenesis, mechanism, and function. Cell 116:281–297
7. Huang JC et al (2007) Using expression profiling data to identify human microRNA targets. Nat Methods 4:1045–1049
8. Carrington JC, Ambros V (2003) Role of microRNAs in plant and animal development. Science 301:336–338
9. Dai R, Ahmed SA (2011) MicroRNA, a new paradigm for understanding immunoregulation, inflammation, and autoimmune diseases. Transl Res 157:163–179
10. Chen X et al (2008) Characterization of microRNAs in serum: a novel class of biomarkers for diagnosis of cancer and other diseases. Cell Res 18:997–1006
11. Fichtlscherer S et al (2010) Circulating microRNAs in patients with coronary artery disease. Circ Res 107:677–684
12. Wang H, Peng W, Ouyang X, Li W, Dai Y (2012) Circulating microRNAs as candidate biomarkers in patients with systemic lupus erythematosus. Transl Res 160:198–206
13. Zhao H et al (2010) A pilot study of circulating miRNAs as potential biomarkers of early stage breast cancer. PLoS One 5:e13735
14. Wang S-T, Li C, Liu L (2009) miRNA microarray technology in miRNA profiling. Curr Bioinform 4:141–148

15. Cheng Yongqiang LZ, Yucong W, Yongshan F (2010) MicroRNA detection. Prog Chem 22:1509–1517
16. Chen C et al (2005) Real-time quantification of microRNAs by stem–loop RT–PCR. Nucleic Acids Res 33:e179
17. Pan X, Murashov A, Stellwag E, Zhang B (2010) Monitoring microRNA expression during embryonic stem-cell differentiation using quantitative real-time PCR (qRT-PCR). In: Zhang B, Stellwag EJ (eds) RNAi and microRNA-mediated gene regulation in stem cells. Humana Press, Totowa, NJ, pp 213–224
18. Udvardi MK, Czechowski T, Scheible W-R (2008) Eleven golden rules of quantitative RT-PCR. Plant Cell 20:1736–1737
19. Rong H et al (2011) MicroRNA-134 plasma levels before and after treatment for bipolar mania. J Psychiatr Res 45:92–95
20. Peltier HJ, Latham GJ (2008) Normalization of microRNA expression levels in quantitative RT-PCR assays: identification of suitable reference RNA targets in normal and cancerous human solid tissues. RNA 14:844–852
21. Schmittgen TD, Livak KJ (2008) Analyzing real-time PCR data by the comparative CT method. Nat Protoc 3:1101–1108
22. Livak KJ, Schmittgen TD (2001) Analysis of relative gene expression data using real-time quantitative PCR and the 2–ΔΔCT method. Methods 25:402–408
23. Zhao S et al (2011) MicroRNA-126 regulates DNA methylation in CD4+ T cells and contributes to systemic lupus erythematosus by targeting DNA methyltransferase 1. Arthritis Rheum 63:1376–1386
24. Alexander T et al (2013) A3.22 upregulated microRNA-182 expression is associated with enhanced conventional CD4+ T cell proliferation in SLE. Ann Rheum Dis 72:A21
25. Luo X et al (2013) The role of miR-125b in T lymphocytes in the pathogenesis of systemic lupus erythematosus. Clin Exp Rheumatol 31:263–271
26. Stagakis E et al (2011) Identification of novel microRNA signatures linked to human lupus disease activity and pathogenesis: miR-21 regulates aberrant T cell responses through regulation of PDCD4 expression. Ann Rheum Dis 70:1496–1506
27. Pan W et al (2010) MicroRNA-21 and microRNA-148a contribute to DNA hypomethylation in lupus CD4+ T cells by directly and indirectly targeting DNA methyltransferase 1. J Immunol 184:6773–6781
28. Lu MC et al (2013) Decreased microRNA(miR)-145 and increased miR-224 expression in T cells from patients with systemic lupus erythematosus involved in lupus immunopathogenesis. Clin Exp Immunol 171:91–99
29. Liu Y et al (2013) MicroRNA-30a promotes B cell hyperactivity in patients with systemic lupus erythematosus by direct interaction with Lyn. Arthritis Rheum 65:1603–1611
30. Fan W et al (2012) Identification of microRNA-31 as a novel regulator contributing to impaired interleukin-2 production in T cells from patients with systemic lupus erythematosus. Arthritis Rheum 64:3715–3725
31. Divekar AA, Dubey S, Gangalum PR, Singh RR (2011) Dicer insufficiency and microRNA-155 overexpression in lupus regulatory T cells: an apparent paradox in the setting of an inflammatory milieu. J Immunol 186:924–930

Chapter 16

Microarray Technology for Analysis of MicroRNA Expression in Renal Biopsies of Lupus Nephritis Patients

Weiguo Sui, Fuhua Liu, Jiejing Chen, Minglin Ou, and Yong Dai

Abstract

Systemic lupus erythematosus (SLE) is a complex autoimmune disease, which predominantly occurs in females and is characterized by autoantibody production against a host of nuclear self-antigens and deposition of proinflammatory immune complexes in the organs including kidney glomeruli. MicroRNAs are small noncoding intracellular RNAs that modulate gene expression at the posttranslational level. Microarray technology is in widespread use for analysis of microRNA (miRNA) gene expression because of its flexibility and accurate high throughput. RNA microarray technology is based on nucleic acid hybridization between a mixture of labeled RNA targets and their corresponding complementary probes. This article offers a technological overview of microarray technology for analysis of microRNA gene expression in kidney biopsies from SLE patients.

Key words Systemic lupus erythematosus, SLE, Microarray, MicroRNA, Gene expression

1 Introduction

Systemic lupus erythematosus (SLE) is a complex autoimmune disease predominantly affecting females and usually characterized by both the production of autoantibodies specific for a host of nuclear antigens and the presence of pathogenic immune complex deposits in the vascular tissues and organs, including the kidney [1, 2]. In particular, kidney involvement in SLE patients is relatively common and often associated with a poor outcome.

The pathogenesis of lupus is unclear and recent studies have shown the potential contribution of several miRNAs to the aberrant regulation of signaling pathways and autoimmune genes in lupus, providing new insights into its development [3]. MiRNAs are noncoding RNAs about 22 nt in length and, as intracellular RNAs, have been shown to modulate or fine-tune gene expression at the posttranslational level [4–6]. As the identity and function of novel miRNAs are revealed, it is becoming clear that their role in regulating biological processes can influence the development and intensity

Paul Eggleton and Frank J. Ward (eds.), *Systemic Lupus Erythematosus: Methods and Protocols*, Methods in Molecular Biology, vol. 1134, DOI 10.1007/978-1-4939-0326-9_16, © Springer Science+Business Media New York 2014

of autoimmune disease. Thus miRNA probes could serve as valuable tools both in understanding the pathogenesis of autoimmune disease and as diagnostic or prognostic biomarkers of disease activity. This has led to the investigation of miRNA signature expression patterns in different tissues associated with lupus pathology including the kidney [7–9].

Northern blotting technique, microarray analysis, in situ hybridization, real-time reverse transcription PCR, isothermal rolling circle amplification, and conjugated polymer-based FRET analysis are used as the major methods for miRNA detection and analysis [10, 11]. Microarray technology is also commonly used for analysis of miRNA gene expression because of its flexibility, sensitivity, accuracy, and high throughput. RNA microarray technology is based on nucleic acid hybridization between a mixture of labeled RNA identified as a target and their corresponding complementary probes [12, 13]. To summarize the procedure, total RNA is first isolated from the experimental sample of interest and the RNA fragments uniformly conjugated with a fluorescent dye. During this process, all of the miRNA moieties within that sample will also be labeled. The miRNA is first isolated and then individual miRNA species are identified by hybridizing the labeled miRNA with a microarray, containing locked nucleic acid oligonucleotide capture probes. The conjugated microarray is then scanned for the presence of fluorescent signal corresponding to each miRNA probe within the microarray. Thus, the presence and quantity of individual miRNAs in the target tissue can be ascertained.

Current miRNA microarray technology can probe for the presence of over 3,000 different miRNAs corresponding to those so far identified in mice, rats, and humans and listed in the miRBase 20.0 miRNA database (*see* **Note 1**). Thus, we can use this technology to develop miRNA signature maps in different tissue samples to draw comparisons between different species, organs, and tissues and increasingly, between expression patterns in health and disease.

Here, we focus on microarray technology for the analysis of miRNA gene expression in renal biopsy tissue from patients with lupus nephritis.

2 Materials

2.1 Preparation of Renal Tissue Samples

1. 0.9 % RNase-free saline solution: Weigh 9 g NaCl into a cylinder and make up to 991 ml with DEPC-treated water (*see* **Note 2**). Autoclave and store at 4 °C.
2. RiboGuard™ RNase Inhibitor (Epicenter, USA).

2.2 RNA Isolation

1. TRIzol® Reagent (Invitrogen Life Technologies).
2. Chloroform.

3. Isopropyl alcohol.
4. 75 % ethanol: Add 78.9 ml 95 % ethanol and 21.1 ml DEPC-treated water to a beaker, mix and transfer to a cylinder, and store at 4 °C.
5. RNase-free water.

2.3 Assessing RNA Yield and Quality

1. TE buffer: 10 mM Tris–HCl pH 8.0, 1 mM EDTA. Add 5 ml 1 M Tris–HCl (pH 8.0; *see* **Note 3**) and 1 ml 0.5 M EDTA (pH 8.0; *see* **Note 4**) to a cylinder and make up to 500 ml with ddH_2O. Autoclave and store at 4 °C.
2. 10× MOPS running buffer: 0.2 M MOPS (pH 7.0), 0.05 M sodium acetate, and 0.02 M EDTA. Weigh MOPS (41.86 g) and $NaOAc.3H_2O$ (4.10 g) into a beaker together with 40 ml 0.5 M EDTA (pH 8.0), mix and add DEPC-treated water to about 900 ml, adjust to pH 7.0 with NaOH, and add DEPC-treated water to 1 l. Store at room temperature and protect from light.
3. Formaldehyde.
4. NorthernMax® Formaldehyde Load Dye (Ambion).
5. Ethidium bromide.
6. Agarose.
7. RNase-free water.

2.4 miRNA Labeling Procedure

miRCURY LNA™ microRNA Hy3 Power labeling kit (Cat. #208031-A, Exiqon, Denmark)

Kit Components:

Hy3™ fluorescent label	24 reactions
Labeling enzyme	48 μl
Nuclease-free water	500 μl
2.5× labeling buffer	250 μl
Positive control	24 μl

2.5 Isolating the Labeled miRNA Sample

The mirVana™ miRNA isolation kit (Ambion, USA) was used to isolate and purify labeled miRNA samples.

Kit components:

40 filter cartridges

80 collection tubes.

miRNA wash solution 1, wash solution 2/3, lysis/binding buffer, miRNA homogenate additive, Acid-Phenol:Chloroform.

Gel loading buffer II.

Elution solution.

2.6 miRNA Array Hybridization

miRCURY™ Array microarray kit (Exiqon).

Kit Components:

Microarray slide (three slides)	
2× hybridization buffer	4×0.5 ml
20× salt buffer	2×125 ml
10 % detergent solution	2×15 ml

Bioarray LifterSlip cover slide (Ambion, Austin, TX).

Hybridization chamber II (Corning Inc., Corning, NY).

2.7 miRNA Array Scanning and Analysis

The Axon GenePix 4000B microarray scanner is used to scan the microarray, and the data is analyzed with GenePix pro V6.0 software.

3 Methods

Total RNA is isolated from renal tissue needle biopsy samples with TRIzol according to the manufacturer's instructions, quantified by UV absorbance at 260 and 280 nm ($A_{260/280}$) and its concentration and quality assessed by gel electrophoresis. Total RNA is then labeled with the fluorescent Hy3™ probe using the miRCURY LNA™ microRNA Hy3™ Power labeling kit. The miRNA is isolated from the total RNA sample with a mirVana™ miRNA isolation kit, washed, and hybridized to a microarray slide with the miRCURY LNA™ Array microarray kit (*see* **Notes 5–6**). Scanning is performed with the Axon GenePix 4000B microarray scanner and the data analyzed by GenePix Pro 6.0 (Fig. 1).

3.1 Preparation of Renal Tissue Samples

1. Renal cortex biopsies (≈0.3 mm^3) obtained from aspirated needle biopsy are immediately washed with sterile 0.9 % NaCl (RNase-free), dipped in RiboGuard™ RNase Inhibitor according to the manufacturer's instructions, and stored at 4 °C overnight (*see* **Notes 7–9**).
2. The RNAse inhibitors were removed by washing and the biopsies stored at −80 °C.

3.2 RNA Isolation with TRIzol® Reagent (Invitrogen)

1. Tissue samples are homogenized in 1 ml of TRIzol Reagent per 50–100 mg of tissue with a power homogenizer (*see* **Note 10**) and the homogenized samples incubated in a water bath for 5 min at 15–30 °C to permit complete dissociation of nucleoprotein complexes.
2. A 0.2 ml aliquot of chloroform is added per 1 ml of TRIzol Reagent, and the sample tubes capped securely and shaken vigorously by hand for 15 s, further incubated at 15–30 °C

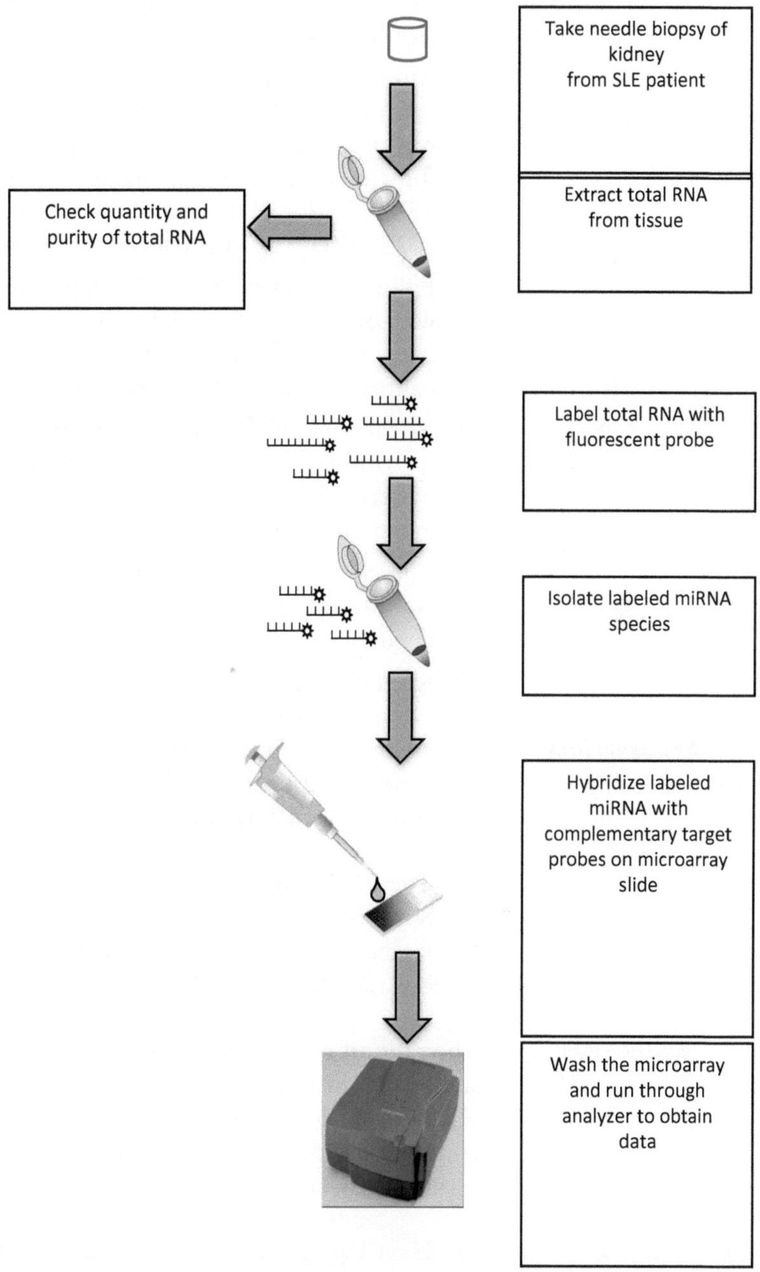

Fig. 1 Schematic diagram outlining the extraction, purification, and analysis of microRNA from SLE renal biopsies. Total RNA is isolated from renal tissue needle biopsy samples with TRIzol. The total RNA is then labeled with the fluorescent Hy3™ probe using the miRCURY LNA™ microRNA Hy3™ Power labeling kit. The miRNA is isolated from the total RNA sample with a mirVana™ miRNA isolation kit, washed, and hybridized to a microarray slide with the miRCURY LNA™ Array microarray kit. Scanning is performed with the Axon GenePix 4000B microarray scanner and the data analyzed by GenePix Pro 6.0

for 2–3 min, and centrifuged at 12,000 × *g* for 15 min at 4 °C (*see* **Note 11**).

3. After the transfer of the upper aqueous phase containing the RNA to a fresh tube (*see* **Note 12**), the RNA is precipitated by mixing in 0.5 ml of isopropyl alcohol per 1 ml of TRIzol used for the initial homogenization, followed by incubation at 15–30 °C for 10 min, and the sample pelleted by centrifuging at 12,000 × *g* in a microfuge for 10 min at 4 °C (*see* **Note 13**).
4. Following aspiration of the supernatant, the pellet is washed with at least 1 ml of 75 % ethanol per 1 ml of TRIzol Reagent used for the initial homogenization, vortexed to mix and centrifuged at 7,500 × *g* for 5 min at 4 °C.
5. At the end of the procedure, the RNA pellet is air-dried for 5–10 min (*see* **Note 14**) and dissolved in RNase-free water, by passing the solution a few times through a pipette tip and incubating for 10 min at 55–60 °C.
6. The concentration and purity of RNA can be determined by NanoDrop® ND-1000 (*see* **Note 15**) according to the manufacturer's instructions.
7. RNA can be stored at −80 °C.

3.3 Assessing RNA Yield and Quality

An absorbance at A_{260} of 1 is equivalent to 40 ng RNA/μl. The concentration of RNA is therefore calculated by multiplying the A_{260} value × 40 ng/μl, e.g., RNA is suspended in 20 μL DEPC water and 1 μl is used for measurement, A_{260} = 65.003.

The RNA concentration = 65.003 × 40 ng/μl = 2,600.12 ng/ μl.

Since there are only 19 μl of the prep left after sacrificing 1 μl to measure the concentration, the total amount of remaining RNA is 19 μl × 2,600.12 ng/μl = 49.4 μg.

3.3.1 Total RNA Purity

The ratio of A_{260} to A_{280} values is a measure of RNA purity, and it should fall in the range of 1.8–2.1. Even if an RNA prep has an A_{260}:A_{280} ratio outside this range, it may function well in common applications including Northern blotting, RT-PCR, and RNase protection assays.

3.3.2 Denaturing Agarose Gel Electrophoresis

1. Heat 1 g agarose in 72 ml water until dissolved and then cool to 60 °C. Add 10 ml 10× MOPS running buffer and 18 ml 37 % formaldehyde (12.3 M).
2. Pour the gel and allow it to set. The wells should be large enough to accommodate at least 25 μl.
3. Remove the comb and place the gel in the gel tank. Add enough 1× MOPS running buffer to cover the gel by a few millimeters.
4. Prepare the RNA sample: to 3 μg RNA, add 3× volumes Formaldehyde Load Dye. Ethidium bromide can be added to

the Formaldehyde Load Dye at a final concentration of 10 μg/ml. Heat denature samples at 65–70 °C for 15 min.

5. Load the gel and electrophorese at 5–6 V/cm until the bromophenol blue (the faster-migrating dye) has migrated at least 2–3 cm into the gel.
6. Visualize the gel on a UV transilluminator (*see* **Note 16**).

3.4 RNA Labeling with Hy3™ Fluorescent Dye

1. Place all kit components on ice to thaw for 15–20 min. Mix thoroughly by vortexing followed by brief centrifugation and combine reagents as follows:

Component	Volume
2.5× labeling buffer	8 μl
Hy3™ fluorescent label	2 μl
Labeling enzyme	2 μl
RNA	5 μg
Nuclease-free water	(To total volume) 20 μl

2. Incubate on ice for 1 h and stop the labeling reaction by further incubation for 15 min at 65 °C. Briefly spin the reaction and leave at 4 °C.

3.5 Isolation of Labeled miRNA Species from Total RNA

Small RNAs (<200 nt) including miRNA can be isolated using the mirVana™ miRNA Isolation Kit according to the manufacturer's instructions. The kit can also be used to purify total RNA.

3.6 miRNA Array Hybridization

1. Preparation of Wash buffers (200 ml each):
   (A) 20× salt buffer. (B) 10 % detergent solution. (C) Nuclease-free water.

   Wash buffer A: 20 ml A; 4 ml B; 176 ml C

   Wash buffer B: 10 ml A; 190 ml B

   Wash buffer C: 2 ml A; 198 ml B
2. Add a volume of 2× hybridization (10 μl) buffer to the labeled sample (10 μl).
3. Incubate at 95 °C for 3–5 min and then on ice for 2 min.
4. Centrifuge for 2 min at max speed.
5. Clean a Bioarray LifterSlip coverslip using 70 % ethanol.
6. Pipette 10 μl distilled water into humidifying well at each end of chamber base.
7. Place slide, printed array side up, in base.
8. Place a Bioarray LifterSlip coverslip slide over the spotted area and add 20 μl of the target preparation by pipetting into the gap between the slide and the Bioarray LifterSlip

coverslip. The capillary effect draws the solution underneath the coverslip.

9. Place cover of hybridization chamber over base by aligning base posts with cover indentations. While maintaining chamber in a horizontal plane, snap a metal retaining clip onto each side of the chamber.
10. Place the hybridization chamber in hybridization systems to hybridize the microarray for 16–20 h at 56 °C.
11. Remove retaining clips; carefully lift off chamber top. Remove array/coverslip assembly from chamber.
12. Wash at 60 °C in Wash buffer A until the Bioarray LifterSlip coverslip falls off.
13. Wash briefly at room temperature in Wash buffer B and wash in a new Wash buffer B at RT for 2 min.
14. Wash in Wash buffer C at room temperature for 2 min.
15. The slide is dried by centrifugation for 5 min at 200 × *g*.

3.7 miRNA Array Scanning and Analysis

1. Scanning is performed with the Axon GenePix 4000B microarray scanner. The 635 nm laser is used.
2. The images are saved as TIF files. Analyze the data in GenePix Pro 6.0 and save the results as Excel files.
3. Data Analysis:
   (a) The intensity of green signal is calculated after background subtraction and four replicated spots of each probe on the same slide have been averaged.
   (b) We use the median normalization method to obtain "normalized data," normalized data = (Foreground − Background)/median; the median is 50 % quantile of microRNA intensity which is larger than 50 in all samples after background correction.
   (c) After normalization, the statistical significance of differentially expressed miRNA is analyzed by Student's *t*-test (*see* **Note 17**).

4 Notes

1. For full details of the microRNA database, go to: http://www.mirbase.org/.
2. 0.1 % DEPC-treated water. Add 0.1 ml DEPC to 100 ml of the ddH_2O to be treated and shake vigorously to bring the DEPC into solution. Let the solution incubate for 12 h at 37 °C and autoclave for 15 min to remove any trace of DEPC.
3. To obtain a 1 mol/l Tris–HCl (pH 8.0) solution, weigh 121.1 g Tris and transfer to 1 l beaker, add about 800 ml

ddH$_2$O to dissolve it, and mix and adjust pH with HCl. Make up to 1 l with ddH$_2$O and autoclave. Store at 4 °C.

4. 0.5 M EDTA (pH 8.0): weigh 18.61 g EDTA, transfer to a cylinder, add about 90 ml DEPC-treated water, and mix and adjust the pH to 8.0 before adding DEPC-treated water to 100 ml. Autoclave and store at room temperature.
5. Current miRNA arrays have over 3,000 probes for all miRNAs from human mouse and rat species on miRBase database.
6. LNA™ technology—locked nucleic acids are modified oligonucleotide capture probes that have improved thermostability allowing a uniform melting temperature to be applied to all the probes in the miRNA microarray.
7. Experiments should be conducted in a dedicated area, and in particular, RNA isolation should be performed in a laminar flow cabinet wiped with alcohol and RNase solution before each experiment.
8. If plastic consumables cannot be guaranteed RNase-free by the manufacturer, they should be soaked with 0.1 % DEPC water overnight before use. Glass and iron utensils should be heated in an oven at 160 °C for 4 h and rinsed thoroughly with RNA-free water and autoclaved to remove any RNase enzyme.
9. Change gloves frequently during the experiment.
10. The sample volume should not exceed 10 % of the volume of TRIzol Reagent used for homogenization.
11. Following centrifugation, the mixture separates into a lower red, phenol–chloroform phase, an interphase, and a colorless upper aqueous phase. RNA remains exclusively in the aqueous phase. The volume of the aqueous phase is about 60 % of the volume of TRIzol Reagent used for homogenization.
12. Don't take the interphase.
13. The RNA precipitate, often invisible before centrifugation, forms a gel-like pellet on the side and bottom of the tube.
14. Do not dry the RNA by centrifugation under vacuum. It is important not to let the RNA pellet dry completely as this will greatly decrease its solubility.
15. Be sure to zero the spectrophotometer with the DEPC-treated water used for sample suspension.
16. The 28S and 18S ribosomal RNA bands should be fairly sharp, intense bands (size is dependent on the organism from which the RNA was obtained). The intensity of the upper band should be about twice that of the lower band. Smaller, more diffuse bands representing low molecular weight RNAs (tRNA and 5S ribosomal RNA) may be present. It is normal to see a diffuse smear of ethidium bromide staining material migrating

between the 18S and 28S ribosomal bands, probably comprised of mRNA and other heterogeneous RNA species. DNA contamination of the RNA preparation (if present) will be evident as a high molecular weight smear or band migrating above the 28S ribosomal RNA band. Degradation of the RNA will be reflected by smearing of ribosomal RNA bands.

17. We perform an analysis using Student's *t*-test in SPSS statistics software to test if the miRNA levels in two comparable groups are expressed in different amounts at a statistically significant level. We use samples obtained from healthy subjects as a control. The chip company also provides an internal control.

References

1. Pan Y, Sawalha AH (2009) Epigenetic regulation and the pathogenesis of systemic lupus erythematosus. Transl Res 153:4–10
2. Te JL et al (2010) Identification of unique microRNA signature associated with lupus nephritis. PLoS One 5:e10344
3. Dai R, Ahmed SA (2011) MicroRNA, a new paradigm for understanding immunoregulation, inflammation, and autoimmune diseases. Transl Res 157:163–179
4. Bartel DP (2004) MicroRNAs: genomics, biogenesis, mechanism, and function. Cell 116: 281–297
5. Huang JC, Babak T, Corson TW et al (2007) Using expression profiling data to identify human microRNA targets. Nat Methods 4:1045–1049
6. Carrington JC, Ambros V (2003) Role of microRNAs in plant and animal development. Science 301:336–338
7. Dai Y et al (2009) Comprehensive analysis of microRNA expression patterns in renal biopsies of lupus nephritis patients. Rheumatol Int 29:749–754
8. Wang H et al (2012) Circulating microRNAs as candidate biomarkers in patients with systemic lupus erythematosus. Transl Res 160: 198–206
9. Dai Y et al (2007) Microarray analysis of microRNA expression in peripheral blood cells of systemic lupus erythematosus patients. Lupus 16:939–946
10. Wang S-T, Li C, Liu L (2009) miRNA microarray technology in miRNA profiling. Curr Bioinform 4:141–148
11. Yongqiang C et al (2010) MicroRNA detection. Prog Chem 22:1509–1517
12. Ehrenreich A (2006) DNA microarray technology for the microbiologist: an overview. Appl Microbiol Biotechnol 73:255–273
13. Huang Y et al (2011) The discovery approaches and detection methods of microRNAs. Mol Biol Rep 38:4125–4135

Chapter 17

Laboratory Tests for the Antiphospholipid Syndrome

Charis Pericleous, Vera M. Ripoll, Ian Giles, and Yiannis Ioannou

Abstract

Antiphospholipid syndrome (APS) is an autoimmune disorder characterized by recurrent vascular thrombosis (VT) and/or pregnancy morbidity (PM) in the presence of persistent antiphospholipid antibodies (aPL), detected by lupus anticoagulant (LA), anticardiolipin (aCL) antibody, and/or anti-β_2 glycoprotein I (aβ_2GPI) antibody assays. These aPL, considered to be diagnostic markers and pathogenic drivers of APS, are a heterogeneous group of antibodies directed against anionic phospholipids, phospholipid-binding plasma proteins, and phospholipid–protein complexes. Although APS is currently considered as a single disease, it presents with a wide range of clinical symptoms and biological characteristics. The clinical diagnosis of APS in a patient with symptoms and signs is dependent upon the presence of a persistently positive result in an aPL assay. The tests recommended for detecting aPL are the standardized enzyme-linked immunosorbent assay (ELISA) to detect aCL and aβ_2GPI and clotting assays for LA performed according to the guidelines of the International Society on Thrombosis and Haemostasis [1, 2]. This chapter describes the standard laboratory test for the diagnosis of APS discussing the clinical and theoretical aspects of LA, aCL, and aβ_2GPI assays.

Key words Antiphospholipid syndrome, Lupus anticoagulant, Anticardiolipin antibody, Anti-β_2 glycoprotein I antibody

1 Introduction

The antiphospholipid syndrome (APS), characterized by the persistent presence of circulating antiphospholipid antibodies (aPL), remains the commonest cause of acquired hypercoagulability [3] and the most important treatable cause of recurrent miscarriage [4]. Pathogenic aPL target plasma proteins, mainly β_2-glycoprotein I (β_2GPI), that bind anionic phospholipids (PL). Considered a regulator of coagulation and fibrinolysis, β_2GPI cross-links anionic PL on the surface of target cells such as platelets and endothelium; aPL in turn bind β_2GPI, promoting a prothrombotic and proinflammatory phenotype (Fig. 1) [5, 6]. Classification criteria for

Charis Pericleous and Vera M. Ripoll have contributed equally to this chapter.

Paul Eggleton and Frank J. Ward (eds.), *Systemic Lupus Erythematosus: Methods and Protocols*, Methods in Molecular Biology, vol. 1134, DOI 10.1007/978-1-4939-0326-9_17, © Springer Science+Business Media New York 2014

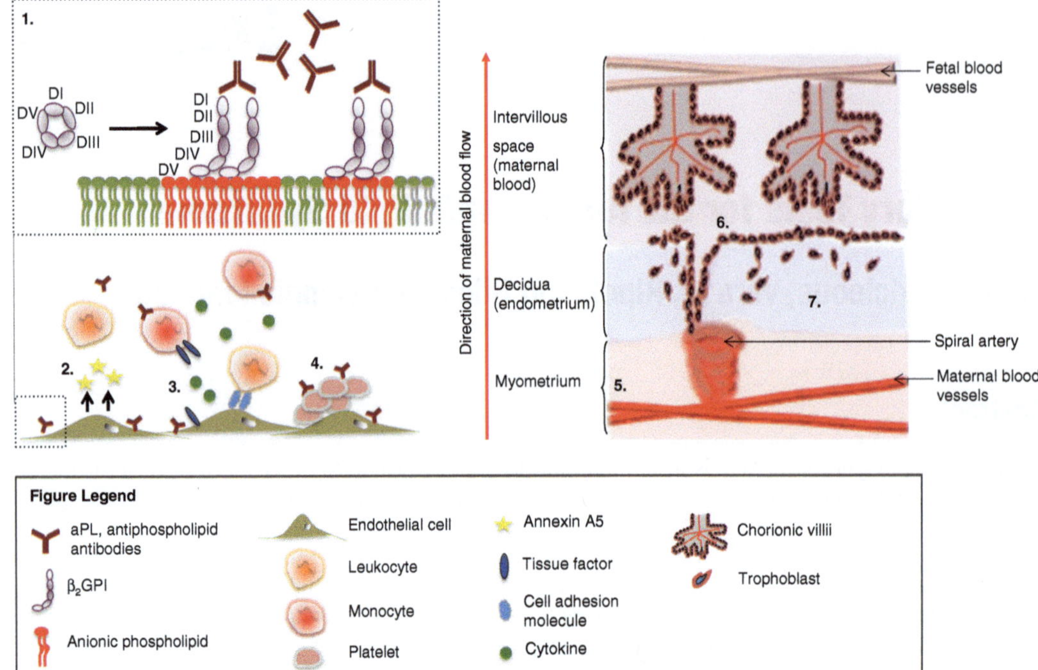

Fig. 1 Summary of the key pathogenic effects of aPL. (*1*) β_2GPI naturally exists in a closed, circular form. Upon encountering anionic PL on the surface of damaged or apoptotic cells, β_2GPI adopts its open fishhook form and binds PL via domain V (DV), while DI is now free to interact with pathogenic aPL. One antibody molecule cross-links two β_2GPI molecules, inducing a prothrombotic and proinflammatory phenotype. aPL promote thrombosis by (*2*) disruption of the cellular anticoagulant annexin-V shield; (*3*) upregulation of cell adhesion molecule expression on endothelial cells, thus allowing leukocytes to bind to the endothelium; and expression of tissue factor and cytokine release by endothelial cells and monocytes. (*4*) aPL also bind to platelets via PL-proteins such as β_2GPI or prothrombin, promoting platelet aggregation. Pregnancy complications in APS can occur as a result of (*5*) placental thrombosis; (*6*) direct effects of aPL on trophoblasts that reduce their ability to proliferate, grow, and invade maternal tissue, thus causing abnormal placentation; or (*7*) direct effects of aPL on endometrial cells to induce a proinflammatory response

APS require that both clinical (arterial and/or venous thrombosis and/or pregnancy morbidity) and laboratory (aPL positivity demonstrated over ≥12 weeks) criteria are present (Table 1) [1].

APS was first described in the early 1980s in patients with systemic lupus erythematosus (SLE); although APS can present in isolation, approximately 50 % of patients also suffer from SLE or other autoimmune diseases. A rare, severe form affecting <1 % of patients is known as "catastrophic APS" which leads to multiple organ failure due to widespread small vessel thrombosis [7].

Current laboratory classification criteria include two direct binding assays measuring antibodies against cardiolipin (aCL), a source of anionic phospholipid and β_2GPI (aβ_2GPI). A third functional assay relies on the ability of aPL to prolong coagulation in

Table 1
Classification criteria for antiphospholipid syndrome[a]

(A) Clinical criteria		
Vascular thrombosis	≥1 Clinical episodes of (1) Arterial or (2) Venous or (3) Small vessel thrombosis in any tissue or organ	Confirmed by imaging, ultrasound, or histopathology
Pregnancy morbidity	(1) ≥1 unexplained death(s) of a morphologically normal fetus ≥10 weeks of gestation or (2) ≥1 premature birth(s) ≤34 weeks of gestation or (3) ≥3 consecutive spontaneous abortions before 10 weeks of gestation	Normal fetal morphology is documented by ultrasound or direct examination of fetus
(B) Laboratory criteria		
Lupus anticoagulant (LA)	Present in plasma on ≥2 occasions at least 12 weeks apart	Detected according to ISTH guidelines [41, 42]
Anticardiolipin antibodies (aCL)	IgG and/or IgM isotype in serum or plasma at medium or high titer (>40 G/MPL units or >99th percentile) on ≥2 occasions at least 12 weeks apart	Measured by standardized ELISA; consensus on assay and standards
Anti-β_2GPI antibodies (aβ_2GPI)	IgG and/or IgM isotype in serum or plasma (titer >99th percentile) on ≥2 occasions at least 12 weeks apart	Measured by standardized ELISA; recommended procedure to be followed but lacking consensus on assay and standards

β_2GPI β_2 glycoprotein I, *CL* cardiolipin, *ELISA* enzyme-linked immunosorbent assay, *GPL* IgG phospholipid units, *MPL* IgM phospholipid units

[a]Adapted from Miyakis et al. [1]. At least one clinical and one laboratory criterion must be met to diagnose APS

various in vitro clotting tests; this effect is known as lupus anticoagulant (LA) [1]. While aCL positivity is strictly β_2GPI-dependent, LA positivity can be attributed to antibodies against β_2GPI or prothrombin [5]. Patients with APS can test positive in one, two, or all three tests for IgG and/or IgM aPL. In this chapter, we provide protocols for performing all three assays, which are the most common aPL assays employed in both the clinical and research setting. Other assays that have been postulated to have diagnostic or prognostic potential include the detection of antibodies to the N-terminal domain of β_2GPI (anti-domain I assay) [8–10], to prothrombin alone or phosphatidylserine/prothrombin complexes (anti-PT and anti-PS/PT assays) [11, 12], and an assay measuring resistance to the anticoagulant effects of annexin-V (annexin-V resistance assay) [13–15], reviewed in [16]. These assays, however, are not in routine clinical use, do not form part of the current classification criteria [1], and are thus beyond the scope of this chapter.

2 Materials

2.1 Components for Detection of Anticardiolipin Antibodies (aCL) by ELISA

1. 96-well PolySorp plates (Nunc).
2. CL solution from bovine heart in ethanol, ≥97 % purity (Sigma-Aldrich).
3. Ethanol (Absolute).
4. Phosphate-buffered saline (PBS), pH 7.4.
5. Fetal bovine serum (FBS).
6. Serum samples diluted 1:50 in 10 % FBS in PBS.
7. Calibrators for the measurement of aCL antibodies IgG and IgM (Louisville APL Diagnostics, Inc.).
8. Anti-human IgG (γ-chain specific) or anti-human IgM (μ-chain specific) alkaline phosphatase antibody (Sigma-Aldrich).
9. Alkaline phosphatase substrate (pNPP Microwell Substrate System, Kirkegaard & Perry Laboratories).
10. Multichannel pipet.
11. Reagent reservoirs.
12. Polypropylene microfuge tubes.
13. Absorbent pads.
14. Spectrophotometer.

Components for Determination of Anti-β_2GPI Antibodies (aβ_2GPI) by ELISA

1. 96-well MaxiSorp plates (Nunc)
2. Human β_2GPI. Purified from serum by Heparin Sepharose chromatography (Louisville APL Diagnostics, Inc.).
3. 0.1 % of Tween in PBS, pH 7.4.
4. 0.5 % of porcine gelatin (Sigma-Aldrich) in PBS.
5. 1 % bovine serum albumin (BSA) (Sigma-Aldrich) in PBS.
6. Serum samples diluted 1:50 in 1 % BSA in PBS.
7. Calibrators for the measurement of aβ_2GPI. For this ELISA, a serum sample from a patient with high aβ_2GPI binding is used (*see* **Note 1** below).
8. Anti-human IgG (γ-chain specific) or anti-human IgM (μ-chain specific) peroxidase antibody (Sigma-Aldrich).
9. Horseradish peroxidase substrate (SureBlue 3,3′,5,5′-tetramethylbenzidine (TMB) Microwell Substrate, Kirkegaard & Perry Laboratories, KPL).
10. TMB Stop Solution (SureBlue TMB Microwell Substrate, Kirkegaard & Perry Laboratories, KPL).
11. Multichannel pipet.
12. Reagent reservoirs.

13. Polypropylene microfuge tubes.
14. Absorbent pads.
15. Aluminum foil.
16. Spectrophotometer.

2.2 Components for Determining the Presence of Lupus Anticoagulant (LA)

1. Patient and healthy control platelet poor plasma (PPP) prepared from fresh venous blood (9 vol.) in 0.109 M trisodium citrate (1 vol.).
2. Quality control plasmas—normal and abnormal for LA (commercially available).
3. Commercially available dRVVT and aPTT kits (*see* **Note 12**).
4. Distilled water.
5. 0.025 M calcium chloride solution (for some kits).
6. Stopwatch.
7. Semiautomated or automated coagulometer, fibrometer, or electromagnetic water bath.

3 Methods

3.1 Principle of the aCL Assay

Cardiolipin (CL) was originally described as an antigenic target present in the blood of patients with syphilis. Later, it became clear that not all patients with antibodies against CL had syphilis but they occasionally developed thrombotic events [17] and recurrent pregnancy losses [18]. In the early 1950s, antibodies against CL were associated with prolonged whole blood clotting time in patients with SLE, an inhibitory effect referred as the LA [19]. Later, in the 1980s, Hughes reported a correlation between thrombosis, LA positivity, and aCL [20]. These findings led to the definition of aCL or "Hughes syndrome," known today as APS.

CL is an essential component of the inner mitochondrial membrane, an anionic PL composed of two phosphate groups and four fatty acids. Antibodies that bind CL may occur transiently, especially postinfection. These are often of the IgM subtype and bind CL directly. However, pathogenic antibodies that bind CL as seen in APS tend to be IgG and are dependent upon the presence of the PL-binding cofactor β_2GPI [21–23]. It is believed that the antigenicity of CL is driven by its relocation from the mitochondria to the cell surface during death receptor-mediated apoptosis [24]. The aCL found in patients with APS may be of the IgG, IgM, or IgA isotype.

The aCL ELISA method measures the interaction of antibodies present in diluted patient serum to CL bound to the microplate in the presence of bovine serum that contains a source of the β_2GPI cofactor. This method allows the detection of antibodies that bind CL alone and those that bind CL-bound β_2GPI (*see* **Notes 1–3**).

3.2 Methods

1. Coat the test half of a 96-well PolySorp plate with 50 μL/well of 50 μg/mL of CL in pure ethanol.
2. Coat the control half of the plate with 50 μL/well of pure ethanol.
3. Incubate the plate at 4 °C overnight, uncovered.
4. Wash the plate two times with PBS.
5. Block the plate with 100 μL/well of 10 % FBS in PBS. Cover the wells and incubate for 1 h at room temperature.
6. Wash the plate three times with PBS. Tap plate upside down on a clean absorbent pad to remove any remaining wash solution (*see* **Note 4**).
7. Load 50 μL/well of the calibrators and 50 μL/well of the serum samples diluted 1:50 in 10 % FBS in PBS into both the test half and the control half of the plate. Samples should be loaded in duplicates (*see* **Note 5**).
8. Cover the wells and incubate both the calibrators and the serum samples for 60–90 min at room temperature.
9. Wash the plate three times with PBS.
10. Add 50 μL/well of anti-human IgG (γ-chain specific) or anti-human IgM (μ-chain specific) alkaline phosphatase antibody diluted according to manufacturer's recommendations in 10 % FBS in PBS.
11. Cover the wells and incubate the plate for 1 h at room temperature.
12. Wash the plate three times with PBS.
13. Add 50 μL/well of alkaline phosphatase substrate prepared according to the manufacturer's instructions.
14. Cover the wells and incubate the plate at room temperature for 30 and 60 min.
15. Read the plate in a spectrophotometer at 405 nm after 30 min and again after 60 min.
16. Calculate the net optical density (OD) by subtracting the background present in the control half of the plate to the test half of the plate.
17. The standard curve is constructed by plotting the net OD value measured for each calibrator versus its corresponding GPL or MPL units (IgG or IgM phospholipid units). One GPL or MPL unit is defined as the CL-binding activity of 1 μg/mL of an affinity purified IgG or IgM aCL preparation from a standard serum. A standard curve should be constructed each time the assay is performed (*see* **Note 6**).
18. After adjusting the fit of the curve to a logarithmic regression, interpolate the GPL or MPL units of the test samples directly from the standard curve.

19. Positivity is defined by the presence of medium or high titers (i.e., >40 GPL or MPL units or >99th percentile) of IgG and/or IgM phospholipid antibodies (*see* **Note 5**).

3.3 Principle of the aβ_2GPI Assay

A number of reports in the 1990s demonstrated that β_2GPI is necessary for the binding of aCL in the solid-phase immunoassays [22, 25]. β_2GPI, also known as apolipoprotein H, is a 50 kDa glycoprotein present in high concentrations in plasma. It circulates in the serum in a primarily circular and biochemically reduced form [26–28], and upon binding, aβ_2GPI linearizes into the characteristic fishhook shape [26]. This glycoprotein is mainly produced by hepatocytes but also synthesized by fetal astrocytes, as well as intestinal and placental cells [29]. The function of β_2GPI remains largely unknown; however, it is thought to act as an anticoagulant regulator through the inhibition of prothrombinase and factor XII–factor XI activation [30, 31]. β_2GPI consists of five homologous domains; domain V is positively charged, allowing β_2GPI to bind negatively charged phospholipids (*see* Fig. 1). Antibodies directed to N-terminal domain (domain I, DI) are better correlated with venous thrombosis than those directed to other domains or even CL [10, 32]. Anti-DI antibodies can cross-link β_2GPI molecules and thus increase the affinity of β_2GPI for the cell surface, thus lowering the threshold for the activation of endothelial cells and monocytes.

The aβ_2GPI ELISA method measures the interaction of antibodies present in diluted patient serum to human β_2GPI bound to the microplate.

3.4 Methods

1. Coat the test half of a 96-well MaxiSorp plate with 50 μL/well of 4 μg/mL of human β_2GPI in PBS (*see* **Note 7**).
2. Coat the control half of the plate with 50 μL/well of PBS.
3. Cover the wells and incubate the plate at 4 °C overnight.
4. Wash the plate two times with 0.1 % of Tween in PBS.
5. Block the plate with 150 μL/well of freshly made 0.5 % of porcine gelatin in PBS. Allow the gelatin to cool down for a minimum of 20 min at room temperature.
6. Cover the wells and incubate for 60 min at 37 °C.
7. Wash the plate three times with 0.1 % of Tween in PBS. Tap plate upside down on a clean absorbent pad to remove any remaining wash solution (*see* **Note 8**).
8. Load 50 μL/well of the calibrator and 50 μL/well of the serum samples diluted 1:50 in 1 % BSA in PBS into both the test half and the control half of the plate. Samples should be loaded in duplicates (*see* **Notes 9–11**).
9. Cover the wells and incubate both the calibrators and the serum samples for 60 min at room temperature.
10. Wash the plate three times with 0.1 % of Tween in PBS.

11. Add 50 μL/well of anti-human IgG (γ-chain specific) or anti-human IgM (μ-chain specific) peroxidase antibody diluted according to manufacturer's recommendations in 1 % BSA in PBS.
12. Cover the wells and incubate the plate for 60 min at room temperature.
13. Wash the plate three times with 0.1 % of Tween in PBS.
14. Add 100 μL/well of peroxidase substrate (SureBlue TMB).
15. Cover the plate with aluminum foil and incubate the plate at room temperature for 15 min.
16. Stop the reaction with 100 μL/well of stop solution.
17. Read the plate in a spectrophotometer at 450 nm.
18. Calculate the net OD by subtracting the background present in the control half of the plate to the test half of the plate.
19. The standard curve is constructed by plotting the net OD value measured for each calibrator versus its corresponding units (*see* **Note 9**). A standard curve should be constructed each time the assay is performed.
20. After adjusting the fit of the curve to a logarithmic regression, interpolate the units of the test samples directly from the standard curve.
21. Positivity is defined by the cutoff determined in the laboratory (*see* **Note 10**).

3.5 Principle of Determining the Presence of Lupus Anticoagulant (LA)

The International Society on Thrombosis and Haemostasis (ISTH) guidelines for determining LA positivity highlight the need to perform two clotting tests, based on either the extrinsic (tissue factor) or intrinsic (contact) coagulation pathway (Fig. 2). The two recommended tests are the dilute Russell viper venom time (dRVVT, extrinsic pathway) and the activated partial thromboplastin time (aPTT, intrinsic pathway) (*see* **Note 12**). The presence of LA is confirmed if either test (or both) gives a positive result [33, 34]. The principle of the LA test relies on three distinct steps (Fig. 3):

1. Screening: determines prolongation of clotting time in the presence of low PL concentrations.
2. Mixing: pooled healthy control plasma and patient plasma mixed at a 1:1 ratio is tested as per **step 1**. To exclude the possibility that coagulation factor(s) deficiency is responsible for a positive result in **step 1**, addition of normal plasma would partly correct for the prolongation of clotting time observed.
3. Confirmatory: as per **step 1** but with high PL concentrations.

Commercial kits for screening and confirming can be interpreted without the mixing step. Manufacturer guidelines must be stringently followed; common practice is outlined below.

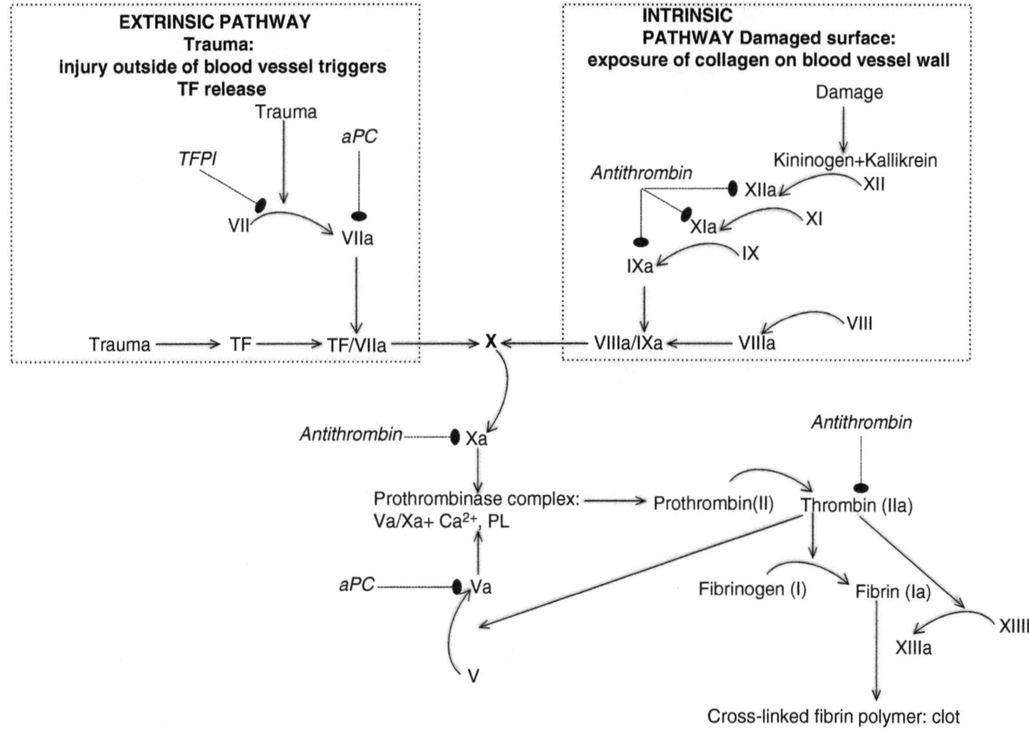

Fig. 2 Summary of the extrinsic (or tissue factor) and intrinsic (or contact) coagulation pathways. *Curved arrows* indicate activation; *blunt end arrows* (and coagulation factors in *italics*) represent inhibition of coagulation (and inhibitors, respectively). *aPC* activated protein C, *Ca^{2+}* calcium ions, *PL* phospholipids, *TF* tissue factor, *TFPI* tissue factor pathway inhibitor

Please note: LA detection in patients on long-term vitamin K antagonists (VKAs) should not be performed as VKAs inhibit the activation of naturally circulating clotting factors, giving false-positive results. LA tests should only be performed 1–2 weeks after discontinuation of treatment or when the international normalized ratio (INR) is <1.5. Patients on low molecular weight heparin can be tested for LA; however, blood should be drawn more than 12 h after the last dose of heparin is administered [34]. The Taipan snake venom time (TSVT) test has been described as an alternative to the dRVVT for patients on VKAs. The TSVT does not interfere with vitamin K-dependent activation of clotting factors, affecting only prothrombin activation [35, 36].

3.6 Methods

1. To obtain PPP, centrifuge blood at 2,000 × *g* for 15 min and transfer plasma to a fresh plastic tube for a second centrifugation at >2,500 × *g* for 10 min. Collect the PPP, taking care not to include any residual pelleted platelets. Test PPP either immediately or quickly freeze at −70 °C or below for future use. Frozen PPP must be thawed rapidly in a 37 °C water bath for 5 min and mixed thoroughly before testing. Residual PPP cannot be refrozen for future LA testing.

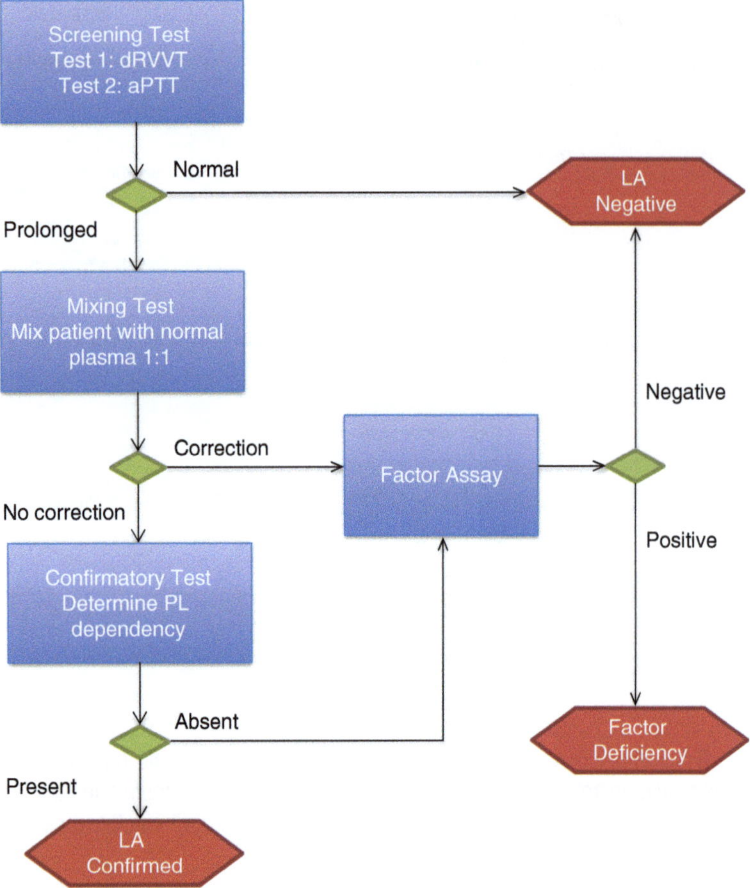

Fig. 3 Lupus anticoagulant test. The diagram shows a flowchart for the investigation of a suspected LA from initial screening to further confirmatory tests. *aPTT* activated partial thromboplastin time, *dRVVT* diluted Russell viper venom test, *PL* phospholipid

2. Vials of commercially available quality control plasmas are available in lyophilized form. Reconstitute in distilled water as stated by the manufacturer (*see* **Notes 13–14**).
3. Commercial kits for clotting tests include vials comprising a mixture of the clotting activation agent (e.g., RVV), PL, and, in most cases, calcium and heparin-neutralizing substances. The mixture either is in lyophilized form and requires reconstitution in distilled water or comes as a ready-to-use solution. Allow the reagent to reach room temperature (18–25 °C) for 30 min prior to use (*see* **Note 15**).
4. Perform LA tests with equal volumes of PPP and reagent (e.g., 100 μL each).
   (a) Semiautomated method: incubate PPP at 37 °C for 2 min in either a glass tube or the reactional cuvette of the coagulation

instrument. In the meantime, pre-warm the kit's reagent in the same manner. Mix reagent well and add an equal volume to PPP (if calcium is not included, add the same volume of pre-warmed calcium solution at this stage, as stated in the kit guidelines). Record the exact clotting time in seconds (e.g., stop of the metal ball indicating clot formation).

(b) Automated method: set the instrument test mode to dispense equal volumes of PPP and well-mixed reagent (±calcium). All components must be pre-warmed at 37 °C for 2 min prior to use (*see* **Note 16**).

5. Compare the patient sample clotting time to the reference healthy control range of the laboratory. Samples are suspected positive for LA when the clotting time exceeds the healthy control range cutoff (*see* **Note 17**).
6. Confirm LA positivity by performing the same test using an excess of PL (*see* **Note 18**).
7. Screening and confirmation tests should not be performed on patients on oral anticoagulants. In some cases, it is possible to perform the same test using a mix of equal volumes of patient and pooled healthy control plasma (*see* **Note 19**).

4 Notes

1. It should be noted that the aCL assay can detect a wide range of aPL antibodies, some with clinical relevance to thrombosis such as aβ_2GPI, and other antibodies with no clinical relevance of which most are associated with infection [37].
2. A weakness of the aCL assay is that it can miss patient antibodies that bind human but not bovine β_2GPI.
3. An initial lack of reference calibrators (e.g., monoclonal versus polyclonal) led to differences in sample results between commercial and in-house assays. Thus sample classification as low, medium, and high positive results could be different depending on the assay used. The introduction, however, of polyclonal calibrators with predefined GPL or MPL units (Louisville APL Diagnostics, Inc.) has allowed comparisons of test results across laboratories [38–43]. As a result, GPL and MPL units are included in APS classification criteria [1].
4. Coated and blocked plates can be kept at 4 °C for up to a month before use.
5. Healthy control samples must be tested in the same manner as patient samples. Take the cutoff for positivity as the value above the 99th percentile of the healthy samples' distribution.

6. It is highly recommended to include a positive and a negative control on each ELISA plate. In the case that the value of the positive control falls outside the predefined percentile, the whole run should be rejected and repeated.
7. The source of purified human β_2GPI may affect how well this assay works. With some sources of human β_2GPI, this ELISA does not give a reliable readout or negligible ODs despite known positive samples. One theory is that β_2GPI is also a substrate for plasmin which causes proteolytic clipping at Lys317–Thr318, and this may affect binding of the protein to negatively charged surfaces [44]. If the purified β_2GPI is clipped in this way, its utility on the standard β_2GPI assay may be compromised.
8. Coated and blocked plates can be kept at 4 °C for up to a month before use.
9. In-house calibrator can be derived from a pool or a single positive patient/s sample/s. An initial 1:50 dilution of the positive sample/s is serially diluted in a 1:1 ratio. Arbitrary activity units of 100, 50, 25, 12.5, 6.25, 3.125, and 1.25 are given.
10. Unlike the aCL ELISA, there are no predefined units to determine positivity in the aβ_2GPI ELISA. Thus we recommend establishing the in-house cutoff level by analyzing at least 200 samples from normal subjects, age and sex matched with the patient population. As per APS criteria guidelines [1], take the cutoff for positivity as the value above the 99th percentile of the healthy samples' distribution.
11. It is highly recommended to include a positive and a negative control on each ELISA plate. In the case that the value of the positive control falls outside the predefined percentile, the whole run should be rejected and repeated.
12. Kaolin-, ecarin-, textarin-based and dilute prothrombin time tests should be avoided due to variability of reagents, poor reproducibility, and/or insensitivity for LA.
13. Quality control plasmas should include both commercially sourced normal and abnormal for LA plasmas. Once reconstituted, such plasmas are stable for 8–24 h at 2–8 °C (depending on manufacturer). Do not freeze.
14. Test both normal and abnormal control plasmas ideally with each test series or with each batch of 40 test samples as a minimum.
15. Once opened, the reaction reagent is usually stable for 24 h at 18–25 °C, 2–7 days at 2–8 °C (depending on manufacturer), or 1 month at –20 °C. Once defrosted, warm to 37 °C and mix well before use. Do not refreeze any residual reagent.

16. When using an automated instrument, dedicated reagent tubing must be used and magnetic stir bars in reservoirs are recommended. Ensure the instrument is cleaned before and after use.
17. Healthy control plasma samples must be tested in the same manner as patient samples. Take the cutoff for positivity as the value above the 99th percentile of the healthy samples' distribution.
18. The confirmatory test must have a separate cutoff to the one used for the screening test. Perform tests with healthy control plasma using both low (screen) and high (confirm) PL concentrations. Record clotting time in seconds and use the following formula to determine the percentage correction for each plasma sample: $[(\text{screen-confirm})/\text{screen}] \times 100$. Calculate the mean of the individual percentage corrections—this is the cutoff value for the confirmatory test.
19. Perform and interpret mixing tests with caution if using plasma from patients on oral anticoagulants. Only carry out the mixing test if the international normalized ratio (INR) is between 1.5 and <3.0. Interpretation of results may still be difficult and the LA titer will be diluted twofold. Of note, the TSVT is increasingly viewed as a useful alternative to detect LA in patients on VKAs; further evaluation is required before its possible inclusion in ISTH guidelines for LA testing.

References

1. Miyakis S, Lockshin MD, Atsumi T, Branch DW, Brey RL, Cervera R, Derksen RH, de Groot PG, Koike T, Meroni PL, Reber G, Shoenfeld Y, Tincani A, Vlachoyiannopoulos PG, Krilis SA (2006) International consensus statement on an update of the classification criteria for definite antiphospholipid syndrome (APS). J Thromb Haemost 4:295–306
2. de Groot PG (2011) Mechanisms of antiphospholipid antibody formation and action. Thromb Res 127(Suppl 3):S40–S42
3. Petri M (2000) Epidemiology of the antiphospholipid antibody syndrome. J Autoimmun 15:145–151
4. Rai RS (2002) Antiphospholipid syndrome and recurrent miscarriage. J Postgrad Med 48:3–4
5. Meroni PL, Borghi MO, Raschi E, Tedesco F (2011) Pathogenesis of antiphospholipid syndrome: understanding the antibodies. Nat Rev Rheumatol 7:330–339
6. Willis R, Pierangeli SS (2013) Anti-beta2-glycoprotein I antibodies. Ann N Y Acad Sci 1285:44–58
7. Cervera R, Piette JC, Font J, Khamashta MA, Shoenfeld Y, Camps MT, Jacobsen S, Lakos G, Tincani A, Kontopoulou-Griva I, Galeazzi M, Meroni PL, Derksen RH, de Groot PG, Gromnica-Ihle E, Baleva M, Mosca M, Bombardieri S, Houssiau F, Gris JC, Quere I, Hachulla E, Vasconcelos C, Roch B, Fernandez-Nebro A, Boffa MC, Hughes GR, Ingelmo M (2002) Antiphospholipid syndrome: clinical and immunologic manifestations and patterns of disease expression in a cohort of 1,000 patients. Arthritis Rheum 46: 1019–1027
8. de Laat HB, Derksen RH, Urbanus RT, Roest M, de Groot PG (2004) Beta2-glycoprotein I-dependent lupus anticoagulant highly correlates with thrombosis in the antiphospholipid syndrome. Blood 104:3598–3602
9. Ioannou Y, Pericleous C, Giles I, Latchman DS, Isenberg DA, Rahman A (2007) Binding of antiphospholipid antibodies to discontinuous epitopes on domain I of human beta(2)-glycoprotein I: mutation studies including residues R39 to R43. Arthritis Rheum 56:280–290
10. de Laat B, Pengo V, Pabinger I, Musial J, Voskuyl AE, Bultink IE, Ruffatti A, Rozman B, Kveder T, de Moerloose P, Boehlen F, Rand J, Ulcova-Gallova Z, Mertens K, de Groot PG (2009) The association between circulating

antibodies against domain I of beta2-glycoprotein I and thrombosis: an international multicenter study. J Thromb Haemost 7:1767–1773

11. Atsumi T, Ieko M, Bertolaccini ML, Ichikawa K, Tsutsumi A, Matsuura E, Koike T (2000) Association of autoantibodies against the phosphatidylserine-prothrombin complex with manifestations of the antiphospholipid syndrome and with the presence of lupus anticoagulant. Arthritis Rheum 43:1982–1993
12. Bertolaccini ML, Atsumi T, Koike T, Hughes GR, Khamashta MA (2005) Antiprothrombin antibodies detected in two different assay systems. Prevalence and clinical significance in systemic lupus erythematosus. Thromb Haemost 93:289–297
13. Rand JH, Wu XX, Lapinski R, van Heerde WL, Reutelingsperger CP, Chen PP, Ortel TL (2004) Detection of antibody-mediated reduction of annexin A5 anticoagulant activity in plasmas of patients with the antiphospholipid syndrome. Blood 104:2783–2790
14. de Laat B, Wu XX, van Lummel M, Derksen RH, de Groot PG, Rand JH (2007) Correlation between antiphospholipid antibodies that recognize domain I of beta2-glycoprotein I and a reduction in the anticoagulant activity of annexin A5. Blood 109:1490–1494
15. Rand JH, Wu XX, Quinn AS, Taatjes DJ (2010) The annexin A5-mediated pathogenic mechanism in the antiphospholipid syndrome: role in pregnancy losses and thrombosis. Lupus 19:460–469
16. Bertolaccini ML, Amengual O, Atsumi T, Binder WL, de Laat B, Forastiero R, Kutteh WH, Lambert M, Matsubayashi H, Murthy V, Petri M, Rand JH, Sanmarco M, Tebo AE, Pierangeli SS (2011) 'Non-criteria' aPL tests: report of a task force and preconference workshop at the 13th international congress on antiphospholipid antibodies, Galveston, TX, USA, April 2010. Lupus 20:191–205
17. Moore JE, Lutz WB (1955) The natural history of systemic lupus erythematosus: an approach to its study through chronic biologic false positive reactors. J Chronic Dis 1:297–316
18. Laurell AB, Nilsson IM (1957) Hypergammaglobulinemia, circulating anticoagulant and biological false positive Wassermann reaction: a study in two cases. J Lab Clin Med 49:694–707
19. Conley CL (1952) Disorders of the blood in disseminated lupus erythematosus. Am J Med 13:1–2
20. Hughes GR (1983) Thrombosis, abortion, cerebral disease, and the lupus anticoagulant. Br Med J 287:1088–1089
21. McNeil HP, Simpson RJ, Chesterman CN, Krilis SA (1990) Anti-phospholipid antibodies are directed against a complex antigen that includes a lipid-binding inhibitor of coagulation: beta 2-glycoprotein I (apolipoprotein H). Proc Natl Acad Sci U S A 87:4120–4124
22. Galli M, Comfurius P, Maassen C, Hemker HC, de Baets MH, van Breda-Vriesman PJ, Barbui T, Zwaal RF, Bevers EM (1990) Anticardiolipin antibodies (ACA) directed not to cardiolipin but to a plasma protein cofactor. Lancet 335:1544–1547
23. Matsuura E, Igarashi Y, Yasuda T, Triplett DA, Koike T (1994) Anticardiolipin antibodies recognize beta 2-glycoprotein I structure altered by interacting with an oxygen modified solid phase surface. J Exp Med 179:457–462
24. Sorice M, Circella A, Misasi R, Pittoni V, Garofalo T, Cirelli A, Pavan A, Pontieri GM, Valesini G (2000) Cardiolipin on the surface of apoptotic cells as a possible trigger for antiphospholipids antibodies. Clin Exp Immunol 122:277–284
25. Matsuura E, Igarashi Y, Fujimoto M, Ichikawa K, Koike T (1990) Anticardiolipin cofactor(s) and differential diagnosis of autoimmune disease. Lancet 336:177–178
26. Agar C, van Os GM, Morgelin M, Sprenger RR, Marquart JA, Urbanus RT, Derksen RH, Meijers JC, de Groot PG (2010) Beta2-glycoprotein I can exist in 2 conformations: implications for our understanding of the antiphospholipid syndrome. Blood 116: 1336–1343
27. Ioannou Y, Zhang JY, Passam FH, Rahgozar S, Qi JC, Giannakopoulos B, Qi M, Yu P, Yu DM, Hogg PJ, Krilis SA (2010) Naturally occurring free thiols within beta 2-glycoprotein I in vivo: nitrosylation, redox modification by endothelial cells, and regulation of oxidative stress-induced cell injury. Blood 116: 1961–1970
28. Agar C, de Groot PG, Morgelin M, Monk SD, van Os G, Levels JH, de Laat B, Urbanus RT, Herwald H, van der Poll T, Meijers JC (2011) Beta(2)-glycoprotein I: a novel component of innate immunity. Blood 117:6939–6947
29. Caronti B, Calderaro C, Alessandri C, Conti F, Tinghino R, Palladini G, Valesini G (1999) Beta2-glycoprotein I (beta2-GPI) mRNA is expressed by several cell types involved in antiphospholipid syndrome-related tissue damage. Clin Exp Immunol 115:214–219
30. Nimpf J, Bevers EM, Bomans PH, Till U, Wurm H, Kostner GM, Zwaal RF (1986) Prothrombinase activity of human platelets is inhibited by beta 2-glycoprotein-I. Biochim Biophys Acta 884:142–149

31. Shi T, Iverson GM, Qi JC, Cockerill KA, Linnik MD, Konecny P, Krilis SA (2004) Beta 2-glycoprotein I binds factor XI and inhibits its activation by thrombin and factor XIIa: loss of inhibition by clipped beta 2-glycoprotein I. Proc Natl Acad Sci U S A 101:3939–3944

32. Galli M, Luciani D, Bertolini G, Barbui T (2003) Anti-beta 2-glycoprotein I, antiprothrombin antibodies, and the risk of thrombosis in the antiphospholipid syndrome. Blood 102:2717–2723

33. Brandt JT, Barna LK, Triplett DA (1995) Laboratory identification of lupus anticoagulants: results of the second international workshop for identification of lupus anticoagulants. On behalf of the subcommittee on lupus anticoagulants/antiphospholipid antibodies of the ISTH. Thromb Haemost 74:1597–1603

34. Pengo V, Tripodi A, Reber G, Rand JH, Ortel TL, Galli M, De Groot PG (2009) Update of the guidelines for lupus anticoagulant detection. Subcommittee on lupus anticoagulant/antiphospholipid antibody of the scientific and standardisation committee of the international society on thrombosis and haemostasis. J Thromb Haemost 7:1737–1740

35. Rooney AM, McNally T, Mackie IJ, Machin SJ (1994) The Taipan snake venom time: a new test for lupus anticoagulant. J Clin Pathol 47:497–501

36. Parmar K, Lefkou E, Doughty H, Connor P, Hunt BJ (2009) The utility of the Taipan snake venom assay in assessing lupus anticoagulant status in individuals receiving or not receiving an oral vitamin K antagonist. Blood Coagul Fibrinolysis 20:271–275

37. Hunt JE, McNeil HP, Morgan GJ, Crameri RM, Krilis SA (1992) A phospholipid-beta 2-glycoprotein I complex is an antigen for anticardiolipin antibodies occurring in autoimmune disease but not with infection. Lupus 1:75–81

38. Harris EN, Gharavi AE, Patel SP, Hughes GR (1987) Evaluation of the anti-cardiolipin antibody test: report of an international workshop held 4 April 1986. Clin Exp Immunol 68: 215–222

39. Harris EN (1990) Special report. The second international anti-cardiolipin standardization workshop/the Kingston anti-phospholipid antibody study (KAPS) group. Am J Clin Pathol 94:476–484

40. Harris EN, Pierangeli S, Birch D (1994) Anticardiolipin wet workshop report. Fifth international symposium on antiphospholipid antibodies. Am J Clin Pathol 101:616–624

41. Pierangeli SS, Stewart M, Silva LK, Harris EN (1998) An antiphospholipid wet workshop: 7th international symposium on antiphospholipid antibodies. J Rheumatol 25:156–160

42. Harris EN, Pierangeli SS (2002) Revisiting the anticardiolipin test and its standardization. Lupus 11:269–275

43. Pierangeli SS, Harris EN (2008) A protocol for determination of anticardiolipin antibodies by ELISA. Nat Protoc 3:840–848

44. Miyakis S, Giannakopoulos B, Krilis SA (2004) Beta 2 glycoprotein I—function in health and disease. Thromb Res 114:335–346

Chapter 18

Isolation, Polarization, and Expansion of CD4⁺ Helper T Cell Lines and Clones Using Magnetic Beads

Lekh N. Dahal, Robert N. Barker, and Frank J. Ward

Abstract

Autoreactive $CD4^+$ helper T cells specific for a range of nucleoprotein-derived autoantigens are an important feature of systemic lupus erythematosus, driving B cell differentiation and autoantibody production and contributing to the inflammatory lesions caused by immune complex deposition. Several peptide epitopes from nucleoprotein antigens have been identified and offer a means selectively to manipulate T cell responses by skewing toward a profile of cytokines that is less pro-inflammatory.

Antigen-specific T cell lines and clones can be useful in the study of helper T cell subsets because their life span is prolonged and many individual cells can be generated, allowing particular phenotypes to be studied in detail. Magnetic beads offer a robust and convenient method for the isolation, polarization, and expansion of T cells, which can be adapted for a broad range of applications.

Key words Helper T cell, T cell line, T cell clone, Magnetic bead expansion, Antigen specificity

1 Introduction

T lymphocyte (T cell) hyperactivity is accepted to be a contributory factor in the underlying disease process of systemic lupus erythematosus, playing a role in driving both autoantibody production and the inflammatory processes associated with immune complex deposition (reviewed in [1, 2]). In particular, $CD4^+$ helper T cells are important for the development of high-affinity autoantibodies by providing antigen-dependent costimulatory signals as well as cytokines that promote cell division and license antibody class switching from low-affinity IgM to higher-affinity IgG molecules in B cells [3]. The precise cytokine profile secreted by different $CD4^+$ helper T cell subsets varies according to the nature of the pathogenic challenge and the particular cues received by T cells from the innate immune system in the early response phase [4]. The first $CD4^+$ helper T cell subsets, T helper (Th)1 and Th2 T cells, were identified several years ago [5] and predominantly

Paul Eggleton and Frank J. Ward (eds.), *Systemic Lupus Erythematosus: Methods and Protocols*, Methods in Molecular Biology, vol. 1134, DOI 10.1007/978-1-4939-0326-9_18, © Springer Science+Business Media New York 2014

Table 1
Summary of CD4⁺ helper T cell subsets

CD4⁺ T cell subset	Differentiating cytokines	Cytokine profile	Probable role in immunity
Th1	IL-12, IFN-γ	IFN-γ	Cell-mediated immunity
Th2	IL-2, IL-4	IL-4, IL-5, IL-13	Extracellular immunity
Th17	IL-6, IL-1β, TGF-β	IL-17A, IL-17F, IL-22	Bacterial and fungal infection
T_{FH}[a]	IL-12, IL-6, IL-21(?)	IL-21, IL-10	Driving B cell responses
Inducible regulatory T cells	IL-2, TGF-β	IL-10, TGF-β	Regulation of effector T cell responses

Differentiation, function, and cellular origin of T_{FH} require further elucidation
[a]T follicular helper cells

secrete IFN-γ and IL-4/IL-5, respectively, but more recently it has become clear that there are more T helper phenotypes, each secreting individual cytokine profiles, which have evolved to provide immunity against particular types of pathogen or other environmental challenge (*see* Table 1). Notably, Th17 T cells that secrete large amounts of IL-17 have been investigated for their role in autoimmune disease [6]. It is likely that more helper T cell subset phenotypes will be defined in future years and could be relevant to lupus disease. Thus, methods to study the precise phenotype and cytokine profiles of CD4⁺ helper T cells in autoimmune disease are therefore important for the study of the individual roles they play in SLE and further, to be able to examine the effects of skewing particular T cell secretion patterns on changing levels of autoantibody development and immune complex lesion formation, which may be useful therapeutically.

In humans and mice, several peptide epitopes have been identified from nucleosomes and other autoantigens that drive CD4⁺ T cell responses [7–11], and because they are central to the autoimmune response, they represent a potential target to manipulate this response, with the advantage of being highly selective. One such peptide, derived from small nuclear ribonucleoprotein U1-70K, has already demonstrated tolerogenic and immunomodulatory properties in SLE patients and murine lupus models and is currently entering phase III clinical trials [12].

In humans, however, there are limitations to studying T cell responses associated with lupus arising from the limited availability of blood samples, making long-term study of a particular T cell response difficult. Traditional methods are useful for generating T cell lines and clones, but these have proved difficult to maintain. A more practical solution for generating T cell lines and clones has become available that relies on culture with magnetic beads coated either with anti-CD4 antibodies to isolate helper T cells or with anti-CD3 and anti-CD28 agonist antibodies to expand them [13]. The techniques allow isolation, polarization, and expansion of a single $CD4^+$ T cell to several billions without the need for an autologous feeder cell population. Prior to expansion, T cells can be first incubated with antigen and polarized with cytokines for the study of particular helper T cell subsets. Expanded T cell populations can also be cryopreserved so that various phenotypic and functional aspects of a particular antigen-specific T cell can be examined when convenient. In addition, autologous B cells, immortalized with Epstein-Barr virus (EBV), can be used as antigen-presenting cells. Together, these factors mean that bead-based expansion of T cells offers a practical solution particularly for human studies in which consistent access to blood samples is difficult.

2 Materials

2.1 Isolation of Peripheral Blood Mononuclear Cells (PBMC) from Blood Samples

Vacuette 9 mL blood collection tubes containing Z serum clot activator (red cap; Greiner bio-one UK).

Vacuette 9 mL blood collection tubes containing lithium heparin (green cap; Greiner bio-one UK).

Lymphoprep™ (density 1.077 g/mL) Axis-Shield (UK).

Sterile Hank's buffered saline solution (HBSS; NaCl 8.0 g/L, KCl 0.4 g/L, KH_2PO_4 0.06 g/L, $NaHCO_3$, $NaH_2PO_4{\cdot}7H_2O$ 0.09 g/L, Glucose 1.0 g/L, $MgSO_4{\cdot}7H_2O$ 0.2 g/L, $CaCl_2{\cdot}2H_2O$ 0.186 g/L, pH 7.1–7.4; Lonza, Wokingham, UK).

Cell culture medium: RPMI 1640 (with phenol red, no Glutamine; Life technologies, UK) supplemented with 100 U/100 μg/mL penicillin/streptomycin, 2 mM L-glutamine, 40 mM HEPES buffer, and 5 % decomplemented, filter-sterilized autologous or AB^+ human serum (*see* **Note 1**).

Swing bucket refrigerated centrifuge that can hold 50 mL tubes.

Sterile 50 mL polypropylene conical tubes (50 mL tubes).

2.2 Isolation of $CD4^+$ T Cells from Peripheral Blood Mononuclear Cells

Dynabeads® CD4 Positive Isolation Kit (contains 4×10^8 beads/mL in phosphate-buffered saline (PBS), with 0.1 % bovine serum albumin (BSA) and 0.02 % sodium azide, and DETACHaBEAD® reagent for disrupting lymphocyte/magnetic bead rosettes (Life Technologies, UK)).

DynaMag™-15 Magnet designed to hold 15 mL tubes (Life Technologies, UK).

Buffer 1: PBS (Ca^{2+} and Mg^{2+} free, Lonza UK) with 0.1 % BSA and 2 mM EDTA, pH 7.4.

Buffer 2: RPMI 1640/1 % fetal calf serum.

2.3 Generation and Expansion of Polarized Antigen-Specific Effector CD4+ T Cells

Sterile cell culture plates including round bottomed 96 well and flat bottomed 48 well plates (Greiner bio-one).

Peptide antigen of interest (typically used over a range of 1–20 μg/mL).

Polarizing cytokines depending on T cell subset of interest.

Cell irradiator (e.g., IBL 437C irradiator for treating blood products).

2.4 Expansion of T Cell Lines and Cloning Using Magnetic CD3/CD28 Beads

384 Well polystyrene cell culture plate with lid, clear, sterile (Greiner bio-one, UK).

Dynabeads® Human T-Activator CD3/CD28 for T cell expansion and activation. Supplied as a suspension containing 4×10^7 Dynabeads®/mL in phosphate-buffered saline (PBS), pH 7.4, w/0.1 % bovine serum albumin (Life technologies, UK).

Cell expansion medium (*see* **Note 2**).

2.5 Long-Term Storage of T Cell Lines and Clones

Nalgene "Mr. Frosty" polycarbonate Freezing Container for 1–2 mL cryogenic tubes.

Sterile cryogenic tubes, 1.5 mL capacity.

Dimethyl sulfoxide (DMSO, Hybri-Max™, sterile-filtered, BioReagent, suitable for hybridoma, ≥99.7 %; Sigma-Aldrich, UK).

Medium for freezing down cells comprising 20 % DMSO in heat-inactivated, filter-sterile (0.2 μM filter) fetal calf serum (FCS) or autologous human serum if available.

3 Methods

3.1 Isolation of Peripheral Blood Mononuclear Cells (PBMC) from Blood with Lymphoprep™

PBMC can be routinely recovered from heparinized blood samples with excellent viability using Lymphoprep™ (Axis-Shield, Oslo, Norway), an isosmotic medium with a density of 1.077 g/mL. Mononuclear cells have a lower cell density compared with granulocytes and red blood cells and so do not sediment through the medium and instead are recovered at the sample: medium interface. All of these cell culture protocols should be performed using standard aseptic technique, preferably in a laminar airflow cabinet.

1. Blood samples are taken from healthy volunteer donors by venipuncture into lithium heparin anticoagulant tubes with local ethical approval and using a standard protocol (*see* **Note 3**).
2. PBMC are prepared from these fresh heparinized blood samples by Lymphoprep gradient.
3. Heparinized blood is diluted 1:1 with HBSS and 25 mL layered onto 15 mL Lymphoprep solution (*see* **Note 4**) in a 50 mL tube and centrifuged at $670 \times g$ (≈1,800 RPM) for 40 min at RT (*with brakes off*).

4. The distinct interface comprising the mononuclear cell fraction is aspirated and washed with HBSS 3 times by centrifugation at 500, 400, and 300 × *g* for 10 min in a fresh 50 mL tube.
5. For cell assays, cell concentration is adjusted to $1–1.25 \times 10^6$ cells/mL and resuspended in RPMI 1640 cell culture medium or further processed to isolate $CD4^+$ T cells (*see* **Note 5**).
6. For serum preparation, blood is collected into a red cap coagulation tube, allowed to clot for an hour at RT, and centrifuged at 800 × *g* for 10 min.
7. The straw colored upper layer of serum is transferred into a 15 mL tube and decomplemented by incubation in a water bath at 56 °C for 30 min before adding to cell culture medium.

3.2 Isolation of $CD4^+$ T Cells from Peripheral Blood Mononuclear Cells

1. $CD4^+$ T cells are isolated from the PBMC using the Dynal® CD4 Positive Isolation Kit according to manufacturer's instructions.
2. After the final HBSS wash (above), the PBMC are resuspended in buffer 1, counted, and adjusted to 1×10^7 cells/mL in a 15 mL tube.
3. The anti-CD4 magnetic beads are added to the PBMC at a ratio of 25 μL per mL of PBMC and incubated at 4 °C with gentle rocking for 20 min.
4. The $CD4^+$ T cells attached to the magnetic beads are recovered by placing in magnet for 2 min.
5. The supernatant containing PBMC depleted of $CD4^+$ T cells is carefully aspirated and discarded.
6. The tube is removed from the magnet and the bead/cell complexes gently resuspended by pipetting in 1–10 mL of buffer 1 (dependent on starting volume of PBMC) before replacing in the magnet.
7. This wash step is performed at least 3 times to ensure optimum purity.
8. After the final wash, the bead/cell complexes are resuspended in 100 μL buffer 2 (dependent on starting volume of PBMC).
9. The beads are removed from the $CD4^+$ T cells by adding 10–100 μL of the DETACHaBEAD® reagent (dependent again on starting cell volume) and incubating for 45 min with gentle rocking.
10. The 15 mL tube is transferred to the magnet for 1 min and the supernatant containing the $CD4^+$ T cells transferred to a fresh 15 mL tube.
11. The detached T cells are washed by making up to 10 mL with buffer 2 and centrifuging at 400 × *g* for 10 min.
12. The $CD4^+$ T cells are resuspended in cell culture medium containing 5 % autologous or AB^+ serum.

3.3 Generation and Expansion of Polarized Antigen-Specific Effector CD4+ T Cells

1. Antigen-specific Th1 effector cell lines are generated by incubating CD4+ T cells (0.5×10^6 cells/mL) in the presence of 1×10^6 irradiated antigen-presenting cells (APC; *see* **Notes 6, 7**), the peptide antigen (usually at a concentration of 1–20 μg/mL), and human rIL-12 at 5 ng/mL.
2. To ensure that T cells are polarized toward the Th1 effector T cell phenotype, anti-IL4 and anti-IL17A antibodies should also be added at 5 μg/mL (*see* **Note 8** for other polarization options).
3. The cell cultures are incubated for 9 days at 37 °C, 5 % CO_2.
4. From day 6, cultures are supplemented with recombinant cytokines only.
5. After 9 days, cells from replicate wells are combined, washed with HBSS twice by centrifugation at $300 \times g$ for 10 min, and the CD4+ T cells re-isolated with the Dynal® CD4 Positive Isolation Kit.
6. If APC are available, the CD4+ T cells are restimulated as above with fresh irradiated APC, antigen, cytokines, and anti-cytokine antibodies.
7. After a further 6-day incubation, the majority of cells in the effector T cell line will be antigen-specific, at which point T cell clones can be isolated and expanded.

3.4 Expansion of T Cell Lines and Cloning Using Magnetic CD3/CD28 Beads

1. Following 2 rounds of stimulation with antigen and polarizing agents (cytokine and anti-cytokine antibodies), antigen-specific T cells can be isolated and cloned.
2. Replicate wells of antigen-specific T cells are combined and washed twice by centrifugation at $300 \times g$ for 10 min with HBSS, resuspended in complete medium and counted.
3. A limiting dilution series is set up to generate CD4+ T cell suspensions at 2×10^4, 2×10^3, 2×10^2, and 2×10^1 cells/mL in RPMI 1640 cell culture medium + 5 % autologous or AB+ serum.
4. These cell suspensions are diluted 1:1 with culture medium containing irradiated APC (2×10^6 cells/mL) and antigen at optimum concentration (e.g., 1–20 μg/mL).
5. The cell suspensions are added in 30 μL aliquots to wells in sterile 384 well cell culture plates (*see* **Note 9**).
6. Some wells containing only APC should be set up to discriminate background irradiated cells from clonal cell growth.
7. Outer wells are ringed with sterile dH_2O and the cells incubated at 37 °C, 5 % CO_2 for a period of up to 12 days.
8. From day 4, plates can be carefully checked for potential clones using an inverted microscope.

9. On day 5, each well is supplemented with a further 20 μL of RPMI 1640 cell culture medium, pre-warmed to 37 °C (total vol. = 50 μL).
10. After 10 days there should be good evidence of clonal growth.
11. To expand potential candidate clones, 25 μL of clone cell suspension can be added to 2 replicate wells in a round bottomed 96 well plate.
12. To the clone cell suspensions, 75 μL cell expansion medium, pre-warmed to 37 °C, is overlaid and the cells re-incubated at 37 °C, 5 % CO_2.
13. Cells can then be observed over a period of up to 3 weeks for signs of growth (it can take up to 3 weeks for some clones to expand sufficiently).
14. Once good active growth is established, cells can be split and transferred into more wells and finally, 48 well plates containing 1 mL cell expansion medium.
15. From this point on cells can be divided when necessary—fast growing clones need to be split 1:4 every 3 days or so, but slower growing clones can be split every 6 days or so.
16. When enough cells from a potential clone are generated, they are counted and cryopreserved at an ideal number of 5×10^6 cells/mL.
17. Some idea of clonality can be obtained using T cell receptor Vβ chain analysis (*see* **Note 10**).

3.5 Long-Term Storage of T Cell Lines and Clones

Long-term storage of T cell lines and clones is an important part of the cloning process, and it is important that the procedure is optimized to ensure that these valuable clones retain high levels of viability. For any period of more than 2 days, it is best to freeze the cells and to store them at −70 °C for up to 2 weeks and under liquid nitrogen for longer periods of time.

1. Aspirate cells to be stored from cell culture plates into a 15 mL tube and wash twice with 4 °C HBSS by centrifuging at 350 × *g* for 10 min.
2. Resuspend the pellet (1×10^7–2×10^7 cells/mL) in heat-inactivated, filter-sterile FCS or autologous human serum cooled to 4 °C.
3. Allow the cell suspension to incubate on ice for 20 min, reducing their activity and consequent absorption of DMSO.
4. Add an equal volume of freezing medium containing 20 % DMSO in FCS (or autologous serum) dropwise to the cell suspension, gently swirling the mix by hand.
5. Transfer 1 mL aliquots to sterile, clearly labeled sterile 1.5 mL cryovials and place in freezing container (e.g., a Mr. Frosty) with an isopropyl alcohol reservoir (*see* **Note 11**).

6. Place freezing container in typical −70 to −80 °C mechanical freezer for 24 h.
7. After 24 h, the cryovials can be transferred to a suitable liquid nitrogen storage container.
8. To thaw the T cell clones, remove them from the liquid nitrogen container and immerse into a 37 °C water bath while trying to avoid direct contact with water (*see* **Note 11**).
9. Immediately aspirate the cell suspension into a sterile 50 mL tube and make up to 50 mL with warmed HBSS (37 °C).
10. Wash twice with warmed HBSS by centrifuging at 350×*g* for 10 min.
11. Resuspend in warmed RPMI 1640 cell culture medium, count using a hemocytometer, and adjust to required cell concentration.

4 Notes

1. Serum and plasma used in cell culture media are routinely heat-treated for 30 min at precisely 56 °C in a water bath to inactivate the range of complement components contained within them. Frozen serum should be allowed to thaw slowly in a refrigerator and then brought to room temperature before incubation in the water bath at 56 °C.

   While this protocol is routinely used in our laboratory to decomplement serum with no associated problems, there is some debate suggesting that heat inactivation of fetal calf serum, if used, is unnecessary. Studies of FCS heat inactivation indicate that for most cell types it offers little or no advantages for cell growth and usually results in decreased growth rates, when the heat inactivation protocol is performed at an optimum temperature of 56 °C. At higher temperatures or longer incubation periods, detrimental effects of FCS heat inactivation on subsequent cell growth were clearly apparent. It is important therefore, that heat inactivation protocols used to decomplement FCS should be strictly defined and followed closely to avoid unfavorable effects on cell growth (Invitrogen, Expressions 1995, Vol. 2 Issue 2. p 11).
2. Cell expansion medium comprises complete RPMI 1640 medium supplemented with 5 % autologous serum, IL-2 at 100 U/mL, and 2 μL/mL Dynal T cell expander beads (Dynabeads® CD3/CD28 T Cell Expander kit). IL-2 can be substituted with IL-15 (50 ng/mL) if so desired. There is some evidence that T cell clones are slightly less prone to apoptosis when IL-15 is used in place of IL-2 [14], although in practice we have not observed any significant advantage. IL-2 is also a lot cheaper.

3. Collection of blood samples, particularly from patients or study group volunteers, should adhere closely with local and national regulations regarding ethics. In essence, protocols used to collect blood and the volume to be taken should be strictly defined prior to any study. A blood sample volume of up to 50 mL is considered reasonable from most adults, but a recovery period of at least 2 weeks should be considered before any further request for another blood sample in order to allow the volunteer's blood composition to be restored. In the UK, an application for ethical permission must be approved before any scientific or clinical study with patient blood or tissue samples can commence. The application must clearly define how blood samples will be collected, logged, processed, recorded, and stored to ensure that each stage of the study is performed ethically and without detriment to the patient or participant's well-being. In the UK, full details can be obtained from the National Research Ethics Service (http://www.nres.nhs.uk/about-the-national-research-ethics-service/). Blood samples should be collected by a trained phlebotomist. Nonclinical scientists can receive phlebotomy training from their local hospital.
4. Lymphoprep is an isosmotic medium with a defined density of 1.077 g/mL and therefore it is important to use it at room temperature (≈20 °C), rather than at 4 °C, which would increase solution density rendering it less efficient. To obtain the best yield, blood samples should be diluted 1:1 with a physiological saline solution (e.g., sterile HBSS or PBS (2 mM EDTA) + 5%FCS) before being applied to the Lymphoprep.
5. A typical yield of PBMC from a 50 mL blood sample provided by a healthy donor will range from 0.5 to 1.5×10^6 cells/mL (or a total of $2.5–7.5 \times 10^7$ cells in a 50 mL blood sample). Patients with lupus, however, are quite often lymphopenic and therefore PBMC yields from blood samples can be very low, typically $0.4–1.0 \times 10^6$ cells/mL. This should be taken into account when planning experiments.
6. Cells are typically irradiated at a level of 30Gy. While irradiation prevents cell proliferation very effectively, it does not necessarily prevent or even reduce secretion of cytokines from some cells. Thus it is always important that suitable controls are used to ensure that any cytokines of interest are originating from T cell lines and clones rather than APC.
7. A key problem with using human cells is lack of availability. Where possible, use fresh blood to isolate PBMC as a source of antigen-presenting cells, but an alternative is to immortalize autologous human B cells with Epstein-Barr virus. This is a reasonable strategy although B lymphocytes are not as efficient at presenting antigen as other immune cells such as dendritic cells. Further, they secrete large amounts of IL-10, which should be taken into account in experimental protocols.

B lymphocytes can be transformed with EBV naturally present supernatants taken from the B95-8 cell line derived from the cotton-top tamarin monkey (*Saguinus oedipus*; ECACC cat. no. 85011419).

8. To polarize $CD4^+$ T cells toward the Th2 T cell phenotype, $CD4^+$ T cells should be incubated in the presence of an antigen (1–20 μg/mL) and irradiated APC (as described in Subheading 3.3) in the presence of rIL-4 at 20 ng/mL and anti-IL-12 at 5 μg/mL. To polarize $CD4^+$ T cells toward the Th17 T cell phenotype is more complicated: $CD4^+$ T cells should be incubated in the presence of an antigen and irradiated APC, as above, together with IL-6 (10 ng/mL), IL-1β (10 ng/mL), TGF-β1 (5–10 ng/mL), IL-23 (10 ng/mL), and the neutralizing antibodies anti-IL-4 (5 μg/mL) and anti-IFN-γ (5 μg/mL).
9. A dilution series is set up to generate $CD4^+$ T cell suspensions at 2×10^4, 2×10^3, 2×10^2, and 2×10^1 cells/mL in cell culture medium, which are further diluted 1:1 with irradiated APC and added to the wells of a 384 well microplate in 30 μL aliquots. Theoretically, this dilution series should provide a cell frequency of 300, 30, 3, and 0.3 per well, respectively. It is important to have many replicate wells for each dilution series—150 replicate wells is a reasonable number for screening. The most desirable clones are likely to be found in wells with lower cell frequency as these are more likely to be truly clonal, i.e., all cells derived from a single cell. For us the best compromise between frequency of "hits" and clonality is typically from wells where cells are added at a concentration of 1×10^2 cells/mL. It is also important to have a few wells that contain just irradiated APC, as during the first few days of incubation, it helps to distinguish potential clones from non-proliferating APC.
10. Once a potential $CD4^+$ T cell clone has been obtained, it should be analyzed by flow cytometry to confirm that it is indeed a $CD3^+CD4^+$ T cell before any further work with the clone. The cytokine profile of activated cells can also be checked in ELISA following stimulation of washed, resting clones with anti-CD3/CD28 beads. True clonality is fairly laborious to confirm, but analysis of T cell receptor Vβ chain usage can provide some reassurance that potential clones are truly clonal and not derived from more than one cell. Kits such as the IOTest® Beta Mark Kit (Beckman Coulter) are designed for quantitative determination of the TCR Vβ repertoire of human T lymphocytes by flow cytometry, but they can also be used qualitatively to examine whether, as would be expected, all T cells from a single clone express the same Vβ gene segment. Antigen-specific responses can also in some case also be investigated using class II tetra or pentamers by flow cytometry, if commercially available.

11. The advantage of specially designed freezing containers is that they provide a uniform cooling rate of 1 °C per minute, which is the best way to cryopreserve cells and thus to ensure maximum cell viability. When freezing cells down in cryovials, tighten the caps only very gently. When the cryovials are recovered from the liquid nitrogen store at a later date, it will be easier to release the pressure caused by expanding nitrogen gas and the cryovials will be less likely to explode!

    The rigid vial holders in these freezing containers are buoyant and can be used to thaw the cells in a 37 °C water bath, preventing direct contact with water, which is a potential source of contamination (especially mycoplasma!).

References

1. Rahman A, Isenberg DA (2008) Systemic lupus erythematosus. N Engl J Med 358: 929–939
2. Clark DN, Markham JL, Sloan CS, Poole BD (2012) Cytokine inhibition as a strategy for treating systemic lupus erythematosus. Clin Immunol 148:335–343
3. Coffman RL, Lebman DA, Rothman P (1993) Mechanism and regulation of immunoglobulin isotype switching. Adv Immunol 54: 229–270
4. Iwasaki A, Medzhitov R (2010) Regulation of adaptive immunity by the innate immune system. Science 327:291–295
5. Mosmann TR, Coffman RL (1989) TH1 and TH2 cells: different patterns of lymphokine secretion lead to different functional properties. Annu Rev Immunol 7:145–173
6. Korn T, Bettelli E, Oukka M, Kuchroo VK (2009) IL-17 and Th17 cells. Annu Rev Immunol 27:485–517
7. Kaliyaperumal A, Michaels MA, Datta SK (1999) Antigen-specific therapy of murine lupus nephritis using nucleosomal peptides: tolerance spreading impairs pathogenic function of autoimmune T and B cells. J Immunol 162:5775–5783
8. Kaliyaperumal A, Michaels MA, Datta SK (2002) Naturally processed chromatin peptides reveal a major autoepitope that primes pathogenic T and B cells of lupus. J Immunol 168:2530–2537
9. Kang HK, Michaels MA, Berner BR, Datta SK (2005) Very low-dose tolerance with nucleosomal peptides controls lupus and induces potent regulatory T cell subsets. J Immunol 174:3247–3255
10. Monneaux F, Briand JP, Muller S (2000) B and T cell immune response to small nuclear ribonucleoprotein particles in lupus mice: autoreactive CD4(+) T cells recognize a T cell epitope located within the RNP80 motif of the 70K protein. Eur J Immunol 30:2191–2200
11. Wu HY, Ward FJ, Staines NA (2002) Histone peptide-induced nasal tolerance: suppression of murine lupus. J Immunol 169:1126–1134
12. Muller S (2012) Synthetic peptides as tools for diagnosis and therapeutic strategies to treat systemic lupus erythematous. Autoimmun Rev 11:799–800
13. Levine BL, Bernstein WB, Connors M, Craighead N, Lindsten T, Thompson CB, June CH (1997) Effects of CD28 costimulation on long-term proliferation of CD4+ T cells in the absence of exogenous feeder cells. J Immunol 159:5921–5930
14. Waldmann TA, Dubois S, Tagaya Y (2001) Contrasting roles of IL-2 and IL-15 in the life and death of lymphocytes: implications for immunotherapy. Immunity 14:105–110

Chapter 19

Meta-analysis as a Diagnostic Tool for Predicting Disease Onset and/or Activity in Systemic Lupus Erythematosus

Isabel Cottrell, Asma Khan, Sidra Maqsood, Jemma Thornes, and Paul Eggleton

Abstract

Systemic lupus erythematous (SLE) is a relatively rare disorder with prevalence rates between 5 and 50 per 100,000 population. This means performing any epidemiological analysis in a specific research center is difficult, due to the low number of cases within any one location. There is a need for biomarkers and diagnostic aids to monitor SLE disease activity and severity prior, during, and after treatment. Many specialist lupus clinics worldwide have published trials following in detail small numbers of patients that have been monitored for a disease biomarker, e.g., an autoantibody against a self-molecule in prospective and retrospective studies. They have then attempted to correlate autoantibody levels against an autoantigen with disease activity, e.g., nephritis development. The results are often inconclusive with the conclusion "the autoantibody may be useful in monitoring disease activity." Meta-analysis is a statistical technique that can be used for combining the findings of multiple studies to add power to any tentative conclusion proposed by individual studies. Here, we describe a method for analyzing biomarkers of interest as predictors of disease activity, using anti-C1q autoantibodies as an example.

Key words Autoantibodies, First component of complement-C1q, Sensitivity, Specificity, Forest plots, Nephritis

1 Introduction

As a chronic autoimmune disease, SLE presents with numerous immunological abnormalities causing inflammation in multiple organs and systems [1]. Detection and monitoring of a number of serum antibodies against nuclear components Ro, La, SM, and double-stranded DNA are used as aids to the diagnosis of SLE [2]. Anti-dsDNA autoantibodies are routinely found in 70–80 % of SLE patients [3] but may be absent in 20 % of SLE patients. There is interest in monitoring other autoantibodies to other host antigens in parallel to dsDNA, including C1q, nucleosome, and histone components [4, 5], in a view to increase the sensitivity and specificity of diagnostic assays for SLE.

Paul Eggleton and Frank J. Ward (eds.), *Systemic Lupus Erythematosus: Methods and Protocols*, Methods in Molecular Biology, vol. 1134, DOI 10.1007/978-1-4939-0326-9_19, © Springer Science+Business Media New York 2014

In addition to diagnosis, with lupus there is a need for diagnostic tests that can measure specific organ involvement in a patient to aid clinical decision-making [6]. But few biomarkers have been validated to aid both diagnosis and disease activity simultaneously, which has frustrated drug companies who have few means of monitoring and validating drug efficacy and clinical outcome of responders vs. nonresponders. The genes that have been studied intensely as possible biomarkers encode for serum components of complement, C1q, C4, and C2 in particular. The lack of these genes in patients makes them very susceptible to developing lupus. Therefore, autoantibodies to these proteins may inhibit the essential bio-function of these proteins increasing a patient's risk of developing SLE and possibly going on to develop kidney disease. To date, a combined positive dsDNA antibody and renal biopsy result remains the best way to diagnose nephritis in a patient. Over the past 20 years, a number of small patient studies have implicated a number of autoantibodies, measured by enzyme-linked immunosorbent assay (ELISA) and other immunoassays, as being potential biomarkers for developing SLE and/or lupus nephritis.

Here, we provide a method for dealing with the practical difficulties of assimilating data from a number of studies with small patient numbers, in order to make a rational decision regarding the effectiveness of monitoring a specific autoantibody for diagnosis or disease activity purposes. In this example, we have performed a meta-analysis on anti-C1q as an example to evaluate the monitoring of anti-C1q as an accurate diagnostic test for predicting the onset of lupus nephritis in SLE patients.

2 Materials

It is necessary to conduct a systematic retrieval of all studies from the literature that may contain original lab-based data employing the method of choice. In this example, autoantibodies for C1q were first identified and an immunoassay developed in 1984; therefore, this acts as a starting point for potential retrieval of data [7, 8].

2.1 Literature Search

1. *The question:* Decide on a specific question to answer. You may have subsidiary questions, or these may arise during the analysis. We asked the question "*Do anti-C1q antibodies act as a predictor of an SLE patient developing nephritis?*" Talk to a statistician to see if your question is realistic or achievable.
2. *Patient and controls:* In order to address the question, consider the patient groups and controls required. In this example, we looked for papers that included SLE patients with no history of nephritis, compared with patients who had a history of lupus nephritis (to determine if patients who had a history of nephritis had more or less anti-C1q autoantibodies). We also looked for

papers that included SLE patients with and without active nephritis, at the time of anti-C1q measurements (to determine if anti-C1q antibodies occurred with greater prevalence during bouts of active nephritis). Control groups are important to include and can consist of healthy controls and non-SLE autoimmune controls.

3. *Online libraries:* The search should be as comprehensive as possible. Obtain advice from your institute librarians as to what access you have. In this example, we screened from within the search window of EndNote X4.0.2—PubMed, Web of Science, TS National Library of Medicine, USA Annual Reviews, ScienceDirect, Medline (EBSCO), Biomed Central, BMJ Journals, Cambridge Journals, EBSCO EJS, Oxford Journals, Medline (Ovid), NHS Evidence, AMED (EBSCO), and the Exeter Health Library online journal collection to ensure all relevant articles were retrieved.
4. *Search terms:* This can be very subjective and the wrong choice of words may omit relevant articles. Here, we extracted articles on the use of C1q immunoassays to detect anti-C1q autoantibodies in SLE patients with and without nephritis, using the search terms *nephritis*, *lupus*, and *C1q*. Keep search terms reasonably general to avoid unintentionally excluding studies.
5. *Obtaining papers:* Obtain all the full papers from the search. This is important, an abstract often appears to provide promising data, but the detail is lacking in the full manuscript and vice versa. To obtain the papers, use electronic online access libraries for speed of delivery. Request paper copies and/or PDF formats via library inter-loan requests and online publishing sites. Normally, only positive data gets published, but look for negative data too and do not exclude it from the study.
6. *Language:* Do not exclude papers based on language alone; a paper in Mandarin, Spanish, or Arabic may contribute important data for the analysis as much as an English-language article.

3 Methods

3.1 Study Selection and Criteria

1. *Generation of abstracts:* Organize several members of staff to perform the study selection. Ideally get two independent pairs of researchers to screen the literature abstracts based on the search terms. Next, collate the two independently generated lists and obtain the papers. Then decide on which studies to exclude based on chosen exclusion criteria decided upon in advance (Fig. 1). Assess the quality of each selected study using a quality assessment tool, such as quality assessment of diagnostic accuracy studies (QUADAS) [9].

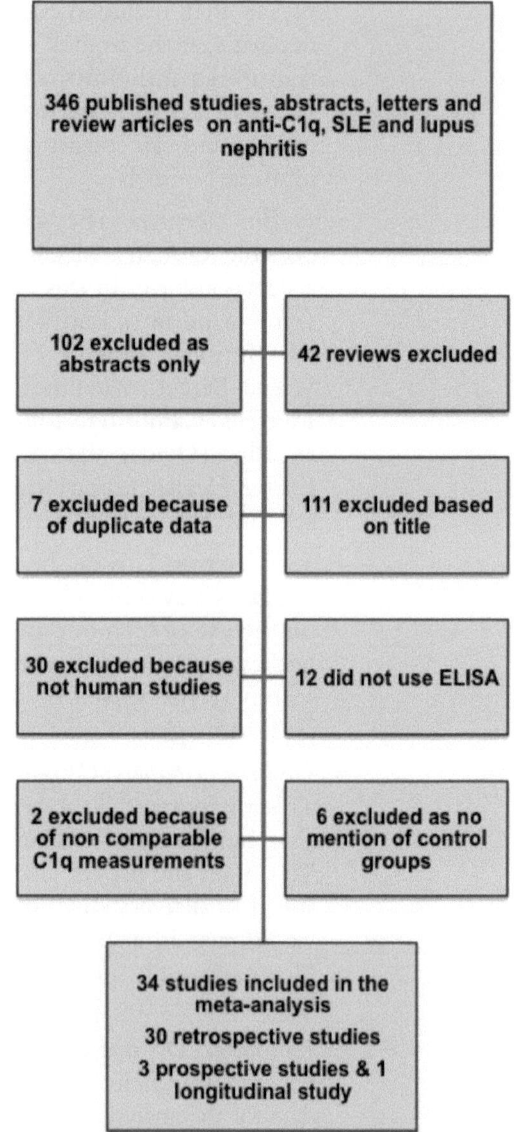

Fig. 1 Flow chart of reasoning for excluding publications from the anti-C1q analysis

2. *The reference test:* Decide on a diagnostic test that is comparable in all studies. In this example, we chose to investigate anti-C1q autoantibodies measured only by ELISA irrespective of manufacturer of the assay (Fig. 2), and not by other immunoassay techniques, e.g., radioimmunoassay (*see* **Note 1**).
3. *Patient selection:* SLE studies must only be included if patients have had their disease diagnosed using internationally recognized diagnostic criteria. The American College of Rheumatology classification criteria developed in 1982 and revised in 1997

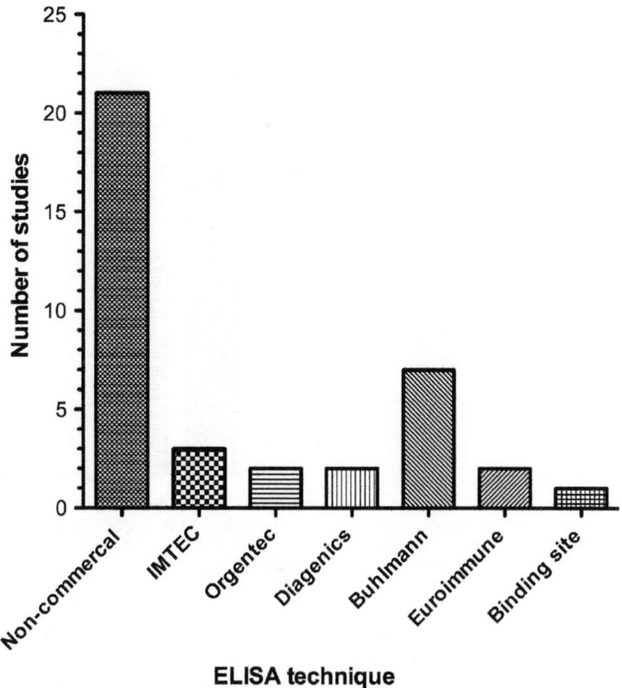

Fig. 2 The number of studies included that used various forms of ELISA to detect anti-C1q antibodies in SLE patients. Despite a single reference test being chosen to perform a meta-analysis, different studies will invariably choose different commercial or noncommercial variants to obtain results

are frequently used [10, 11]. However, a number of other indices have been developed including SLE Disease Activity Index (SLEDAI), European Consensus Lupus Activity Measurement (ECLAM), and British Isles Lupus Assessment Group (BILAG) index, and these are also acceptable to include in an analysis alone or in combination with one of the other indexes (Fig. 3).

4. *Selection of "gold standard":* When investigating a diagnostic or screening test, ensure selected papers have used a well-recognized confirmatory method of diagnosing the disease (Fig. 4). This is necessary as it acts as metric for determining sensitivity and specificity of the assay (*see* **Note 2**), as well as the predictive values for positive and negative results (*see* **Note 3**).

5. *Construction of a multiplex 2×2 format tables:* Extract relevant data from the manuscripts, number of patients tested, number of patients with disease testing positive (true positive) and negative with the test (false negative), patients with no disease testing positive (false positive) and negative (true negative) with the test. Compile a table in a spreadsheet (Table 1) using selected software (*see* **Note 4**). Using this raw data, calculate

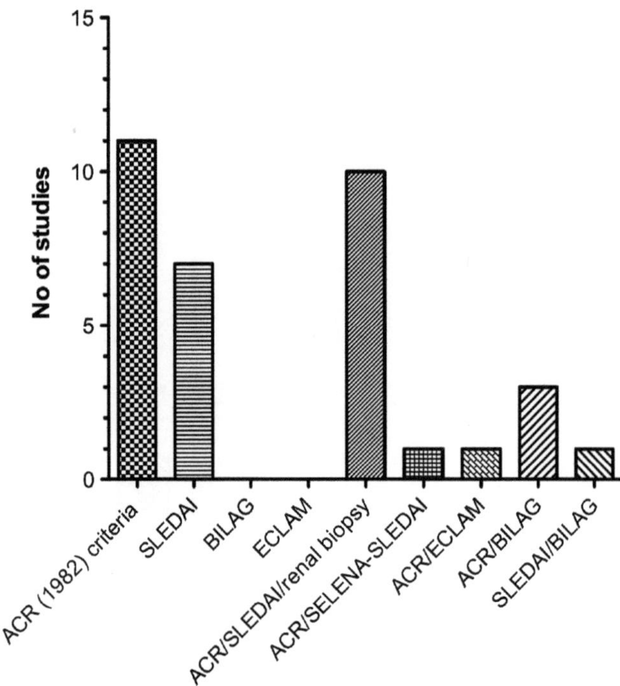

Fig. 3 The frequency of various indices used to assess SLE disease activity while measuring anti-C1q autoantibodies. When performing a meta-analysis involving SLE, various research groups preferentially use the disease activity index routinely used in their institute or combinations thereof

the sensitivity, specificity, and positive and negative predictive values for each study. Some studies may provide these values but omit to give patient numbers, and these may have to be excluded from the study, or contact the authors directly for the values.

6. *Risk and odds ratio:* Calculate the risk ratio (RR) of developing the disease relative to presenting with a positive diagnostic test result. To do this, extract data from your spreadsheet constructed in Table 1. Use a software program, e.g., GraphPad Prism, Meta-Disc, or STATA, to perform this (*see* **Note 4**). Also calculate the odds ratio (OR) for comparison (Table 2).
7. *Construction of a forest plot:* Using the RR or OR data, create a new spreadsheet in GraphPad (Fig. 5) or similar statistical software (*see* **Note 5**) and generate a graphical summary of RR or OR with 95 % CI of all the studies.
8. *More complex meta-analysis of the studies:* This can then be completed with the guidance of a statistician. These can include risk differences, hazard ratios, likelihood ratios, and diagnostic odds ratios and the overall heterogeneity of the selected studies and how this impacts on the overall results.

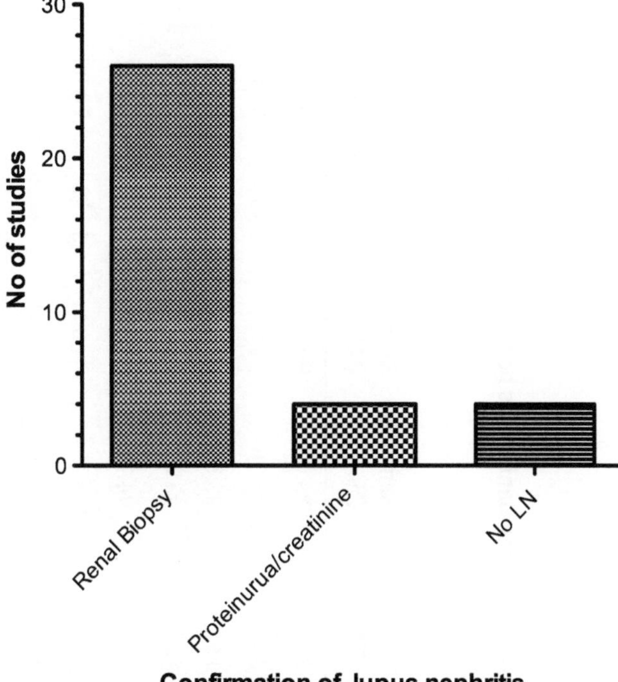

Fig. 4 The use of a "gold standard" to confirm lupus nephritis in SLE patients with anti-C1q autoantibodies. In this example, of the 27 studies examined, 23 studies confirmed nephritis by renal biopsy, 2 studies monitored proteinuria and creatinine levels, and two studies found no evidence nephritis

4 Notes

1. Having decided on selecting one method to analyze, the different researchers may have used ELISAs manufactured by different companies or developed their own "in-house" method. This makes data difficult to compare unless data has been normalized and presented as ELISA units or compared to a "gold standard." What one group considers a positive result, another may consider negative. Consequently, some data may have to be groups in a sub-cohort.
2. When a "gold standard assay" has been employed to confirm disease status, both the specificity and sensitivity of the assay can be calculated if the authors themselves did not do so. The sensitivity of the assay is defined as the % of patients with disease who test positive and is calculated: Sensitivity = true positives/(true positives + false negatives). The specificity of the assay is judged by accurately predicting which individuals that are truly negative for the disease test negative and is calculated: specificity = true negatives/(true negative + false positives).

Table 1
Construction and presentation of data in a tabulated "2 × 2" format in the assessment of anti-C1q autoantibodies being biomarkers for nephritis in SLE patients

Selected references and year of publication	Total patients	Active LN and +ve anti-C1q (TP)	Active LN and −ve anti-C1q (FN)	No LN and +ve anti-C1q (FP)	No LN and −ve anti-C1q (TN)	Sensitivity (%)	Specificity (%)	+ve Predictive value (%)	−ve Predictive value (%)
Bernstein (1994) [12]	60	4	26	3	27	13.00	90.00	57.00	51.00
Moroni (2001) [13]	59	20	3	3	33	86.96	91.67	86.95	91.66
Oelzner (2003) [14]	45	14	5	10	16	73.68	61.54	58.30	76.10
Marto (2003) [14]	77	32	11	18	16	74.40	47.10	64.00	59.25
Trendelenburg (2006) [15]	64	36	2	9	17	94.74	65.38	80.00	89.47
Zabaleta-Lanz (2006) [16]	46	7	9	19	21	43.75	70.00	26.92	70.00
Moroni (2009) [17]	228	NK	NK	NK	NK	80.50*	71.00*	NK	NK
Matrat (2011) [18]	23	13	10	NK	NK	78.30*	84.00*	56.00	70.00

TP true positive, *FN* false negative, *FP* false positive, *TN* true negative, *LN* lupus nephritis, +ve positive, −ve negative, *PV* predictive value, *NK* not known
Sensitivity and specificity equations: % Sensitivity = TP/(TP + FN) × 100: % Specificity = TN/(TN + FP) × 100
Predictive value equations: % Positive predictive value +ve PV = TP/(TP + FP): % Negative predictive value −ve PV = TN/(TN + FN) × 100
*Patients with active LN at time of testing

Table 2
Use of data in a tabulated "2 × 2" format to construct the risk ratio and odds ratio of anti-C1q autoantibodies being biomarkers for nephritis detection in SLE patients

Selected references and year of publication	Total patients	Active LN and +ve anti-C1q (TP)	Active LN and −ve anti-C1q (FN)	No LN and +ve anti-C1q (FP)	No LN and −ve anti-C1q (TN)	Risk ratio (95 % CI)	Odds ratio (95 % CI)
Bernstein (1994) [12]	60	4	26	3	27	1.2 (0.58–2.3)	1.4 (0.28–6.8)
Moroni (2001) [13]	59	20	3	3	33	10.4 (3.5–31.2)	73.3 (13.5–399)
Oelzner (2003) [14]	45	14	5	10	16	2.5 (1.1–5.6)	4.48 (1.2–16.3)
Marto (2003) [14]	77	32	11	18	16	1.6 (1.0–2.6)	2.59 (1.0–6.8)
Trendelenburg (2006) [15]	64	36	2	9	17	7.8 (2.0–28.4)	34.0 (6.6–174)
Zabaleta-Lanz (2006) [16]	56	7	9	19	21	0.89 (0.3–2.1)	0.86 (0.2–0.3)

TP true positive, *FN* false negative, *FP* false positive, *TN* true negative, *LN* lupus nephritis
Definitions: risk ratio = the risk of developing disease (nephritis in this example) related to being positive for diagnostic test (anti-C1q antibodies in this example); odds ratio = a measure of the strength of association between two binary values. In this example, the odds of a patient with nephritis being positive for anti-C1q antibodies, compared to the odds of a patient without nephritis being positive for anti-C1q antibodies

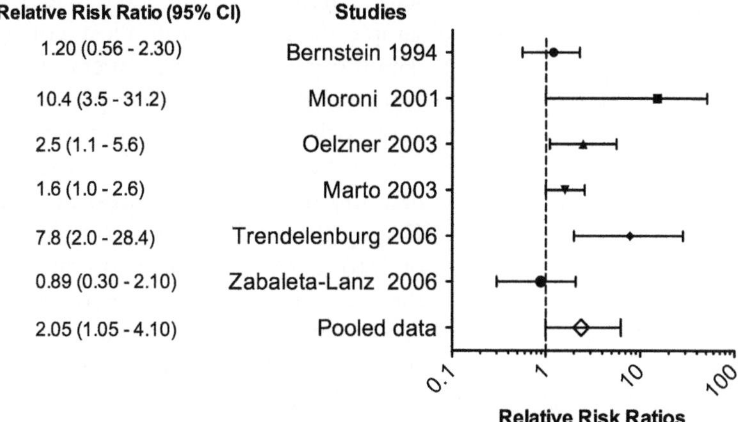

Fig. 5 Example of a forest plot of individual and pooled risk ratios that compared the risk of having nephritis in the SLE patients with and without anti-C1q antibodies. The findings from each individual are shown with 95 % CI (*horizontal lines*). The combined effect of all the selected studies is displayed as an open diamond. The vertical dotted line represents a "no-difference" guideline. The pooled data to the right of the vertical line indicates an ~twofold increase in relative risk of developing nephritis if the patient has anti-C1q antibodies, than SLE patients without anti-C1q antibodies in these selected examples

3. If the sensitivity and specificity of the assay have been or can be calculated, then the positive and negative predictive values of the diagnostic assay under test can also be calculated. The positive predictive value is an indicator of the probability of a patient positive for the test actually having a disease (e.g., nephritis). This is calculated as follows: true positive/(true positive + false positive). The negative predictive value is based on a patient being negative for a test and not actually having a disease and is calculated as true negatives/(true negatives + false negatives).
4. Extract the raw data from the selected papers for 2 × 2 table construction. The sensitivity, specificity, negative and positive predictive values, risk ratio, and odds ratio of the study can be obtained by entering the individual data set from each study into a GraphPad Prism spreadsheet. Selected "new data + graph" from the "create a new spread sheet" menu. Select table style "survival" and create. In the first two "Y" columns, add disease options (e.g., nephritis, no nephritis). In the first two "X" rows, add test result options (e.g., anti-C1q +ve, anti-C1q negative) and insert data. Open "Analyse" menu and select "Contingency tables analysis" and select "Chi-square (and Fisher's exact) test." In the pop-up Parameter box, select Fisher's exact test, two-tailed, 95 % CI, and select additional calculations—OR, RR, sensitivity, specificity, and predictive values.
5. In your GraphPad project file, click on drag menu "new" and select "new data table" and select "column" and select "use sample data." This will allow you to select how the column data is organized. Select "meta-analysis" (forest) plot and click "create." Remove the example data and replace with your own data, with each column representing a different study. Add the RR to the second row of each study and insert the CI in the first and third rows. A forest plot of the data will be created. Change the *x*-axis to a log-10 scale. Change each plot by clicking on it to represent median and range. Create a new "analysis" of the meta-analysis spreadsheet, select "XY analysis," and select "row means/totals and select median and range." Calculate the median RR with CI for pooled studies and add the data to the forest plot.

Acknowledgement

We thank Dr. Obioha. C. Ukoumunne of the University of Exeter Medical School, Exeter University, for the useful discussions and for reading the manuscript.

References

1. Gilboe IM, Kvien TK, Husby G (2001) Disease course in systemic lupus erythematosus: changes in health status, disease activity, and organ damage after 2 years. J Rheumatol 28:266–274
2. Liu CC, Manzi S, Ahearn JM (2005) Biomarkers for systemic lupus erythematosus: a review and perspective. Curr Opin Rheumatol 17:543–549
3. Watts R (2006) Auoantibodies in the autoimmune rheumatic diseases. Medicine (Baltimore) 34:441–444
4. Gussin HA, Tselentis HN, Teodorescu M (2000) Noncognate binding to histones of IgG from patients with idiopathic systemic lupus erythematosus. Clin Immunol 96: 150–161
5. Hermanova Z, Zadrazil Z, Dostal C, Olejarova M, Zavada J, Tesar V et al (2010) Anti C1q and antinucleosome antibodies (Ab) in the clinical trial in lupus nephritis. J Clin Rheumatol 16:S67
6. Liu CC, Ahearn JM (2009) The search for lupus biomarkers. Best Pract Res Clin Rheumatol 23:507–523
7. Uwatoko S, Aotsuka S, Okawa M, Egusa Y, Yokohari R, Aizawa C et al (1984) Characterization of C1q-binding IgG complexes in systemic lupus erythematosus. Clin Immunol Immunopathol 30:104–116
8. Uwatoko S, Aotsuka S, Okawa M, Egusa Y, Yokohari R, Aizawa C et al (1984) C1q solid-phase radioimmunoassay: binding properties of solid-phase C1q and evidence that C1q-binding IgG complexes in systemic lupus erythematosus are not bound to endogenous C1q. J Immunol Meth 73:67–74
9. Whiting PF, Rutjes AW, Westwood ME, Mallett S, Deeks JJ, Reitsma JB et al (2011) QUADAS-2: a revised tool for the quality assessment of diagnostic accuracy studies. Ann Intern Med 155:529–536
10. Tan EM, Cohen AS, Fries JF, Masi AT, Mcshane DJ, Rothfield NF et al (1982) The 1982 revised criteria for the classification of systemic lupus erythematosus. Arthritis Rheum 25:1271–1277
11. Hochberg MC (1997) Updating the American College of Rheumatology revised criteria for the classification of systemic lupus erythematosus. Arthritis Rheum 40:1725
12. Bernstein KA, Kahl LE, Balow JE, Lefkowith JB (1994) Serologic markers of lupus nephritis in patients: use of a tissue-based ELISA and evidence for immunopathogenic heterogeneity. Clin Exp Immunol 98:60–65
13. Moroni G, Trendelenburg M, Del Papa N, Quaglini S, Raschi E, Panzeri P et al (2001) Anti-C1q antibodies may help in diagnosing a renal flare in lupus nephritis. Am J Kidney Dis 37:490–498
14. Oelzner P, Deliyska B, Funfstuck R, Hein G, Herrmann D, Stein G (2003) Anti-C1q antibodies and antiendothelial cell antibodies in systemic lupus erythematosus – relationship with disease activity and renal involvement. Clin Rheumatol 22:271–278
15. Trendelenburg M, Lopez-Trascasa M, Potlukova E, Moll S, Regenass S, Fremeaux-Bacchi V et al (2006) High prevalence of anti-C1q antibodies in biopsy-proven active lupus nephritis. Nephrol Dial Transplant 21:3115–3121
16. Zabaleta-Lanz ME, Munoz LE, Tapanes FJ, Vargas-Arenas RE, Daboin I, Barrios Y et al (2006) Further description of early clinically silent lupus nephritis. Lupus 15:845–851
17. Moroni G, Radice A, Giammarresi G, Quaglini S, Gallelli B, Leoni A et al (2009) Are laboratory tests useful for monitoring the activity of lupus nephritis? A 6-year prospective study in a cohort of 228 patients with lupus nephritis. Ann Rheum Dis 68:234–237
18. Matrat A, Veysseyre-Balter C, Trolliet P, Villar E, Dijoud F, Bienvenu J et al (2011) Simultaneous detection of anti-C1q and anti-double stranded DNA autoantibodies in lupus nephritis: predictive value for renal flares. Lupus 20:28–34

INDEX

Paul Eggleton and Frank J. Ward (eds.), *Systemic Lupus Erythematosus: Methods and Protocols*, Methods in Molecular Biology, vol. 1134, DOI 10.1007/978-1-4939-0326-9, © Springer Science+Business Media, New York 2014

P

Q

R

S

T

W

MIX
Papier aus verantwortungsvollen Quellen
Paper from responsible sources
FSC® C105338

If you have any concerns about our products,
you can contact us on
ProductSafety@springernature.com

In case Publisher is established outside the EU,
the EU authorized representative is:
Springer Nature Customer Service Center GmbH
Europaplatz 3, 69115 Heidelberg, Germany

Printed by Libri Plureos GmbH
in Hamburg, Germany

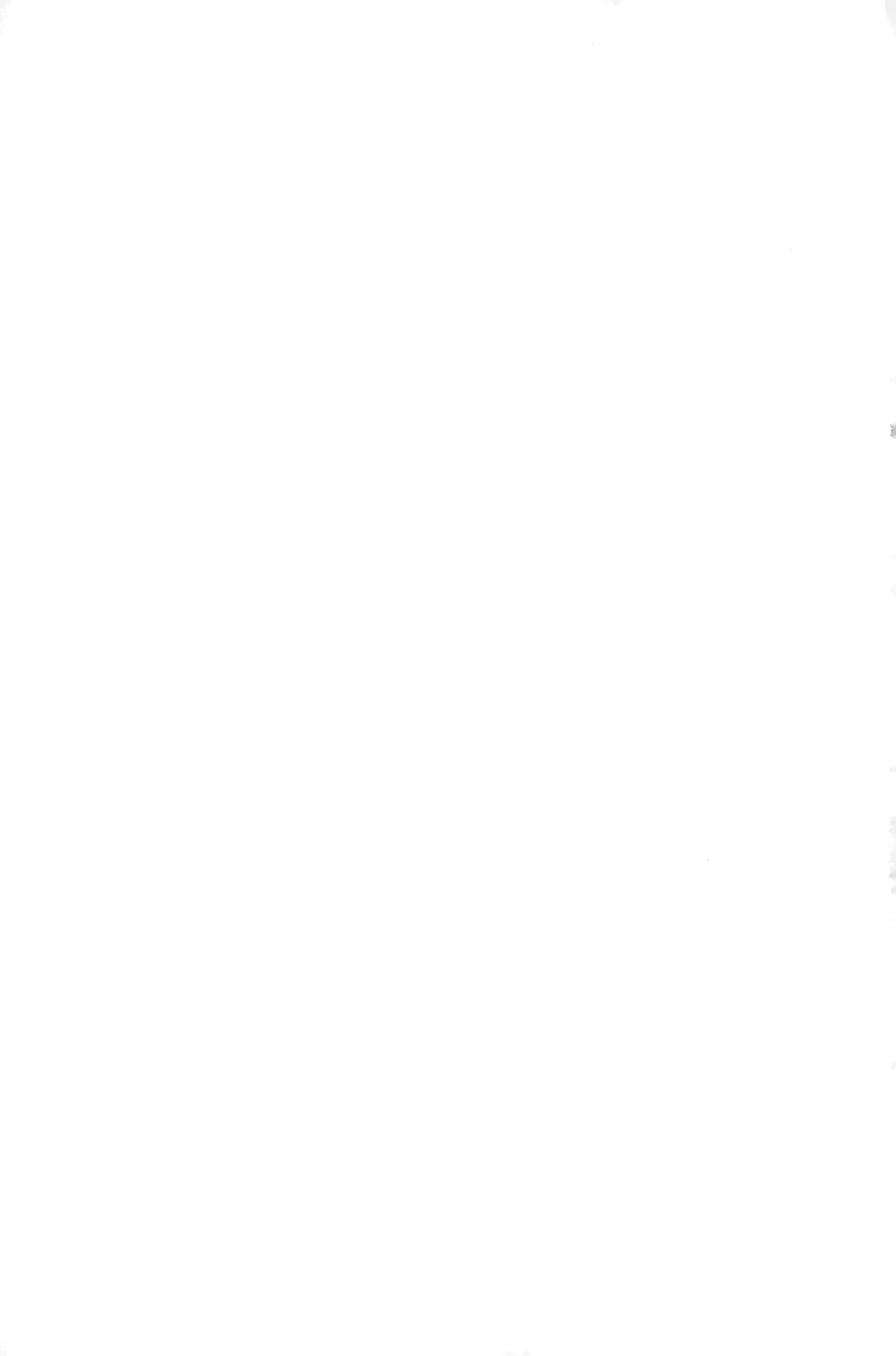